HOW TO STAY HEALTHY
WITH
HOMOEOPATHY

Rajendra Tandon is the author of *The Homoeopathic Guide to Family Health*, a bestseller since it was published in 1989. That classic has been translated into Hindi and Urdu. Tandon has been studying homoeopathy in depth for the last thirty years. He has tried more a large number of medicines on himself and on others and watched their healing effects carefully. All this observation is reflected in his writing in this book. His writing reflects his no-nonsense approach to the subject and every word is marked with precision and reader friendliness.

books by the same author

Bhartrihari: Atha Sringarashatakam
Bhartrihari: Atha Vairagyashatakam
Bhartrihari: Atha Nitishatakam
Kalidasa: The Meghadootam

HOW TO STAY HEALTHY WITH HOMOEOPATHY

A Quick Reference Manual for Improving
Your Family's Health

RAJENDRA TANDON

Rupa & Co

For my elder brother, Jagdish Tandon,
in loving gratitude. As a young man
he worked hard and sacrificed his comforts
and the comforts of has wife and children
so that I could study uninterrupted and succeed. How would I ever
repay his debet?

To my loving wife Swarn who has been patient with my long writing
bouts when I tend to forget everything else. For me her forbearance is
priceless and a source of great emotional and physical comfort.
It is to Swarn's credit that she made me seriously interested in the
study of homoeopathy.

Contents

HOMOEOPATHY

SYMPTOMS AND THEIR REMEDIES

THE FACE   62

THE EYES   73

THE EARS   112

THE MOUTH, THE LIPS, THE TONGUE, AND THE PALATE   124

THE TEETH AND THE GUMS   132

THE MALE GENITAL SYSTEM   290

THE RECTUM AND THE ANUS   307

THE STOOL   320

THE LOCOMOTOR SYSTEM   332

MATERIA MEDICA 491

PREFACE

It was a chilly December morning of 1979. A liveried bearer brought a tray with my morning tea and biscuits to the veranda of my room at the Secunderabad Club. He also brought red roses in a vase and laid the tray and the flowers with the sophistication and expertise of a man used to doing even such an ordinary chore with finesse.

In that instant, something happened. I exclaimed to my colleague who was sitting in the chair opposite, "Avatar, I can smell the roses! My sinus has been cured."

"What medicine have you been taking?" Avatar asked excitedly.

"Pulsatilla 30," I answered.

Both of us were familiar with homoeopathy and its medicines in a rudimentary manner. I told him how since my childhood I had suffered from a blocked nose, a bland discharge of yellow-green mucous and how no other system of medicine had been able to cure me of my chronic cold.

I had chosen my medicine on my own after studying the available books on homoeopathy and filtering one medicine after another according to my symptoms until I zeroed on Pulsatilla 30. It was fifteen days since I had started the treatment. This morning I could smell the fragrant roses, a faculty denied to me for years because of a stuffed nose.

The discharge from my nose had stopped a few days earlier. I continued taking the medicine for a few days more because mine was a chronic problem. The return of the sense of smell proved the efficacy of the medicine beyond all doubt.

Since childhood, I had suffered from chronic dysentery, mostly mucous, at other times with blood. Large ayurvedic mixtures prescribed by the Raja-Vaidya at Patiala did not help much. In later years, drugs given by the doctors in the Central Government Health Scheme helped but a few days later the symptoms returned.

In 1976 when I started taking an interest in homoeopathy, I searched for a cure for my chronic dysentery. I selected Merc Sol 200 as the medicine that suited my symptoms. Seven days and twenty-eight doses later, the chronic dysentery disappeared, almost never to return with any severity. Now, although rarely, whenever I sense the symptoms making a show, one or two doses of the medicine are all that is required.

Early morning in May 1980, I was awakened by my friend, S.R. Jha, commissioner of Income Tax, Bombay, who had come to attend a conference in Delhi. "R.K., can you come with a doctor to our guest house to look at S.Y. Gupte who has been vomiting and running to the toilet every few minutes?"

I was with Jha and Gupte in fifteen minutes.

"Where is the doctor?" asked Jha.

"I have the medicine. Gupte should take it now. I shall sit and watch for an hour. If I fail, we need hospitalisation for which arrangements have been made."

I administered a dose of Veratrum Alb 1000 to Gupte, a dear friend. His retching stopped. Soon, he was fast asleep. In the afternoon, to my surprise, he arrived at the conference room at Vigyan Bhavan.

The number of such stories is endless. Every homoeopath has his repertoire.

However, the proof of the pudding lies in eating.

Try for yourself. Start using this book. Persist with the effort at differentiating the symptoms and their remedies. The rewards are handsome.

I do not want to make any tall claims for homoeopathy. It does not cure every malady. However, for that matter, which system does?

No surgical procedures are available in homoeopathy. No pathological laboratories work for the homoeopaths. No sonography. Neither 2-D echo nor angiography. No MRI. No CT scans.

Yet, there is substantial relief available in homoeopathy for hundreds of ailments. Try Apis 200 or 1000 in cases of severe eye inflammation, whether Trachoma or Conjunctivitis. Relief sets in no time. Administer a mixture of Cimicifuga 200, Bryonia 200, and Cicuta 200 to a person suffering from Cervical Spondylosis. He will soon bless you.

Homoeopathic medicines are inexpensive. They have no side effects. They are easily available. This book makes their choice easy if you can identify the symptoms precisely.

To perform this feat you do not have to be a trained doctor. If you carefully go through the subchapters under various body parts where I have described the symptoms in detail, even at the cost of repetition, you will soon learn to identify the symptoms your patient is exhibiting. Once you have reached that stage, the choice of the medicine is automatic.

For instance, for chronic sinusitis when the mucous is flowing outwards, Pulsatilla is the remedy. Where ropy, tough, green mucous flows inwards, Kali Bichrome is the medicine of choice.

Blood dysentery requires Merc Cor 30. Mucous dysentery responds to Merc Sol 200. Mucous dysentery with pain in the thighs can be tackled with Rhus Tox 200.

I have highlighted the distinctive symptom that can identify a remedy throughout the book. These are manifestations apparent to our senses. None can have a problem in understanding them.

I have pointed out when you need urgent medical advice. Do not ignore these warnings. Our purpose is to alleviate suffering. Whatever system is best suited and at hand, ought to be used.

I reiterate that anytime you are in doubt about either the nature of the sickness or you face difficulty in zeroing upon symptoms, please consult a qualified physician or surgeon as the occasion demands.

This book has been organised in a user-friendly manner. Symptoms and remedies are given under the various body parts in sub-chapters titled with the common *nomenclature of the disease* or sensations like *pain, burning, sweating* or even body parts such as *thighs*. A reader can reach his problem by looking at the chapter index.

The section on Materia Medica deals in detail with forty-seven carefully selected remedies. This part is valuable reading for anyone who is interested in understanding the core of the homoeopathic system. For an exhaustive study of Materia Medica refer to books written by J.T. Kent, Dr. William Boerick or Dr. E.B. Nash mentioned in the

Bibliography. All these treatises and many others are a source of priceless information. For me, reading these books has been a rewarding experience.

Please read Dr. Samuel Hahnemann's *Organon of Medicine*, often. He was a pioneer, a genius and a great writer. He had the courage of his convictions and explained his theories of homoeopathy boldly and fearlessly to a disbelieving fraternity of doctors.

I acknowledge my debt to Dr. Samuel Hahnemann, and to other great pioneers like Dr. C. Hering, Dr. T.F. Allen, Dr. J.T. Kent, Dr. William Boerick, and Dr. E.B. Nash. Their learned writings have been an inspiration.

For selection of symptoms, I have taken guidance from whatever original sources I could tap. There is an unavoidable reliance on original symptoms as recorded by the "Provers" and tabulated by Dr. S. Hahnemann, his colleagues and successors.

I have suggested a list of remedies that can be kept handy in every home. Another small list of remedies that can be carried by a traveller on his journey inland or abroad will be found at the end of the book.

An interesting section in this book is *'A Short Circuit to Selection of Remedies/ A Repertory for Instant Reference in Home, Office and for Travellers.'* This provides you with the essence of the book in a few pages. Make a copy and carry it with you wherever you go to work or for pleasure.

I believe that homoeopathy is a significant system of healing within its limitations. It is suited to all, the old, the young, the rich or the poor, men or women, people in developed countries or in the underdeveloped ones. India, the United Kingdom, most European countries, Latin American countries, use homoeopathy on a vast scale. The USA, where the system flourished a hundred years ago, is catching up.

Besides being inexpensive, homoeopathic remedies give relief fast. If in an acute case you do not get relief within a reasonable period, please recheck your choice of remedy. In a chronic case, the chosen remedy takes time to take effect.

My reply to those critics of homoeopathy who say that homoeopathic medicines cannot be tested in a laboratory is, "Every day they are tested in millions of effective doses in the human body, the most complicated laboratory designed by nature. Is that not enough evidence of the efficacy of the system?" May be one day we will have tools to scientifically test the efficacy of the minute homoeopathic dose. Until then let doubt not assail our faith in a proven system of healthcare.

In any case, homoeopathy has outlived its detractors for two centuries. Everyday it grows stronger! That is reason enough to raise a homoeopathic toast to the health of mankind.

In the making of this book my daughter, Bindu has helped me tirelessly with reading and suggestions. It was a labour of love. I record my thanks and appreciation.

My editor at Rupa, Sanjana Roychoudhury, has edited this book with her customary smile and dedication. Our interactions on e-mail have been thought proroking and inwariable fruitful. I express my gratitude to her

My publisher, and his son Kapish Mehra have taken immense interest in this project. So has Mrs. Mehra. She is barely interested in Homoeopathy. Sincere thanks to all three of them.

R.K. Tandon
Mumbai
January, 2007

HOMOEOPATHY

HOMOEOPATHY, THE SYSTEM, ITS ORIGIN, AND PRACTICE

Homoeopathy is a system of medicine in which symptoms of a sickness are treated with medicinal substances, which, if taken in their pure form, will cause similar symptoms to appear. This is an apparent contradiction. However, in practice this principle of 'like cures like' has worked to the satisfaction of the patients all over the world since the time of Dr. Samuel Christian Hahnemann. [11 April 1755-2 July-1843.]

Dr. Hahnemann, a German physician was a practicing allopath when he, dissatisfied with the prevalent mode of medical diagnosis and treatment, after considerable thinking and experimentation, formulated the basic principles of the system of homoeopathic cure.

Dr. Hahnemann strived to know why a particular substance was used to cure a particular sickness. He did not get a satisfactory answer from his teachers, from eminent doctors of the time or from textbooks.

In 1790, Dr. Hahnemann started an experiment to test China, a drug made from Peruvian bark and used for treating periodic fevers and other ailments. He found that he could make himself sick by taking, twice a day, four drachms of the medicine, in pure form. He noted that many different symptoms of diseases which were being treated with China appeared in his body.

It struck Dr. Hahnemann that in a healthy person China developed symptoms similar to the ones it was used to cure in a sick man. He reasoned that this could be true of other substances as well.

However, there was a catch. Pure arsenic kills by poisoning the system. How could it be administered to take care of cases of food poisoning? A bee sting causes inflammation. How will it take care of swelling, heat, and pain? Pure mercury was known to generate several symptoms of decay. Wherein did lie hidden its goodness to treat decay in various parts of the body?

Dr. Hahnemann started administering pure substances diluted in a scientific manner and soon discovered that the basic premise of his theory was correct. With dilution which he called potencization, the learned doctor obtained startling results by way of cures. This became the second principle of the homoeopathic system.

Dr. Hahnemann wrote: *"This remarkable change in the qualities of natural bodies develops the latent, hitherto unperceived, as if slumbering, hidden, dynamic powers which influence the life principle change the well being of animal life. This is affected by mechanical action upon their smallest particles by means of rubbing and shaking and through the addition of an indifferent substance, dry or fluid. This process is called dynamizing, potencizing [development of medicinal power] and the products are dynamizations or potencies in different degrees."*

Potencization is not to be confused with simple dilution. The latter does not develop the hidden curative qualities of a substance.

During experiments conducted on human volunteers it was further found that higher the potencization, the greater is the curative force generated. I have experienced this efficacy of higher potencies, say of Veratrum Alb 1000 in cases of profuse rice water stools with retching, vomiting, of Calcarea Fluorica 1000 in case of calcaneal spur, of Rhus Tox 1000 in case of sciatic pain, of Bryonia 200 in bronchitis, of Antimony Tart 1000 in mucous that has settled in the lungs and does not come out and in several other situations.

Dr. Hahnemann's experiments revealed another valuable principle of homoeopathy. Besides known medicinal substances, potencization converted several inert substances like wood charcoal, sand, lime etc. into efficacious medicinal substances. Carbo Veg, a medicine of tremendous benefit under several conditions, is made out of charcoal ash. Silicea is made out of sand.

I have stated earlier that so many pure substances can cause serious sickness if administered as such. I referred to arsenic, a known poison. Homoeopathy uses dozens of natural or animal poisons to cure. The secret of cure lies in potencization. The adverse properties of a substance are neutralized by this process. To put it differently, potencization brings out the curative quality in such measure as to totally overwhelm the inherent adverse properties.

Homoeopathy does not use any substance unless it has been proved. By proving, we mean administering a pure substance to healthy human beings, observing, and meticulously recording the effects produced in them. Thousands of such trials have been made and their records have been published. The entire system has been built around those observations and records. If an adverse effect is noticed uniformly and repeatedly, it can be cured by the substance that generated it. This adverse effect is called a *leading symptom*.

Homoeopathy uses natural substances sourced from mineral, herbal, and animal kingdom. The drugs are manufactured in a manner that does not render them toxic. There are no side effects of homoeopathic drugs. Their shelf-life, if stored carefully, is long.

HOMOEOPATHIC REMEDIES
STORAGE AND DOSAGE

1. Store medicines in airtight phials. Keep them away from sunlight, heat, and moisture. Perfumes and other substance with strong odours ought not to be stored nearby.
2. Keep a number of medicines handy in your home. Wooden or plastic boxes are available for this purpose. A select list of medicines most often used follows.
3. Ask your chemist to make phials of 2 drams each. I prefer pill size 20. Pills are easy to handle as against liquids.
4. The medicines are good for years unless discolouration occurs.
5. Your chemist will label the medicines on the bottle. Ask him to add the date of packing. You can add small labels on the top for quick selection. For convenience, arrange the medicines alphabetically.
6. Put the cap back tightly after using a phial.
7. Keep all medicines out of the reach of children.
8. Take 4 to 8 pills on a dry tongue as a dose. [The number of pills depends on your psychological satisfaction. A large number taken at a time constitutes one dose only.] Let the pills dissolve on the tongue. Do not use water. When taking the medicine in liquid form, keep the drops rolling on the tongue for a few seconds. The purpose is to let the medicine enter the bloodstream immediately.
9. In acute cases, where the sickness comes suddenly and flares up fast, the first few doses can be safely taken at thirty minutes interval.

However, as the symptoms stabilize, reduce the dose to four times a day. Discontinue the medicine gradually as the cure occurs.

10. In chronic cases, medicines with higher potencies are recommended. At the outset, two doses can be safely taken during a day. Later reduce the dose to one. Stop when the cure has occurred.

11. An aggravation may occur if a wrong medicine has been chosen or too many doses have been administered. *Do not panic.* Stop taking the medicine. The aggravation will subside. In case the aggravation is of the disease for which the medicine was administered, it is a proof of cure.

12. For children use 30 potency ordinarily. Nevertheless, a higher potency will do no harm. Just reduce the number of doses.

13. *At times it happens that a medicine after showing good results, stops leading to a cure. In such cases, increase the potency to the next.*

14. If no improvement occurs and the patient does not feel better after the first few doses, it is time to think whether the medicine has been carefully chosen.

MEDICINE CHEST FOR YOUR HOME WITH A FEW QUICK REFERENCE SYMPTOMS

Keep this carefully selected medicine chest handy. It can save you many a visit to a doctor and expense.

The listed medicines have several uses. Reference is available in the chapters on various systems and parts of the body, and in the Materia Medica part of this volume. What is given here is more like a lighthouse beam.

A reverse chart will be found at the end of this book. It is called repertory. Therein the quick reference medicines are listed against names of sickness or prominent symptoms.

	Medicine	Quick reference symptoms
1.	Abies Nigra 200	**Obstruction in the oesophagus**. As if an egg is lodged in the cardiac end of the stomach.
2.	Aconite Nap 30	**Acute, sudden** cold, fever, hoarse, dry croupy cough etc. Anything on **exposure to dry cold air. Numbness. Tingling**. Great remedy in ailments of children with other well-chosen medicines.
3.	Allium Cepa 200	**Burning, smarting in the eyes**. Bland flow from the eyes. Copious, acrid discharge from the nose. Hoarseness. **Tickling in the larynx**.
4.	Aloe 200	**Loss of control in passing stool** which is

expelled with flatus or urine. Lumpy, watery, gel like, yellowish stool. Pulsating pain around navel. Burning in anus.

5. Antim Crud 200 **Indigestion with sour eructation.** Nausea, retching, vomiting after food.
Foul wind downwards.

6. Antim Tart 1000 **Asthma. Bronchitis. Rattling cough.** Mucous lodged in chest. Inability to take it out. Rattling can be heard in other rooms.

7. Apis 200 **Swelling anywhere.** Red rosy hue. Stinging pain. **Insect bites.**
Inflammation of the eyelids. **Severe trachoma. Violent conjunctivitis. Uvula swollen.**

8. Argentum Nitricum 200 **Acidity with cutting pain** in the centre of the ribs. Hiatus hernia.
Ulceration of the stomach with pain radiating in all directions.
Green spinach like stool in diarrhoea.

9. Arnica 200 In **injuries,** physical or emotional, acute or chronic.
Angina pectoris. [Always carry with you.]

10. Arsenic Alb 200 **Food poisoning.** Indigestion. **Typhoid.**
Burning pain in eyes, in throat, in stomach, in rectum.
Oozing eczema.

11. Arundo 200 **Acute burning, itching in palate, nostrils, gums, eyes with unbearable discomfort.**
Hay fever. **Onset of cold.**

12. Belladonna 200 Great remedy for children.
Heavy congestion. **Heat, redness, throbbing and burning anywhere.** Skin **bright red,** shining. **Severe tonsillitis.**
Violent attack. Sudden onset.

13. Bryonia 200, 1000 **Bronchitis. Hacking cough** with pain in the centre of the ribs.
Arthritic pain worse on movement.

Discomforts of the **knee joint**. Constipation. **Stool hard, dry**, as if burnt.

14. Calendula ointment

A most remarkable healing agent applied locally. For **bruises, injuries**. Open wounds, ulcers, parts that do not heal. Rough skin.

15. Camphor 30 and mother tincture. Drops on a clean cloth to smell.

In **cholera, collapse**. Icy coldness of the whole body. Pulse small and weak. Besides smelling, 30 potency doses every 15 minutes.

16. Cantharis 200. Mother tincture for local application as often as possible.

Burns. Scalds. Great medicine for this emergency. Relieves pain. Heals the skin. Administer pills and apply diluted tincture on affected skin.

Intolerable, constant urging to urinate. Urine burns, scalds.

17. Carbo Veg 200

The finest medicine available for **acidity.** Indigestion. **Lack of appetite**. For weakness resulting from perennial sickness.

18. Chamomilla 30

Irritable, peevish child. Pain, diarrhoea during **dentition.**

19. China off 200

Flatulence.

Weakness following **loss of liquids** from the body for any reason such as cold or haemorrhage.

Intense **throbbing of head and carotids. Intermittent fevers**.

20. Cimicifuga 200. Great remedy for cervical spondylosis. Use with Bryonia.

Cervical spondylosis. Giddiness. Stiffness and contraction in neck and back. **Pain in shoulder blades.**

Rheumatic pains in muscles of back and neck. Pain in lumbar and sacral region, down thighs and through hips.

21. Cocculus 200

Travel sickness.

22. Coffea Cruda 200

Insomnia. Cannot sleep at the right hour.

23. Colocynthis 200

Agonizing pain in abdomen causing patient to bend double.

Sensation of cutting, twisting, grinding, contracting, and bruised; as if clamped with iron bands.

Dysenteric stool renewed each time by least food or drink. Jelly like stool. Musty odour.

24. Cuprum Met 200   **Epileptic fit**. Jerking and twitching of muscles. Coldness of hands. Clenched thumbs. Spasms beginning in fingers and toes.
Cramps in palms, in calves and toes.

25. Drosera 200   **Whooping cough**. Paroxysms rapidly following each other. Can scarcely breathe. Chokes. Asthma when talking.

26. Dulcamara 200   Colds on **exposure to damp, cold weather**. Stuffs up when there is cold rain.
Winter coughs, dry, teasing.
Whooping cough, with excessive secretion of mucous.

27. Eupatorium Perf 200   **Pain deep in the bones**, a consequence of another sickness. Aching pain in the back. Aching in bones of extremities with soreness in chest.
Influenza with great soreness of muscles.

28. Euphrasia 200   **Catarrhal conjunctivitis.**
Discharge of acrid matter.
Sticky mucous on cornea.

29. Gelsemium 200   **Onset of influenza. Severe body pain.**
Pain in the temple extending into ear and wing of nose, chin.
Congestion in the back, centre of the skull as if it is being **tightened by a steel band.**
Vertigo with the above sensation.
Dullness, languor, **listlessness many days in advance.**
Pain from throat to the ear.

30. Glonoine 200   **Heat stroke**. Surging of blood to head and heart. Throbbing.
Vertigo on assuming upright position.
Collapse. Feeble heart. Angina pectoris.
Wiry, small pulse. Pallor.

31. Hepar Sulph 200   **Abscess. Pain as if a needle is being thrust** deep through flesh.

Tendency to suppurate.

Pus on tonsils: white patches. Stabbing pain on empty swallowing.

Discharge of **fetid pus** from anywhere on the body.

32. Hypericum 200

Injuries to nerves, especially of fingertips and toes. Severe pain.

Spinal concussion. Injury to coccyx in a fall.

33. Ipecac 200

Nausea for any reason. **Vomiting.**

Asthma.

Sore throat with a sensation of **heaviness.**

Wheezing. Cough incessant and violent with every breath.

34. Kali Bichrome 200

Sinusitis. Pain in sinuses, bones above the eyes, in the eyeballs and behind the ears.

Can never clear throat of **sticky, green mucous flowing downwards.** Trying to do so every morning.

Profuse, yellow expectoration, very glutinous and sticky, coming out in a **long, stringy, and tenacious mass.**

35. Kreosotum 200

Painful dentition.

Rapid decay of teeth, with spongy, bleeding gums.

36. Lachesis 200

Tonsils inflamed with a **purple colouring.** Cutting pain. Difficult empty swallowing.

37. Ledum 200

Anti tetanus. Punctured wounds.

Anal fissures.

38. Lycopodium 200

Indigestion with flatus. Eating ever so little creates fullness.

Incomplete, burning eructation rising to pharynx.

Haemorrhoids painful to touch.

39. Merc Cor 30

Iritis.

Throat red, swollen, painful, intensely inflamed. **Uvula swollen**. Swallowing painful. Pain in postnasal spreading to ears. Burning pain.

Tenesmus of bladder, of stool. A 'never get done' feeling.
Blood dysentery.
Ulcers that do no heal.

40. Merc Sol 200   **Fetid odour** from mouth. **Gums inflamed, spongy, recede easily.**
Thick, yellow discharge from ears. Pain in the ears.
Tonsillitis. Pus formed but not much pain.
Pain and swelling of **nasal bones,** with **fetid, greenish ulceration**. Thick or running coryza.
Mucous dysentery.

41. Millefolium 200   Various types of **haemorrhages. Blood bright red.**
Nosebleed. Blood from bowels, in urine, from haemorrhoids, while coughing.

42. Natrum Mur 200   **Blinding headache**, as if a thousand little hammers were knocking on the brain
Violent, **fluent coryza**. Cold commencing with sneezing.
Numbness. Palms hot and perspiring.
Malarial fevers.

43. Nitric Acid 200   **Splinter pain in blisters in the mouth**.
Bleeding ulcers. Ulcers on the soft palate. Bloody saliva.
Bleeding, spongy gums. Teeth coming loose.

44. Nux Vomica 200   **Hangover.** Effects of heavy drinking. Vertigo with momentary loss of consciousness.
Constipation. Frequent, ineffectual urging to stool. Constant uneasiness in the rectum.Itching, blind haemorrhoids.
Sleeplessness early morning, from around 3 a.m.

45. Podophyllum 200   Profuse, **gushing, offensive, yellow, green, stool with jelly like mucous.**
Prolapse of rectum before or after stool.

46. Pulsatilla 30   Thick, profuse, **yellow, bland discharge** from anywhere, eyes, ears or nose etc.

Chronic cold. Sense of smell lost. Nose stuffed. **Otorrhoea**. Catarrhal otitis. Mucous full of pus coming out in bronchitis.

Indigestion, flatulence because of **overindulgence in heavy food.**

47. Ratanhia 200

Anal fissures with constriction, burning like fire. **Oozing** at anus.

Rectum aches as if full of **broken glass**.

48. Rhus Tox 200, 1000

Muscular pains temporarily better on movement.

Strain.

Mucous dysentery with pain in thighs.

Sciatica on the left side.

49. Ruta 200

Eyestrain followed by headache. Eyes red hot and painful sewing, reading, using a PC, or doing fine needlework.

Pain and stiffness in **wrists and hands, in bones of feet and ankles.**

50. Sepia 200

Constipation. Large, hard stools. Dark brown, round balls **glued together with mucous**. Feeling of a ball in the rectum.

In females, **bearing down sensation** as if everything would escape through vulva.

51. Silicea, 200

Long lasting suppuration in any part of the body.

Stinging pain on swallowing. **Chronic cases**.

Anal fistula. Fissures and haemorrhoids, painful, with spasm of the sphincter.

Abscesses, boils, old fistulous ulcers.

To expel **foreign bodies in tissues anywhere**.

52. Sulphur 200

Dry, scaly, unhealthy skin. Every little injury suppurates.

Itching, burning, worse scratching, and washing.

Burning in soles and hands at night. Hot, sweaty hands.

Revives the effect of medicine already taken.

Complaints that relapse. *When carefully selected remedies fail to act, especially in acute cases.*

53. Veratrum Alb 1000 **Collapse with extreme coldness**, blueness, and weakness. **Cold sweats**.

Copious vomiting and nausea.

Cholera. Cramps in extremities.

Uncontrollable rice water stools with retching.

SELECTION OF REMEDY
GUIDING PRINCIPLES

Sometime in 1980, on way to my office, as I reached the door of my garage in Bharti Nagar, New Delhi, I saw a middle-aged woman sitting near the next gate with her leg bare and oozing a sticky liquid. I asked her what had gone wrong. She told me that she had been suffering from chronic eczema·of the skin and felt miserable.

I returned home, prepared a small phial of Arsenic 200, and asked the patient to take 4 pills on dry tongue, 4 times a day for a few days.

I met her after about a week sitting at the same spot and basking in the winter sun with her leg covered this time. I asked her if she had been taking the medicine regularly.

"I finished the medicine in two days. The pills were tiny," she answered.

"Come in the evening and take some more medicine," I said.

"I do not need any. My leg is dry and clean."

Even I was astonished.

I examined her leg. Not only had the oozing disappeared, but also healthy skin had formed all over.

It was a skin problem. If you refer the chapter on '*The Skin*', reach the sub-chapter titled '*Eczema*', you will notice the following entry:

'Suppressed, chronic eczema. Oozing holes with offensive discharge.' Arsenic Alb 200.

That is precisely how you select your remedy.

- Ask the patient about the state of his mind. Ask him to describe in his own words what is being experienced by him while suffering from a particular sickness. Besides, note what is apparent and write it on a piece of paper in minute detail. Slight differences in symptoms can lead to the choice of a different remedy.
- Go to the chapter dealing with the affected part of the body.
- Look at the list of contents. You will find the name either of the disease or of the symptom or both.
- Turn to the relevant page and go through all the symptoms listed. You will soon reach the precise symptoms that you noticed or those which have been described by the patient.
- Fill in the gaps in information by asking questions based on the symptoms as indicated against various remedies. Narrow down the specifics by excluding very general symptoms.
- Quite often, the symptoms require more than one remedy. Bronchitis requires Bryonia. However, if green mucous is coughed out, Pulsatilla too has to be given. If the chest rattles with phlegm which cannot be taken out, Antim Tart has to be added. There is no harm in giving more than one remedy together or separately at short intervals so long as the remedies do not clash. [Refer chart of inimical remedies].

Homoeopathic treatment is based on an overall understanding of the symptoms in the mind and body created by a sickness.

Dr. Hahnemann had, based on extensive research, concluded that symptom-similarity is the curative method of medically curable diseases. He wrote in paragraph twenty-five of the *Organon of Medicine*:

"——that medicine which , in its action on the healthy human body, has demonstrated its power of producing the greatest number of symptoms similar to those observable in the case of disease under treatment, does also, in doses of suitable potency and attenuation, rapidly, radically, and permanently remove the totality of symptoms of this morbid state,——and change it into health.——all medicines cure,

*without exception, those diseases whose symptoms most nearly resemble
their own and leave none of them uncured."*

This indicates the importance of symptoms in the diagnosis and
treatment in homoeopathy. I shall illustrate this with examples from the
chapter on *The Digestive System*, sub-chapter, *Indigestion*.

Indigestion from overeating and eructation as soon as food is taken,
indicates Antim Crud.

In Carbo Veg, eructation is not there but indigestion is accompanied
by acidity.

Acidity with pain needs Argentum Nitricum. Please notice the
change and the addition of pain to acidity.

Indigestion leads to flatulence. The abdomen is bloated like a tent.
We choose China.

Indigestion with flatus moving downwards requires Lycopodium.

When nausea is the most prominent symptom, Ipecac comes in.

These symptoms are easily distinguishable. That is how you choose
your remedy.

In chronic cold, bland, green mucous flowing outwards indicates
Pulsatilla. The same mucous going inwards and getting sticky, responds
to Kali Bichrome.

The tonsils are purple in colour. You require Lachesis. The tonsils
are red and inflamed. Belladonna is indicated. Tonsils are inflamed with
pus patches on them. On empty swallowing, there is stabbing pain. Use
Hepar Sulph.

Thus, the choice of the correct remedy is a matter of observation
and concentration on differences between the indications of different
remedies.

With practice, concentration, and experience, it would not be
difficult for you to arrive at the correct remedy. Try to notice minute
differences. They play an important role.

For acute problems, repeat medicines in a low potency such as 30,
every fifteen minutes or half an hour until the patient stabilises.
Thereafter raise the potency as indicated and administer four times a
day.

In chronic cases, the selected remedy has to be administered in a
high potency such as 1000 or 10000, once or twice a day for quite a

few days, even weeks. Recovery sets in slowly, imperceptibly until a cure occurs.

If recovery stops midway, it is time to raise the potency to the next level.

If an aggravation occurs, stop medication. Cure has set in.

Absence of amelioration indicates choice of a wrong medicine. Normally, if the medicine has been correctly chosen, the patient starts feeling better after a few doses, often after a single dose.

Administration of drugs ought to be stopped as soon as a cure has occurred. Taper the dosage gradually over two or three days. Using a drug beyond this limit can aggravate the malady which you set out to cure.

SYMPTOMS AND THEIR REMEDIES

THE BRAIN, THE MIND, THE EMOTIONS, AND THE HEAD

Lord Byron, the English poet, called the brain 'the dome of thought, the palace of the soul'. He was right. Our mind, our conscience, our soul [if you believe in one], reside in the brain.

The 'brain' is an anatomical term which means that part of the central nervous system which is encased in the cranium of man and other vertebrates and which consists of grey and white matter. It controls and coordinates all mental and physical activity. It is the centre of the thinking universe of human beings, of their mind and of their intellect. The brain makes thinking, willing, and feeling, perceiving and experiencing emotions possible.

'Mind' has been defined in Dictionary of the English Language as 'the agency or part in a human or other conscious being that reasons, understands, wills, perceives, experiences emotions etc.'

The American Heritage Dictionary defines 'mind' as 'the human consciousness that originates in the brain and is manifested especially in thought, perception, emotion, will, memory and imagination'. It is the 'collective conscious and unconscious processes in a sentient organism that direct and influence mental and physical behaviour'.

Basically, 'mind' is an intangible faculty that the anatomical 'brain' exercises and that has been equated with intelligence. Thus awareness, reasoning, understanding, will power to express emotions, to take decisions, to love, to hate, to feel and express anger, to take notice or to ignore, all these and other qualities of the human beings are attributable to their having a 'mind of their own'.

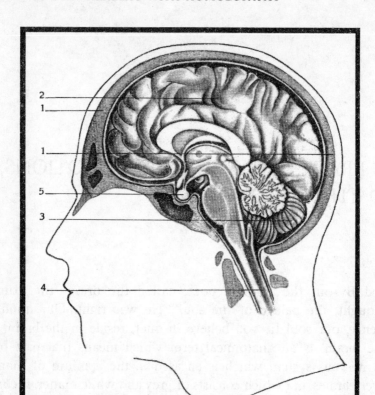

1. Cranium [Skull bone]. 2. Cerebrum. 3. Cerebellum.
4. Spinal cord. 5. Pituitary gland. (Secretes several hormones)

'Memory' is a faculty of the mind but anatomically it is the brain that provides the storage for experiencing and retaining data thereof.

The faculty to reason is an intellectual exercise and is different from 'feeling'. Intellect too is exercised by the 'mind' using the 'brain' as a physical medium.

'Emotions' result from complicated interaction between sensory information reaching the brain and processes of remembering and evaluation.

It is the 'mind', which experiences 'emotions'. The latter create physical changes in the body. Our hair stand on end when we are frightened or excited. The emotion of love makes the heart beat faster. Smiling, laughing, feeling sorrow, expressing shock, fear, hatred, or attraction, all these activities flow from emotions flowing from the mind.

The 'mind' does all this through the physical agency of the 'brain'. The body reacts. It expresses, obeying the commands from the control centre in the brain. "Tis the mind that makes the body reach", wrote Shakespeare in *The Taming of the Shrew*. That is why so many maladies in the following chapter relate to not the physical 'brain' but to disturbances in the intangible 'mind'.

The outer layer of the grey matter that covers the surface of the cerebral hemisphere is known as 'cortex'. Different areas of the cortex carry out different functions. However, in complex functions, for example, learning, more than one area of the cortex is involved. It is like teamwork.

'Cerebral cortex' processes complex information like music, emotions, and data. That is why we call it the 'higher' part of the brain.

Different parts of the cortex look after different functions such as coordinating complex movement sequences, like playing on a piano, [premotor cortex], and sending signals to muscles to cause voluntary movements, [motor cortex].

Other areas look after sensations in the skin, muscles and joints, [primary sensory cortex], analysis of the sensory data, formation of images and analysis of the same, [visual association cortex], interpretation of the spoken and written language, [Wernicke's area], detection of discrete qualities of sound, of its pitch and volume, [primary auditory cortex], recognition of words and melodies, [auditory association cortex], and aspects of behaviour and personality, [prefrontal cortex].

On each side of the body, movement is controlled and touch is sensed by the motor and sensory cortices of the part of the brain on the opposite side.

The word 'head' indicates the upper part of the body in man, which contains the brain, eyes, ears, nose, and mouth. The head is joined to the body by the neck. In lay terms, head is the seat of the mind, the brain, the intellect.

Outside information is conveyed to the brain via the nerves. In turn, the brain issues directions to the muscles to react to the information thus conveyed and be mobile. This too is done through nerves.

The spinal cord serves as a conduit for the nerves leaving the brain.

The brain depends on a continuous supply of oxygen through thousands of blood vessels. Permanent damage can be caused to the brain cells, if, for any reason, the blood supply is stopped for more than two minutes.

If a blood vessel bursts or is choked by internal narrowing, the victim suffers a stroke resulting in paralysis, loss of mental faculties and sometimes death. That is why I have sounded a warning for immediate medical help, even hospitalization, in quite a few of the following sub-chapters.

The versatility of the human brain is infinite. Man's creativity in art, literature, music, mathematics, and sciences, is witness to this. The storing capacity of the brain is amazing. No computer has so far exceeded, or even equalled the intellectual or other functions of the brain. The human recall of the past happenings is incredible.

How does the brain control the human body, is an enigma.

When a person changes his behaviour adversely and for no reason, it is a sign of mental illness. Our upbringing trains us to distinguish between right and wrong. A mental illness can change all that.

The patients suffering from mental illnesses require our sympathy. Give it in full measure. Remember the plaint of King Lear when he was let down by those on whom he had showered all his wealth:

"O let me not be mad,
Sweet heaven!
Keep me in temper;
I would not be mad"!

Here is the cry of a brave man who felt that he was going to lose his mental balance. Quite probably, the mentally sick feel the same. Listen to them. In this, perhaps, might be found their cure.

'A sound mind in a sound body', wrote Juvenal, the Roman satirist, almost two thousand years ago. This dictum is as true today as it ever was. As pointed out in the following sub-chapter, *Memory/the Problems of* to keep our mind in balance and healthy, the same diet and the same exercise have to be undertaken as are necessary for, say, keeping the heart in a sound condition.

Meditation is one of the most effective means to keep our mind at peace and in balance. Any system of meditation is good. It is easy. It costs nothing. Just sit down in a quiet corner of your house, close your eyes, and banish all thought. Breathe deep and exhale chanting 'OM' [pronounced 'aum'], in a measured tone, prolonging the exhalation as long as possible. Do it for thirty minutes or more, every day, at the same time. Take the telephone off the hook. Controlling the thought will be difficult, to begin with. However, with passage of time you will succeed. In any case, if the mind wanders, do not feel guilty. Bring it back to concentrate on the movement of your breath.

Two thousand years ago, Bhartrihari, a king turned hermit and poet, advised us to lead a life of equanimity. He put down his ideas on meditation in the following words:

"I wait for the moment when, sitting in the lotus pose on a Himalayan rock on the banks of the Ganges, contemplating the Supreme Being, I shall be lost in a meditative trance.

"I shall be so impervious to my surroundings that the aged deer, roaming free in the jungle, will fearlessly needle my body with the edges of their horns.

"At that moment, after making a continuous effort according to the prescribed meditation techniques, I shall be submerged in the deep and relaxed mental state of the great yogis wherein all the external senses and their experiences are no longer relevant".

The Vairagya Shatakam, Shloka 41.

You do not have to leave everything and go to a jungle to meditate. You can do it in your home. However, the basic rules are the same.

Visualisation can be a fascinating aspect of your meditation. Close your eyes. Think of pleasant journeys, such as to a garden in bloom, to a stunning waterfall, to green countryside, to a bird sanctuary, to any place you have experienced or would like to experience and that gave you peace of mind.

Climb a mountain. Marvel at the snow covered peaks.

Look at a rainbow, moving your sight from one end to the other end.

Walk in the woods. Listen to the bird song.

Sit by a gushing stream. Listen to the song of the waves on a see shore. Fly with the sea gulls into the unknown.

Float on a cloud. Be one with nature. 'Stand and stare' in your imagination.

Welcome the rays of the sun entering your body and overtaking you in your entirety. Feel their golden, healing warmth in each nook and corner of your body. Relax your muscles one by one as the sunrays travel and touch them. Think that your tension, your pains are disappearing.

"The mind can weave itself warmly in the cocoon of its own thoughts, and dwell a hermit anywhere", wrote J.R. Lowell in 1869. Turn inwards. Listen to relaxation music. Be a hermit in your home. Alternatively, go to a park nearby.

To improve concentration, meditate, do *Pranayama* and yoga.

Spend time in pleasant company.

Develop a hobby such as gardening.

Read selected enlightening literature, particularly poetry.

The requirement of medicine will become secondary if you exercise self-control through good thoughts and noble deeds. Be pleasant to everyone. Do not think ill of others. Forgive even your enemies. Barter feelings of hatred with feelings of love.

On the field of Kurukshetra, Krishna advised Arjuna to develop an attitude of equanimity, to look at sorrow and joy with indifference and stay firm. For many a problem of the brain, this still holds good.

Be happy. Laugh. You may not need medicine.

ABSCESS OF THE BRAIN

A life-threatening emergency. Seek medical help immediately.

A collection of pus caused by bacterial or fungal infection. Brain tissue swells around the abscess-filled pocket. The patient feels pressure inside the skull.

It is often caused by a sudden attack of otitis media, a dental abscess, or infection in the sinuses.

Symptoms: Severe headache in the morning, worse lying down. Nausea, vomit. As the pus forms, temperature rises. Seizures can occur. If left untreated, the patient can become unconscious and ultimately lapse into a coma.

Distinguishing symptoms of the patient	Medicine and potency
• Abscess formed because of injury.	
• **First aid on concussion.**	Arnica 200
• **Throbbing and burning pain**. Symptoms develop fast.	Belladonna 200
• Otitis media.Tearing pain in the middle and external ear. **Delirium.**	
• **Clouded perception. Loss of memory.** Patient depressed, confused, sad. Auditory vertigo.	Crotalus H 200
• **Blood oozing** from ears.	
• Discharge of fetid **pus with shooting pain.** Temperature.	Hepar Sulph 200
• Inflammation of the middle ear leading to brain abscess.	Myristica 200

ALOPECIA/ BALDNESS

Loss of hair can occur in any part of the body. However, hair loss on the scalp is most worrying, cosmetically at least. These days it can be treated surgically by transplantation and quite successfully too. Consult a specialist.

Distinguishing symptoms of the patient	Medicine and potency
• Hair turns grey at a young age. Starts falling.	Phosphoric Acid 200
• Itching of scalp. Dandruff. Hair falling in large bunches.	Phosphorus 200, once a day.
• Hair dry, falling. Dandruff white and scaly.	Thuja 200

AMNESIA

Loss of memory because of injury to the head, excessive intake of alcohol, epileptic fit, or a brain tumour. Emotional upsets can also cause amnesia.

Distinguishing symptoms of the patient	Medicine and potency
• **Absent minded.** Weak memory. Senses of sight, of hearing weak. Old age.	Anacardium 200
• Lack of self-control. Aversion to work.	
• **Confusion of thoughts.**	Lycopodium 200
• Wrong spellings, wrong words, wrong syllables.	

ANGUISH/GRIEF

Anguish is agonizing physical or mental pain that can originate due to several reasons. Grief is deep mental anguish caused by bereavement or unbearable loss.

Besides medicine, seek relief in meditation, spiritual studies, and religion.

Distinguishing symptoms of the patient	Medicine and potency
• Desires to cry but cannot. Melancholic. **Internal grief**.	Ammonium Mur 200
• Apprehends loss.	
• Trauma of **grief, new or old,** of loss human or financial.	Arnica 200. **A great pick up.**
• Wants to be left alone. Morose. Nervous.	
• Does not want to be touched.	
• **Restless** due to grief.	Arsenic Alb 200
• Exhausted after even a slight exertion.	
• Debility all over owing to grief.	
• Aggravation at night.	
• **Hysterical**. Joy and sorrow alternate.	**Ignatia 200**
• Sighs, sobs. Has suffered disappointment.	

ANOREXIA NERVOSA

Some young persons have a misconception that they are overweight, even though they are not. They strive to lose weight by means fair or foul, in sheer ignorance of the debilitating effects of this strategy. They exercise excessively, diet, even vomit or take laxatives. This effort can be life-threatening in some cases. In almost all cases, it creates a hormonal imbalance that can affect growth and later lead to menstruation disorders in women.

Homoeopathy provides a way out as given below.

However, simultaneously, **consult a dietician and a physician if serious symptoms have developed and the patient refuses to understand the gravity of her self-inflicted malady. Psychological therapy too is desirable.**

Distinguishing symptoms of the patient	Medicine and potency
• **Lost appetite**. Does not like the look of food. The simplest of food distresses.	Carbo Veg 200. Take four times a day for a few months.

• **Persistent sensation of nausea**. Self-induced vomiting.	Ipecac 200. Treatment takes a long time.
• Vomits food, blood, mucous, bile.	
• **Nausea not relieved by vomit**.	
• Weight loss accompanied by irregular menstruation. **Pain in sacrum**.	Nux Vomica 200
• Patient sullen, irritable.	

APOPLEXY/STROKE

If an interruption of blood supply to a part of the brain occurs, due to either haemorrhage, or cerebral thrombosis or a blood clot, forming elsewhere, travelling to the brain [cerebral embolism], it leads to a loss of bodily functions.

Symptoms: The symptoms develop rapidly and include paralysis and numbness on one side of the body in a limb or limbs, inability to perform delicate tasks, which, otherwise, the limbs perform as a matter of routine, blurry vision or loss of vision in one eye, slur in speech, vomit, and vertigo.

Symptoms vary according to the part of the brain affected by the stroke.

It is an emergency. Seek medical advice immediately. Hospitalisation is necessary.

Distinguishing symptoms of the patient	Medicine and potency
• **Paralysis of the left side** of the face, left arm, left leg.	Allium Cepa 200 **All medicines for a few weeks.**
• **Caused by physical injury**. Head hot, body cold. Entire body aches.	Arnica 200. First medicine when the cause is injury.
• **Dilated pupils**. Pulse full, rapid. **Face red** and head congested.	Belladonna 200. In case of sudden attack, use
• Sudden, acute attack.	30 potency dose every 15
• On exposure to cold air.	minutes until situation is under control.

• **Right side of the face** affected. Right arm. Right leg.	Causticum 200
• **Difficulty in speaking, writing, reading**.	
• **Paralysis of tongue, vocal cords, eyelids, face, bladder, and extremities**.	
• **Left-side facial paralysis.**	Lachesis 200
• Cerebral **apoplexy**. Pupils **dilated**.	Opium 1000. One dose per week.
• Jaw droops. Coma. Face dusky, red.	
• Pulse slow, laboured.	

CATAPLEXY

Symptoms: Strong emotions such as fear, mirth, anger or sorrow, can at times cause a collapse of posture. The patient falls to the ground although he is conscious. The head slumps forward and the jaw droops.

These attacks come off and on and a complete cure may not be possible.

Distinguishing symptoms of the patient	Medicine and potency
• **Collapse of posture**.	Cannabis Indica 30 or Mother tincture, 15 drops,
• **Hallucination**. Exaggeration of duration, of time and extent of space.	diluted in water, at a time.
• Unbounded happiness. **Laughter not controllable.**	
• Terrible **depression**.	
• Rapid changes in mood. Emotional excitement.	

COLLAPSE

A loss of consciousness for several reasons.

Distinguishing symptoms of the patient	Medicine and potency
• Collapse for any cause other than death. • **External surfaces cold**, though patient throws off all the covering.	Camphor, mother tincture. Five drops on sugar to be administered every five minutes.
• Collapse in a patient who has been **perennially sick**. • State of collapse **in cholera, in typhoid**. Face puffy, **blue**. Pulse imperceptible. • **Imperfect oxygenation.** • **Last stage** of a sickness with copious **cold sweat, cold breath, cold tongue.** Voice lost.	Carbo Veg 200 Continue for 8 weeks.
• **Epileptic collapse**. Jerking and twitching of muscles. **Eyes fixed**, staring, sunken, glistening, and turning upwards. • Face pale. Lips blue. **Jaws contracted**. **Foam** at the mouth. • Fingers stiff, turned. **Cramps in calves, in soles**. • Unconsciousness.	Cuprum Met 200
• **Collapse in surgical shock**. • Acute vomit and diarrhoea of thin, **copious, rice water stool**. Cholera. **Gastroenteritis**. • Cold sweat on the forehead. Face pale or blue. • Cramps in extremities.	Veratrum Alb 1000

CONCUSSION

An injury to the head that results in unconsciousness. Its complete impact is known only when the patient returns to consciousness.

Symptoms: A partial loss of memory, lack of mental coordination. Confusion. Nausea. Dizziness. Headache.
Seek medical counsel.

Distinguishing symptoms of the patient	Medicine and potency
• **First remedy in any injury on the head.** In recent cases as well as chronic cases where the effects of injury appear a long time after the injury was suffered.	Arnica 200
• **Resulting in convulsions**.	Cicuta 200
• In a **chronic case** where Arnica has proved ineffective.	
• Of the brain which **feels compressed**.	Hypericum 200
• **Fractured skull**.	Use Arnica simultaneously
• Injury to nerves.	in fractures.

CONGESTION, OF BRAIN, OF HEAD

Accumulation of excessive blood or tissue fluid in blood vessels or organ.

The symptoms have been given below.

Distinguishing symptoms of the patient	Medicine and potency
• **Any surging of blood to the brain.**	Glonoine 200
• First inflammatory stage.	
• **Throbbing, undulating sensation** as if the brain is moving in waves. Fullness. Pain.	

- **Sensation of a rush of blood to the heart**.
- Relief in open air; by application of cold water. He wants his head uncovered.
- Least movement aggravates.
- Worse in warmth. Worse lying down.
- **Throbbing** and **fullness**, but less intense.   Belladonna 200
- Better bending head backwards.
- Better by pressure on head.
- Worse by head uncovered.
  Worse lying down. Any motion aggravates.
- Less disturbance of heart action.
- Goes beyond first stage.

CONVULSIONS/EPILEPTIC FIT/SEIZURE

Sudden, abnormal electrical activity of the brain leads to convulsions.

Symptoms: The body stiffens and breathing becomes irregular, to begin with. An uncontrolled movement of the limbs and the trunk occurs. Mental confusion and disorientation follow. A variety of symptoms are exhibited such as, the head and the eye turning to one side, twitching on one side of the face, foaming at the mouth, numbness, grimaces, an experience of unusual smells and sounds.

In petit mal seizures, the child lies with eyes open and staring, out of touch with his surroundings. He later forgets all about the episode.

Distinguishing symptoms of the patient	Medicine and potency
• Cerebral congestion in children.	Belladonna 200
• Sudden.	
• **Intense heat, redness, throbbing**. The child jumps in sleep.	
• From concussion of brain.	Cicuta 200
• **Frightful distortions**. The patient is violent.	

• Epilepsy with moaning, **howling**. **Limbs curved**. Cramps in calves and feet.	
• Caused by **worms. Twitching limbs**.	Cina 200
• Left foot in spasmodic motion.	
• Inward jerking of the fingers of the right hand.	
• **Epilepsy**. Violent pain.	Cuprum Met 200
• Unconsciousness.	
• Convulsions beginning in fingers, palms and toes. **Cramps**.	
• **Foam** at the mouth. **Face distorted**. **Contraction of jaws. Lips blue**.	

DEBILITY

The state of being weak or feeble. Infirmity owing to several causes. Symptoms are indicated below against the respective remedies.

Distinguishing symptoms of the patient	Medicine and potency
• **Debility all over**. Sudden. Exhaustion after the slightest exertion.	Arsenic Alb 200
• **Restlessness** mental and physical. Anguish.	
• **Body always freezing**.	
• Debility in **asthma, in typhoid, in malaria, coryza, food poisoning**.	
• Aggravation at night.	
• **Never ending sickness**. Never a full recovery.	Carbo Veg 200. To be taken four times a day for a few months until the patient feels recovered.
• Deficient supply of oxygen. **Face blue. Skin pale**.	
• **Cold sweat**, cold breath, cold tongue, voice lost.	
• **Chronic indigestion. Acidity**.	

- Caused by **excessive loss of fluids**,   China 200
  mucous or blood, from the body,
  for whatever reason.
- **Debility after intermittent fevers** like
  malaria, typhoid.
- Face pale, sunken eyes.
  Sweats on least motion.
- **Darkness in front of eyes.**
  Ringing sound in ears.
- Loss of memory. Apathetic.
  Indifferent, **low-spirited**.
- Averse to hard work.
- **Anaemia caused by loss of fluids**,   Nat Mur 200
  by menstrual irregularities, by grief.
- Pale, emaciated.
- Depressed. Does not want to be consoled.
- **Throbbing headache**.
- Debility of mind, of body. Mental first,   Phosphoric Acid 30
  physical later.
- **Crushing headache**.
- **Nervous exhaustion**
- **Ravages of acute diseases**, excessive
  grief, haemorrhage, of typhoid.
- Grey hair, early in life.
- Deficient sexual prowess.
- **Blue rings around eyes**.
- Mother deteriorates after nursing.

DELIRIUM

A mental disturbance that is acute, of short duration and usually reflects a toxic state of mind. It is caused by a shortage of supply of oxygen to the brain because of heart failure, or because of damage to the brain or due to nutritional and severe vitamin deficiency.

Symptoms: Visual hallucinations, illusions, excitement, restlessness, delusions. Impaired memory. The patient lacks coherence, is disoriented, loses sleep and tosses in the bed. Rapid eye movement. Speech slurred. Repetitive actions. Bites. Spits. Sheds tears. Sees ghosts, heinous faces, animals, and insects. He is loquacious, sings, laughs, grins, whistles, screams, prays, or swears. He indulges in bodily contortions. His face may turn red, flushed, carotids throbbing. He can be lascivious, talks vulgar, and exposes himself.

> *"The physician in charge of such unhappy people must indeed have at his command an attitude which inspires respect but also confidence; he will never feel insulted by them, because a being that cannot reason is incapable of insulting anyone".*

SAMUEL HAHNEMANN, 1796.

Distinguishing symptoms of the patient	Medicine and potency
• Delirium of **fever, alcoholism**. From cerebral excitement.	Agaricus 200
• **Loquacious**. Shouting, muttering, prophesying, rhyming.	
• **In cerebro-spinal meningitis**. Loquacity.	Apis 200
• Child screams, gnashes his teeth.	
• Worse by heat.	
• **Hallucinations**. Visual illusions. Frightful images. Sense of reality lost.	Belladonna 200
• **Cerebral congestion.**	
• Furious. **Rages, bites, strikes, is violent.**	
• Face, skin red-hot. Hands and feet cold. **Throbbing of carotids.** Arteries visible.	
• **Uncontrollable laughter.** Clairvoyance.	Cannabis Indica 30. Mother Tincture for delirium tremens.
• With epilepsy, mania, dementia.	
• Excessive loquacity.	
• **Amorous frenzy**. Fiery sexual desire.	Cantharis 200
• **Urinary complications present.**	

• Furious. Paroxysms of rage, crying, barking.	
• Sudden loss of consciousness. Face red.	
• **Talks obscene. Uncovers genitals**.	Hyoscymus 200
• Deep stupor and hallucination alternate.	
• Face pale, sunken.	
• Talks in delirium **with eyes wide open**.	Opium 200
• Tremors.	
• **Talks with spirits**. Violent Lewd. Swears, sings, and prays. Tremors.	Stramonium 30

DEMENTIA

As we grow old, there is a marked deterioration in the intellectual and physical condition of the brain. However, there can be other causes such as vitamin deficiency, pernicious anaemia, rarely some brain disorders that may require a proper diagnosis and treatment. Serious cases may require hospitalization.

Symptoms: Disorientation of memory, particularly the memory of recent events. The sense of time is lost. The patient has no interest in life. His concentration is poor. He forgets names. His vocabulary is reduced. He finds it difficult to engage in conversation. He wanders restlessly. Sometimes depression sets in. He stays unclean.

Nothing has been lost. If you use the brain, it will continue to be as active as before. The secret of success is: 'use the brain continuously'.

Indulge in intellectual exercises such as solving crossword puzzles, playing bridge, chess, writing letters to newspapers, actively participating in social and cultural events. Teach your grandchildren. Write poetry or a short story if the muse inspires you.

Distinguishing symptoms of the patient	Medicine and potency
• Impaired memory. **Absent-mindedness**.	Anacardium 200
• Paralytic weakness of limbs.	
• **Deep melancholy**.	
• Loss of memory in **hysteric cases**.	Kali Phos 30

- Loss of interest in life.
- **Night terrors**.
- **Difficult comprehension.**   Phosphoric Acid 30
- Cannot collect his thoughts or find
  the right word.
- Unable to carry on conversation.

DEPRESSION

A morbid sadness, melancholy or dejection. A lowering of spirits, a loss of interest in the normal activities of life.

Symptoms: Diminished energy level. Hopelessness. Shedding tears. Feeling guilty for no reason. Wakes up early and cannot go back to sleep. Cannot concentrate. Cannot take decisions. Loses self-esteem, feels as if she is good for nothing. Fears death. Loses weight. Reduced interest in sex.

Take good care of the depressed person. Give her hope, encouragement and reassurance. Make her feel wanted, loved.

In quite a few cases help and guidance of your doctor is essential.

Distinguishing symptoms of the patient	Medicine and potency
• Great fear, anxiety, without basis.	Aconite 30
• Restlessness.	
• **Numbness**.	
• Indigestion. **Lack of appetite.**	Alfa Alfa, Mother Tincture. 15 drops, five times daily. Induces exhilaration, and a feeling of well being.
• **Mental depression**.	Graphites 200
• Thinks only of **death and salvation.**	
• Mental and physical depression. **Want of nerve power**.	Kali Phos 30
• **Loss of self-confidence**. Melancholy. Afraid to be left alone.	Lycopodium 200

• Failing mental faculties. **Spells wrong**.	
• Depression because of **suffering in chronic diseases**.	Nat Mur 200
• Wants to be left alone to cry.	
• Result of **hangover. Disturbed early morning sleep**.	Nux Vomica 200

ENCEPHALITIS

Seek medical advice.

It is an acute inflammation of the brain caused by viral infection. A rare complication that develops mainly in young children and elderly persons. In mild cases, the symptoms develop slowly.

Symptoms: High fever. Splitting headache. Nausea, vomit. Slurred speech. General body pain. Stiff neck, convulsions, partial paralysis. Impaired memory and loss in hearing faculty.

Distinguishing symptoms of the patient	Medicine and potency
• **Great muscular soreness and** rigidity all over. **Septic** condition. **Fever**. Chill.	Baptista 30. Repeat frequently.
• Delirium. Face besotted. Stupor.	
• Muscular soreness of neck and of shoulders. **Stiffness**.	Gelsemium 200
• **Varying degree of motor paralysis** of muscles around the eyes, throat, larynx, chest, and extremities.	
• Chill up and down the spine.	
• Dizziness, drowsiness, dullness, and trembling.	
• Better, profuse urination.	

EPILEPSY

Look up *Convulsions/epileptic fits/seizure* in this chapter and under *'Convulsion'* in the chapter, *"The Locomotor System."*

FAINTING [SYNCOPE]

A partial or total loss of consciousness, often occurring without warning. It is caused by lack of food or by reduced blood flow to the brain or by a heatstroke. Recurring episodes call for medical help.

Symptoms: A sensation of dizziness or light heartedness followed by partial or total loss of consciousness. Disturbed vision. Numbness or tingling in any part of the body. Epilepsy. Uncontrollable twitching. Stroke. Shortness of breath. Bleeding from the digestive tract. Low blood sugar levels in diabetic patients. Chest pain. Palpitations. Pale face. Fatigued.

Clear the airways in the nose and the throat. Pull the jaw downwards and backwards. If there is no recovery within a few minutes, start artificial respiration.

If there is no pulse, start cardiac message. **In any case, seek a doctor immediately**.

No alcohol to the patient when he comes around. Only sips of water if he asks for it.

Distinguishing symptoms of the patient	Medicine and potency
• Fainting fit because of being **anaemic**. Face pale. Headache.	Acetic Acid 30
• Unquenchable thirst.	
• Faints out of **fear, anguish**, or sudden loss.	Aconite 30
• Due to **concussion**.	Arnica 200
• A result of **shock**. Pulse weak.	Camphor Mother Tincture.
• Icy coldness all over body.	Fifteen drops on sugar every
• **Heat stroke**.	ten minutes.
• Breathlessness	

• Caused by **excessive discharge** from the body. Haemorrhage, menstruation, in fevers, in childbirth.	China 200
• In epilepsy.	Cuprum Met 200
• Heat stroke.	Glonoine 30

HALLUCINATION

It is a serious brain disorder during which a person perceives events that never took place.

Also, refer '*Delirium*' above.

Distinguishing symptoms of the patient	Medicine and potency
• **Frightful visions**.	Absinthium 30
• Loss of memory of recent events.	
• Thinks he is **possessed of two persons**.	Anacardium 200
• Failing memory.	
• Sees varied **kaleidoscopic colours**.	Anhalonium
• Visions of **monsters**, of gruesome figures.	Mother Tincture. Five
• **Pupils dilated**. Vertigo. Headache.	drops. Four times a day.
• **Fantastic illusions**. Touch with reality lost.	Belladonna 200
• Sees ghosts, monsters, and spirits. Sees animals, insects out to hurt him.	

HANGOVER

Unpleasant physical effects following excessive use of alcohol. A let-down, as after a period of excitement.

Distinguishing symptoms of the patient	Medicine and potency
• **Brain clouded** in the morning.	Nux Vomica 200
• Effects of drinking, of late night revelry.	

- Indigestion.
- **Sleepless after 3 a m.**

HEADACHE

Pain in the head, which can be mild or severe. Treat according to symptoms and the type of pain as described below.

However, in *unyielding*, severe, or even mild headaches, seek medical advice. There could be a serious complication.

Distinguishing symptoms of the patient	Medicine and potency
• **On exposure to dry cold wind.** **Burning headache**. Fever.	Aconite 30
• Undulating sensation. Head hot, bursting.	
• Caused by **indigestion**, overeating.	Antim Crud 200
• With vertigo. Belching. **Eructation**.	
• In **half of the head**. Emotional upset.	Arg Nit 200
• Pain in the frontal head. **Eye feels enlarged**. Better on tight bandage or pressure.	
• **Throbbing carotids. Flushed face**.	Belladonna 200
• Pain in temples.	
• **Sun headache**. Blood rushing to head. Worse on leaning forward.	
• **Neuralgic** headache on exposure to cold air	
• Pain worse by light, noise.	
• Congestion caused by suppressed catarrh.	
• **Frontal, splitting** headache. Worse on motion. Early morning.	Bryonia 200
• A full and upset stomach. Nausea. Constipation	
• Pain in **frontal sinuses**. Coryza.	
• Caused by **debility** because of **outflow of liquids.**	China 200

- Bursting. **Intense throbbing of carotids**.
- Vertigo on walking.
- **Distension** in the stomach. Enlarged liver
- **Intermittent fever**.
- **Pain deep in every bone of the skull.**   Eupatorium Perf 200
- Eyeballs sore.
- Feels as if the skull is being **crushed**.
- Feeling of a **band tightening** around the   Gelsemium 200
  skull.
- Muscular soreness of neck, shoulders.
- Because of **tension**.
- Influenza.
- **Sun or heat stroke** headache.   Glonoine 200.
- Skull feels too small for the brain.   First remedy in heat stroke.
  Continuous hammering.
- In **hysteric** persons   Ignatia 200
- As if a nail is being driven through
  the head
- Following **grief or anger.**
- With **nausea.**   Ipecac 200
- Crushing pain in the skull, extending
  to the teeth and the tongue.
- In bones **over the eyebrows**. Pain settles   Kali Bich 200
  in a small spot. Pain in the **eyeballs**
- **Sinus headache**. **Sticky mucous** down
  the throat.
- **Chronic**. From sunrise to sunset   Nat Mur 200
- Nausea.
- **Numbness, tingling** in nose, lips,
  and tongue before the attack.
- **Menstrual**
- Throbbing, blinding headache as if
  a thousand little hammers were
  knocking at the brain.
- In **hangover**. After heavy drinking   Nux Vomica 200
- **Disturbed sleep**
- With haemorrhoids, **constipation**.

• Wandering, stitching pain about the head.	Pulsatilla 30
• Indulging in **heavy food.**	
• During **menstruation**.	
• **Eyestrain.**	Ruta 200
• Heavy drinking.	
• Half headache **in women** at any time.	Sepia 200
On **menopause**. Painful menstruation.	
• Pain in **lower back**. **Overtired housewife.**	
• **Prolapse** of vagina and uterus.	
Painful intercourse.	

HEATSTROKE/SUNSTROKE

Heatstroke is caused by exposure to excessive heat of the sun or otherwise leading to loss of fluids and salts. The body temperature might rises to 40°C.

Symptoms: Headache, nausea, vomiting, excessive sweating, muscle cramps, exhaustion, fatigue; rapid, shallow, noisy breathing, and confused thinking. Even seizures. Dehydration can lower blood pressure. The patient can lose consciousness. He may collapse without treatment.

The moment it is felt that a patient has suffered a heatstroke, he should be shifted to a shady area or into an air-conditioned room. His body should be cooled by wrapping it in sheets soaked in cold water so that loss of fluids can be made up. Replace the wet sheets with dry ones, once the temperature comes down to 38°C. Give the patient diluted fruit juice with a pinch of salt every few minutes.

Send for a doctor at the earliest or, after giving first aid as above, take the patient to the nearest hospital.

Distinguishing symptoms of the patient	Medicine and potency
• Sunstroke. Blood surges to head and heart	Glonoine 200 First remedy.
• Confusion. Giddiness.	
• Cannot lay head on a pillow.	

• **Throbbing carotid.**	Belladonna 200
• **Face flushed**.	
• **Chronic effects** of sunstroke.	Nat Carb 200
Debility. Exhaustion.	
• **Vertigo** from exposure to sun.	
• **Nausea. Vomit. Loose motions**,	Veratrum Alb 200, 1000
white and profuse.	
• Cold sweat on the forehead.	
• Throbbing arteries.	

HYSTERIA

An irrational, uncontrollable, violent outburst of emotion or fear. Its characteristics are exaggerated laughter, weeping, or irritability.

Symptoms: The patient behaves unusually to attract attention or to get out of an unpleasant situation. She loses control over her emotions by morbid self-consciousness, autosuggestion, or by feigning various disorders. Sometimes amnesia or physical deficit, such as paralysis, or a sensory deficit without an organic cause is present.

The problem is more common in women than in men. It recurs.

Distinguishing symptoms of the patient	Medicine and potency
• Weeping and laughing alternately.	Camphora Monobromata 30
• **Loss of consciousness.**	Cicuta 200
• Involuntary twisting and jerking of muscles. **Frightful distortions.**	
• **Effects of grief**, worry, trauma. Sighing, sobbing, and trembling.	Ignatia 200. Excellent in acute cases. Administer Mother
• Sleeplessness and excitement. Alternately sad and happy.	Tincture, ten drops doses at an hourly interval when the attack starts.
• **Chronic cases**. Administer if Ignatia fails.	Nat Mur 200

INSANITY

It is a legal term for mental illness during which the patient is unable to distinguish between right and wrong. He is, therefore, not responsible for his acts in law. Find remedies under the sub chapters '*Delirium*' and '*Mania*' in this chapter.

IRRITABILITY

Distinguishing symptoms of the patient	Medicine and potency
• Fretful, peevish.	Antim Crud 200
• Glutton. **Belching** all the time. **Foul eructation.** Tongue coated thick, milky.	
• Body sore, mind irritable. **Result of any injury.**	Arnica 200
• Has **suicidal tendencies.**	Arsenic Alb 200
• **Anxiety** alternates with **fear**.	
• Every muscle **aches on movement.** Does not want to stir.	Bryonia 200
• Child **peevish, irritable.** Is **teething**	Chamomilla 200
• Older persons cross, spiteful. Cannot bear others.	
• Because of **worms** with **convulsions**. Worse at night.	Cina 30
• Results of **excessive drinking**, of **hangover**, of leading a **fast life.**	Nux Vomica 200
• Sullen. All the time finding faults with others.	

MANIA

Excessive enthusiasm, excitement.
A sort of insanity characterized by great excitement with or without delusions.

Symptoms: Violence in acute stages. Excited for no apparent justification. An obsession, say, for neatness or any other thing. Abnormal behaviour. Bipolar disorders, characterized by profuse and rapidly changing ideas, exaggerated sexuality, gaiety, or irritability. Duration of sleep reduced.

Distinguishing symptoms of the patient	Medicine and potency
• Cannot be at rest. Must move incessantly,	Cannabis Indica 30
• Fears turning insane.	
• **Sexual** mania. Insatiable desire.	Cantharis 200
• Usually with **urinary problems**.	
• **Obscene**, lascivious. **Uncovers genitals.**	Hyoscymus 200
• Violence alternates with stillness.	
• Religious depression. **Fears divine wrath.**	Kali Bromatum 30
• Suicidal. Trembling.	
• Justifies his behaviour declaring that he is carrying out God's commands.	Lachesis 200
• **Ecstatic, prophetic. Revengeful.**	
• Talking incessantly.	
• **Exposes** genitals in public.	Phosphorus 200
• Insatiable sexual appetite.	
• Believes he is in direct communication with God. Acts **devout**, beseeching.	Stramonium 200
• Laughing, singing, seeing ghosts, hearing voices, **talking with spirits**.	
• Philosophical. **Meditating all the time. Unclean**.	Sulphur 200
• Cursing. **Howling all night.**	Veratrum Alb 200
• Violent. **Talks lewd**.	

MELANCHOLY/SAD/HOPELESS/INDIFFERENT

Gloom. Sadness.

Symptoms: Sullenness and outbreaks of violent anger. Pensive reflection or contemplation. Depression of the spirits. Irrational fear. Weariness with life. Unable to sustain mental effort. Indifferent to happiness or to sorrow.

Distinguishing symptoms of the patient	Medicine and potency
• **Fears failure**. Irrational. Nervous apprehension.	Arg Nit 200
• Diarrhoea. Vomit. **Painful acidity**. Hiatus Hernia.	
• **Weary of life**. Has lost all hope.	Calcarea Carb 200
• **Cannot sustain mental effort.**	
• Crushed by **successive illnesses**.	Carbo Veg 200
• **Bemoans deformity** in joints. Rheumatism.	Causticum 200
• **Warts**, too many.	
• **Broken down** constitution. Hence, suspicious, distrustful.	
• **Total debility** caused by **excessive discharges.**	China 200. A 'pick-me-up' medicine.
• Anaemic.	
• **Exhausted housewife**. Overburdened.	Sepia 200
• Lacks stamina. Cannot exert.	
• **After menopause.**	
• Women with uterine problems. **Vagina hurts** during intercourse.	
• **Headache in half the head. Uncontrollable.**	

"What is the use of worrying?
It never was worthwhile.
So, pack up your troubles
In your old kit-bag,
And smile, smile, smile".

GEORGE H. POWELL

MEMORY/PROBLEMS OF

Memory is the mental faculty of retaining and recalling past experience, learning, sights and sounds. Recollection. The process of memorizing. The progress of civilization depends on human memory preserved in various ways. With age, human memory, if not regularly used, loses its sharpness in various ways. A discussion of this loss is available in the sub-chapter, 'Dementia' above.

However, this inevitable decline can be arrested. The human brain has the capacity to learn throughout its life. While medicines as indicated below will certainly help, the greatest resource is your own effort in the use of your brain continuously. Watching television programmes does not help. Reading serious books or good fiction helps. Writing helps even more. So do mind games, crossword puzzles, spell tests. An activity must engage your brain. Passive entertainment is of no use.

Whatever else helps your cardiovascular health, helps in sharpening your brain and its faculties. This includes regular walks, aerobic exercise, swimming, stretching, diet control, social interaction, voluntary welfare work, and regular meditation.

Do not smoke. If you do, give up smoking at the earliest.

According to Dr. Andrew Well*, M. D, diets high in omega-3 fatty acids such as fish and fish oil, walnuts, turmeric, colourful fruits and vegetables, go a long way in keeping your brain healthy.

Distinguishing symptoms of the patient	Medicine and potency
• Forgets **recent events**.	Absinthium 30
• Absent-mindedness **after paralysis**.	Anacardium 200
• Failure because of **injury**, new or old.	Arnica 200
• Forgets names of streets, numbers of houses.	Glonoine 200
• In old people using **wrong words**, wrong **spellings**.	Lycopodium 200

*Clinical professor of medicine at the University of Arizona, writing in the *Time*, on '*You [and your brain] are what you eat*', issue dated January 23, 2006.]

• Forgetfulness with **nervous and physical exhaustion**. Cannot add figures.	Natrum Carb 30
• Instant forgetfulness of the written word.	
• Mental weakness **that follows physical debility**	Phosphoric Acid 30
• Cannot find the right word.	

MENINGITIS

Inflammation of the meninges, membranes that cover the brain and spinal cord, due to a bacterial or viral infection. The viral infection is more common and is not as severe as the bacterial infection. The latter develops rapidly, often within a few hours.

Symptoms: Severe headache. Stiffness and pain in the neck or back. Nausea, vomiting. High fever. Convulsions leading to seizure.

Immediate medical assistance and hospitalization is essential.

The following remedies ought to be taken as first aid according to symptoms.

Distinguishing symptoms of the patient	Medicine and potency
• Delirium. Acute cerebral infection.	Apis 200
• Cries in sleep. Shrill cries of pain.	
• Throbbing carotids. **High temperature.**	Belladonna 200
• **Eyes bloodshot.**	
• **Violent** delirium.	
• Severe headache.	
• **Frightful distortion of limbs** in convulsions. Unconscious.	Cicuta 200
• **Cramps** in the muscles of the **neck and spine**. Bending backwards.	
• Internal chill.	
• Acute attack of **violent convulsions.**	Cup Met 200
• Pain in the brain and the eyes.	
• Dropsy of brain following an acute disease	Nat Mur 200

- **Chronic jerking of head**.
- Tubercular meningitis.

Tuberculinum 200
Start with one dose of this remedy. Follow with other selected medicines.

MIGRAINE

A disease of the nervous system that runs in families. There is recurring headache and the sufferer knows in advance of the onset of migraine. Often it sets in soon on waking when the vision is disturbed by bright spots or zigzag lines.

Symptoms: A feeling of confusion and dizziness accompanied by numbness. These symptoms are soon replaced by a throbbing, severe headache on the side opposite to the one that had experienced numbness. Nausea, vomiting. Anxiety. Mood changes. Dislike of bright light, of noise.

Certain foods can bring an attack of migraine. Consult you physician for proper advice.

Distinguishing symptoms of the patient	Medicine and potency
• **Throbbing carotids. Hot flushed face.** Violent headache.	Belladonna 200
• Better by pressure. Worse by light, noise, jolt, lying down, in the afternoon.	
• Preceded by **unusual loquacity** and excitement.	Cannabis Indica 30
• Shocks through brain. An open and shut feeling.	
• Due to acidity and **sluggishness of liver.**	Chionanthus 30
• In **hysterical** patients.	Ignatia 200
• Begins with a **blur before the eyes** after rest. **Constriction of scalp.**	Iris Veriscolour 200
• Nausea. Vomit of sour **blood-stained bile.**	

- Frontal headache. Worse right temple.
- In children with an **upset stomach.**
- Pressure on and **burning in vertex**   Lachesis 200
  on waking up. Waves of pain.
- **Flickering before eyes**. Vision dim.
- Better warm application.
  Start of menstruation. Worse on
  movement, or after sleep.
- Mostly left side, stinging.   Sepia 200
  pain from **within, and outwards**.
- Nausea, vomit.
- Cold vertex.
- **Worse during menses**, indoors,
  when lying on painful side.

MULTIPLE SCLEROSIS

A disease of the nervous system that is chronic and progressive.

Symptoms: In most cases, it begins with some visual disturbance, blurred vision, and pain beyond the eye. The patient loses co-ordination and control of some limbs. He is clumsy. Loses control over bowel and bladder movement. Emotional depression. More often than not, lighthearted behaviour.

Please seek competent medical advice.

Distinguishing symptoms of the patient	Medicine and potency
- **Trembling, twitching, and jerking**. Hysteria.	Tarentula Hispanica 30
- Hysterical epilepsy.	
- Sensation of crawling ants.	
- Intense sexual excitement.	

NEURALGIA

Symptoms: Severe pain generated by an irritation or compression of a nerve. The pain follows the route of the nerve.

Neuralgia can be the result of an infection, inflammation, exposure to dry, cold air, of fracture of the bone or a slipped disc.

Distinguishing symptoms of the patient	Medicine and potency
• **On exposure to dry, cold air**. Sudden attack.	Aconite 30
• Of face. Tingling in the cheeks and bones. Pain in the jaws.	
• Restlessness. Worse left side.	
• Following amputation or **injury to the nerves.**	Allium Cepa 200
• Cutting-thread pain.	
• **Lips black. Restlessness.** Nightly aggravation.	Arsenic Alb 200
• Pain as if someone is thrusting a needle.	
• Unbearable pain in **teeth, ovaries**, anywhere. Every **nerve cries for relief**.	Chamomilla 200
• **Repeated haemorrhage**, long lactation or intermittent fevers.	China 200
• **Injury to the nerves**, especially in fingers, toes and nails. **Crushed fingertips**.	Hypericum 200
• **Contraction** of the muscles of the eye, ear, ovary, or leg. Excruciating pain.	Mag Phos 200
• **Cramping neuralgia** in face, stomach, abdomen, spinal cord, fingers of writer, pianists, and violinists. **Writer's cramp.**	
• Pain comes and disappears like lightning.	
• Facial neuralgia because of **mental exertion**.	Phosphorus 200
• Of the **fifth nerve.**	Spigelia 200
• **Ciliary neuralgia**. Pain deep into the socket. Eye feels big for the socket.	
• Pain in temple, eye, cheek, jaw, or teeth.	

PARALYSIS AGITANS

An involuntary shaking of hands.

Distinguishing symptoms of the patient	Medicine and potency
• **Involuntary shaking of hands**. Fingertips stiff and numb. Arms weak.	Mag Phos 200

RESTLESSNESS

Marked by a lack of quiet, peace, repose, or rest. Inability to be at rest, to relax, to be still. A feeling of impatience or uneasiness induced by certain maladies, by external coercion or internal turmoil.

Distinguishing symptoms of the patient	Medicine and potency
• In **high-grade fevers**. On exposure to dry cold air. Onset of an inflammatory disease.	Aconite 30
• With **numbness**, tingling.	
• **Tosses in agony**. Worse in the evening.	
• **Restless in** the mind and in the body.	Arsenic Alb 200
• Debility with **burning**.	
• **In low-grade fever** like typhoid.	
• Midnight aggravation.	
• Because of **aching pains,** temporarily better on motion. Pain in **joints**, sheaths, and tendons.	Rhus Tox 200

SCHIZOPHRENIA

Any of a group of serious mental disorders.

Symptoms: The patient lives in a dream world of his own. He withdraws from reality. He is unable to react realistically to situations of sorrow or of joy. He hears voices, sees visions. Quite often, he is violent. His behaviour is odd. He follows an illogical pattern of thinking, has delusions and hallucinations.

Refer '*Delirium*', *Hallucinations*', and '*Mania*' in this chapter.

STROKE

See '*Apoplexy*' above.

THROBBING

Distinguishing symptoms of the patient	Medicine and potency
• **Of carotids. Hot, red, and dry skin**.	Belladonna 200
• Flushed face, glaring eyes.	
• Sudden attack. No thirst.	
• **Occipital** throbbing, synchronous with pulse.	Camphor 200. Begin with Mother
• Eyes staring. **Pupils dilated**.	Tincture, five drops on
• Violent **convulsions**.	sugar every fifteen minutes in case of 'shock.'
• Intense throbbing in the **skull and carotids**.	China 200

THROMBOSIS

Formation of a blood clot in a blood vessel, either artery or vein. Coronary thrombosis leads to the symptoms of a heart attack. A thrombosis in the brain can lead to a stroke. In other parts of the body, thrombosis causes severe pain and discoloration of the skin.

The medicines indicated below help greatly. However, **consult your doctor immediately as the symptoms appear**.

Distinguishing symptoms of the patient	Medicine and potency
• **Angina Pectoris**. Severe pain in left elbow and in the region of the heart	Arnica 200
• **Suffocating constriction** after over-exertion. Skin might turn black or blue.	
• With **one sided paralysis.**	Bothrops 30
• Loss of power of speech, writing, or other faculties.	
• **Skin purple**.	Lachesis 200
• **Left side facial paralysis.**	
• Thrombosis affecting **pelvic region.**	Lilium Tig 200
• Angina Pectoris. Pain in the right arm.	

TUMOUR OF THE BRAIN

An abnormal growth that develops in brain tissue or the meninges of the brain. It requires **immediate medical attention**. A tumour compresses a part of the brain or raises the pressure inside the skull.

Symptoms: Partial loss of vision. Changes in the personality of the patient. A one-sided lack of muscular coordination, epileptic seizures. Vomit. Severe headache, worse in the morning. Slurred speech. Difficulty in reading and writing.

Distinguishing symptoms of the patient	Medicine and potency
• **Vertigo**. Headache on turning the head.	Calcarea Carb 200
• Piercing, stitching pain in the skull.	
• **Icy coldness** in the skull.	
• Sensation as if a **foreign body** is under the scalp.	Conium 200
• Walking difficult. **Staggers**.	
• Scorching feeling at the **top.**	
• Vertigo on turning eyes, lying down, turning in the bed.	

- Brain tumour **with migraine** and
  intense pain.   Thuja 200
- Sweat on forehand and arm.
- Start treatment with this remedy. It might   Tuberculinum 200
  arrest the disease and take care of the
  resultant headache.

VERTEX, PROBLEMS OF

Distinguishing symptoms of the patient	Medicine and potency
• Sensation of **weight**.	Cactus 200
• Weight on top, **icy coldness inside**.	Calcarea Carb 200
• A feeling of **opening and shutting**.	Cannabis Indica 30
• Skull feels **crushed and bruised.**	Ipecac 200
• Pain extends to **teeth** and the **root of the tongue**.	
• Heat on top. Heat inside.	Sulphur 200
• Lump of **ice on top. Cold sweat** on the forehead.	Veratrum Alb 200

VERTIGO

It is a false sensation of moving or spinning, often accompanied by nausea and vomit. It can be experienced in several situations.

Symptoms: An unpleasant sensation of spinning. Inability to stand or straighten the head. In cases of arthritis in the neck, it occurs when the head is turned or tilted.

Distinguishing symptoms of the patient	Medicine and potency
• **Epileptic seizure**.	Absinthium 200
• Worse on rising. **Full of fear**.	Aconite 30

• From **sunlight**. On walking.	Agaricus 200
• Chronic. **A result of injury**, recent or past.	Arnica 200
• Violent vertigo on **climbing steps**. Patient anaemic.	Arsenic Hydro 30
• When **descending**.	Borax 200
• With nausea, worse on **motion**.	Bryonia 200
• With liver disorder.	Chelidonium 200
• In **cervical spondylosis**. The **neck is stiff. Giddiness** on turning.	Cimicifuga 200
• Of mountain climbers. Preceded by **flashes of lightning**.	Coca 30
• Travelling in a motorcar, plane or ship.	Cocculus 200. Take a dose thirty minutes before the journey.
• On seeing flowing or **running water**.	Ferrum Met 30
• Spreading from occiput. A **tight band around the head**.	Gelsemium 200
• From **exposure to sun**.	Glonoine 200
• With **nausea, vomit**.	Ipecac 200
• From use of **intoxicants**. Loss of sleep. Fast life.	Nux Vomica 200
• After **suppressed menses**.	Pulsatilla 30
• Looking up.	Silicea 200

THE FACE

We present ourselves to the world with a pleasant face to make an impression. 'The face is the image of the soul', wrote Cicero in 80 BC. Facial expressions give a man away because the face is an index of the mind and a repository of emotions. The face expresses joy, hatred, compassion, anger, disgust, anguish, or jealousy. The face is also the most significant and prominent surface of the human body. We determine the beauty and temperament of a person firstly by a look at her or his face.

Anatomically speaking, the 'face' is the surface of the front of the head from the top of the forehead to the base of the chin and from ear to ear. The bones and muscles are covered by taut skin. The cranial nerves arising directly from the brain, serve the facial muscles. The disorders of the face relate to skin, bones, muscles, and the nerves.

In the following sub-chapters, attention has been concentrated on the symptoms such as 'burning', 'colour', 'distortion,' 'neuralgia' and 'swelling'. All possible symptoms have been covered. Select your remedy according to the most prominent symptoms.

Quite often, the face reflects the consequences of what is happening in the other parts of the body. A number of nervous disorders show symptoms in the face. Skin disorders like 'erysipelas,' 'urticaria' affect the face. Debility on any account reflects in the face like in a mirror. Cold sweat on the face may be a sign of an impending collapse or heart attack.

Facial numbness comes because of tension in the nerves. Mental tension causes wrinkles because it affects the muscles of the face.

Use medicine where indicated. However, to get a glow on your face, keep your cool under any situation. Avoid use of cosmetics as far as possible. Wash your face with cool water frequently.

Nurture good thoughts and think well of everyone.

Regular exercise considerably delays the formation of wrinkles in young as well as old age.

Smile. Laugh whenever you can. It is a great exercise for the facial muscles, for the throat and the lungs. Besides, it soothes the mind.

Avoid late nights, smoking and liquor. A good night's sleep is essential in order to avoid dark rings around the eyes and to relax the facial muscles.

A diet of nuts, fresh fruit, and green vegetables will make your face healthy.

In 1671 Jean De La Fontaine wrote: "The ruins of a house may be repaired; why not those of a face"? This holds true at any time. Look after your face as you look after a treasure.

BELL'S PARALYSIS

One side of the face droops because of inflammation of or damage to one of the facial nerves. At times, it happens suddenly.

Symptoms: Partial or total paralysis on one side of the face. Difficulty in speaking and eating. The corner of the mouth on the affected side droops. Muscles of the eyebrow and forehead become weak. On the affected side, eyelids cannot be shut. At times saliva dribbles on the affected side. Taste is impaired.

Distinguishing symptoms of the patient	Medicine and potency
• **Acute and violent** attack of facial paralysis. Sudden. Caused by **exposure to dry, cold air** or suppressed perspiration.	Aconite 30
• Facial paralysis, more on **left side**. **Mouth distorted.**	Cadmium Sulphate 200
• **Trembling jaw**. Swallowing difficult.	
• On the **right side.**	Causticum 200
• Pain in facial bones.	
• **Difficulty in opening the mouth**.	
• **Distortion** of facial muscles **around the mouth**.	Gelsemium 200
• Neuralgia of the face.	
• **Difficult to shut the eye**.	
• **Corners** of the mouth **twitch** spasmodically.	Opium 200
• The lower jaw droops. Distortion of the facial muscles.	

BURNING

Distinguishing symptoms of the patient	Medicine and potency
• **Sudden**, terrible burning sensation.	Arsenic Alb 200
• **Restlessness**.	

- Better hot application. Worse cold application.
- Skin **red and swollen**. **Large blisters**. Erysipelas.

Cantharis 200

- **Urinary complications.**
- The patient moans in discomfort.
- **Elevated red patches on the skin**. Urticaria.

Nux Vomica 200

- The patient is **chilly on movement**, on uncovering.
- Outbursts of anger. Dislikes noise or medicines.
- Chronic cases. **Filthy habits.**

Sulphur 200

- Worse washing, at night, in the bed.

COLOUR

Distinguishing symptoms of the patient	Medicine and potency
• **Pale face.** Waxen. Emaciated.	Acetic Acid 30
• Profound **anaemia**. General debility.	
• **Dark rings** around eyes.	
• Red face becomes **deathly pale** on rising.	Aconite 30
• Caused by **exposure** to dry, cold air.	
• Tingling. **Numbness**.	
• Eruptions on cheeks, **yellow, crusty**.	Antim Crud 200
• Looks haggard.	
• Digestion upset. **Stinking eructation**.	
• **Lips black, livid**.	Arsenic Alb 200
• Face pale, yellow, swollen.	
• Restlessness. **Burning** sensation.	
• **Red, bluish**, hot, swollen and **shining** face.	Belladonna 200
• Erysipelas of the face on exposure to cold air.	
• Blue, pale face **in collapse.**	Camphor Mother Tincture.

- Body ice-cold. **Cold sweat**.

15 drops on sugar every 15 minutes.

- **Liver enlarged**. Jaundice.
- Tongue, eyes, urine, skin **yellow.**
- **Urine copious, foaming**.

Cheledonium 30

- **Eyes sunken. Debility** due to excessive discharges. Anaemic.
- **Darkness before eyes**. Ringing sound in ears.

China 200

- Face pale. Around eyes, dark rings.
- **White and bluish rings around mouth**. Red-hot face alternates with sickly pale in children.
- **Worms** inside.

Cina 200

- Pale, **bluish, distorted** face.
- Contraction of jaws. **Foam** at the mouth.
- Fingers **cramped**. Cramps in calves and soles. **Epileptic** attack.

Cup Met 200

- Face **red** with **lips black and swollen.**
- Facial neuralgia, deep in bones.

Merc Cor 30

- **Red, swollen, besotted, stupefied as if drunk**.

Opium 200

- **Blue rings** around eyes.
- Swelling and necrosis of **lower jaw.**
- Tearing **pain in facial bones**.

Phosphorus 200

- **Skin purple**. Urticaria. Large, burning **blotches.**
- **Intense itching** with restlessness.

Rhus Tox 200

- **Yellow blotches**. Saddle like distribution of yellow, brown spots on the nose and the cheeks.
- In women after climacteric or with other uterine problems.

Sepia 200

- Pale, blue, **ice-cold** in **collapse.**
- Gastroenteritis. **Vomit. Rice white**, profuse, **thin stool**.

Veratrum Alb 200

DISTORTION

Distinguishing symptoms of the patient	Medicine and potency
• Distortion and twitching of the left **facial muscles**. • While speaking, left angle of the **mouth** is **drawn upwards** and to the left. • Worse cold weather, laughing.	Tellurium 30

ECZEMA/DERMATITIS

An inflammation of the skin.

Symptoms: Eczema is characterized by redness, itching, and the outbreak of lesions. The lesions may discharge serous matter and become encrusted and scaly.

Eczema is of different types. **Please consult a skin specialist for proper diagnosis**. Most of the time it is a manageable problem.

Distinguishing symptoms of the patient	Medicine and potency
Moist eczema around mouth and chin. Eczema on the **nose**.	Graphites 200

ERYSIPELAS

An acute disease of the skin and subcutaneous tissue.

Symptoms: Localized inflammation and fever. Blisters or cysts full of pus or serum.

Distinguishing symptoms of the patient	Medicine and potency
• Burning, redness and swelling of the skin.	Cantharis 200
• **Urinary complications** present.	
• Large burning blisters.. Small **serum filled**. **cysts** formed in or beneath the skin.	Rhus Tox 200
• **Skin purple**. Pits on pressure.	
• Restlessness.	
• **Intense itching**.	
• Inflammation spreading fast.	

JAWS

Distinguishing symptoms of the patient	Medicine and potency
• **Contraction** of the jaw. **Foam** at the mouth.	Cup Met 200
• Epileptic fit.	
• Jaws clenched in **rigid spasm**. Convulsions and paralysis.	Hydrocyanic Acid 200
• Frothing.	
• Lips pale, blue. **Skin blue**. Paralysis of the lungs.	
• Lower jaw **drooping**.	Opium 200
• **Cracking sound** when chewing.	Rhus Tox 200

NUMBNESS

Distinguishing symptoms of the patient	Medicine and potency
• Face numb. Intense pain like **hot wires** running through. **Tingling.**	Aconite 30 Nothing like it.
• Either on **exposure to dry**, cold air or due to grief or fear.	

- With pain in the **entire right side** of
  the face.   Platina 30
- Bones feel as if being **screwed**. Pain comes
  in **waves**; comes and goes.
- In hysterical women.
- Anaesthetic paralysis.
- Better walking in sunshine, in open air.
  Worse evening.

PAIN/NEURALGIA

Pain extending along the course of one or more nerves.

Distinguishing symptoms of the patient	Medicine and potency
• **Left side**. Restlessness. **Numbness.** • **Hot wires** running through. • Exposure to dry, cold air, due to fear, anguish.	Aconite 30
• Sensation of cold **needles piercing.** • Tearing **pain in cheeks.** • Twitch in facial muscles. • Worse cold air.	Agaricus 200
• **Needle-like** pain in a face that is pale, **yellow, swollen, burning**. • Cases of **malnutrition**. • Restlessness. Worse at night.	Arsenic Alb 200
• **Violent, throbbing** pain. Can see the **carotids throbbing.** • Face **bright red, purple**. Fever. Unbearable twitching. Erysipelas. • Orbital neuralgia in **conjunctivitis.** • Worse right side. Worse on movement.	Belladonna 200
• Pain in facial nerves with the sensation of **an iron band tightening**.	Cactus Mother Tincture, 10 drops

- Spasmodic, violent, unbearable pain. The patient cries. | in water, every hour till pain subsides.
- Face, lips turning **purple**.
- Pain with **hard swelling** in jawbone and cheek. | Calcarea Fluorica 30 for a week or more. Slow acting.
- Intense neuralgia Feels chilly.
- Pain runs through **stomach, teeth and head simultaneously**.
- Facial neuralgia in **epileptic fits. Spasmodic convulsions, cramps**. | Cuprum Met 200
- Pain in cheeks, upper jaw and behind the right ear.
- Worse in women **preceding menses**.
- Worse from exposure to **wet, cold** air. | Dulcamara 200
- From **carious teeth**. After tooth extraction. | Heckla Lava 30
- Neuralgia of the chief facial sensory nerve, and the motor nerve of the **masticatory muscles**. | Lachesis 200
- Left side.
- Face swollen, purple.
- **Left side paralysed**.
- **Face and teeth, running into ears**. Violent pain | Mezerium 30
- Worse cold air, eating. Better near a hot stove.
- Death of cells or tissue [necrosis], **in lower jaw**. | Phosphorus 200
- **Swelling and tearing pain in bones**.
- Numbness in **molar bones**. | Platina 30
- **Right side** of the face numb, tickling.
- Woman hysterical.
- Better in sunshine. Worse evening.
- Pain beginning in occiput, settling in **right eye.** | Sanguinaria 200
- **Temple veins extended.**
- Nausea, vomiting.
- Worse during day.

- Left-side pain in head, **eye, face, zygoma, cheek, teeth, and temple.**   Spigelia 200
- Increases with sunrise and decreases with sunset.
- Pain below frontal eminence and temples. Pain in the fifth nerve.
- Pain violent, throbbing, unbearable.
- **Eyes** feel **too large** for their sockets.

PARALYSIS

Total or partial loss or impairment of the ability to move a body part, usually because of damage to its nerve supply.

Symptoms: Loss of sensation. Inability to perform normal bodily functions by the affected part.

Distinguishing symptoms of the patient	Medicine and potency
• **Left sided** paralysis. Mouth distorted.	Cadmium Sulph 200
• Paralysis of face **on exposure to cold**.	Causticum 200
• Left sided, extending to right, **with neuralgia**.	Lachesis 200

SWELLING

Distinguishing symptoms of the patient	Medicine and potency
• Face swollen, **pale**, yellow.	Arsenic Alb 200
• Needle-like pain.	
• Restlessness, **burning**.	
• Swollen, red hot **and shiny.**	Belladonna 200
• On exposure to cold air.	
• With **hard swelling** of cheek, pain in jaw bone.	Calcarea Fluorica 30

• **Blue, puffy**, pale. Lack of oxygen.	Carbo Veg 200
• **Abscess** in gums.	Heckla Lava 30
• **Upper jaw** bone swollen.	
• **Lips black** and swollen.	Merc Cor 30
• **Face red** and puffy.	
• Red, hot and swollen.	Opium 200
• **Lower jaw drooping**.	
• **Decay** in lower jaw.	Phosphorus 200
• Tearing pain in facial bones.	
• **Blue rings** around eyes.	

TWITCHING

Distinguishing symptoms of the patient	Medicine and potency
• Facial muscles **twitch**. Are **stiff**. • Worse by contact with cold air.	Agaricus 200

IMPORTANT

The following topics relating to '*the Face*' are discussed in the chapters indicated.

Acne: *The Skin*.
Impetigo: *The Skin*
Myasthenia Gravis: *The Extremities*
Rosacea: *The Skin*

THE EYES

We see through our eyes. Hence, our perception of the world depends, normally, on the health of our eyes. Things look yellow to a jaundiced eye.

An old proverb says, "A small hurt in the eye is a great one". Therefore, take good care of your eyes. They truly are precious.

On the outside, eyelids fringed by eyelashes, protect the eye. The eyebrows prevent sweat from running into the eyes.

The lining inside the eyelids is called 'conjunctiva'. It provides the outer cover to the eyeball. It is a site for infection, inflammation, and soreness.

Tears produced by glands clean the eye of any foreign substance. These kill harmful bacteria. These are washed into the throat through a passage in the corner of the eyes near the nose.

'Iris' is the coloured part of the eye in the front. In its centre lies the 'pupil' through which light passes, with its opening adjusting according to the quantity of light entering the eye.

'Cornea' is the external transparent coat of the anterior of the eye. It covers the iris and the pupil. It is part of a sphere, which is superimposed upon the surface of the large sphere, the eyeball.

A lens lies behind the iris. Light passes through it before falling on the 'retina'. The 'retina' forms the innermost lining at the back of the

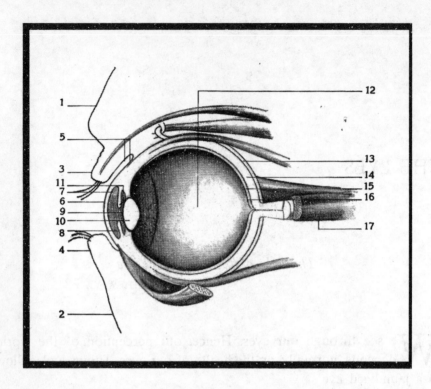

1. Forehead. 2. Cheekbone. 3. Upper eyelid. 4. Lower eyelid.
5. Conjunctiva. 6. Cornea. 7. Aqueous humor. 8. Iris. 9. Pupil.
10. Lens. 11. Ciliary muscle. 12. Vitreous humor. 13. Sclera.
14. Choroid. 15. Retina. 16. Macula. 17. Optic Nerve.

eyeball and is rich in nerves. In a thickness of 0.4 millimetres are located the receptors for the sensation of light. Here the light waves are converted into nerve impulses to be transmitted to the brain for analysis and interpretation.

Mainly, a vitreous humour maintains the shape of the eyeball.

Small muscles surrounding the eyeball control its movement. We can shift with speed from a distant to a close object; adjust from dim to bright light.

Tear glands lubricate the cornea.

The act of seeing is the result of images of objects forming through the pupil on the retina and conveyed from there to the brain. Light rays are converted into nerve impulses. The brain interprets. How? We do not yet know for certain.

For defects in vision, there is no substitute to spectacles or contact lenses.

For other problems of the eye, medicines help.

Besides, take care of your eyes in the following simple ways:

1. Keep the eyes clean. Wash them with cold, running water as often as you can.
2. Do not use your eyes in insufficient light. Do not overuse them. Do not undertake minute tasks when there is not enough light.
3. Protect your eyes while watching television, films in the theatre, working with oxi-acetylene flame or handling fast moving tools in a workshop.
4. Avoid the use of eye-drops, ointments or other direct applications unless advised by your doctor. Homoeopathic medicines taken internally provide an excellent substitute.
5. Do not rub eyes in case of infection or if there is a sensation of ground glass. Rubbing spreads the infection and injures the eye.
6. Exercise the eye muscles at short intervals while working on a computer, while watching television or while reading, writing, or doing any other job where you require the concentration of vision, in order to reduce fatigue and to make them flexible.
7. Keeping the eyes shut for a few minutes offers the best relaxation to the tired eyes. Additionally, consciously tense the surrounding muscles and relax them repeatedly while the eyes are shut.

Versatility of the human eye

"Our visual capabilities are among the most sophisticated of any living creature. We can judge speed and distance well enough to catch a fast moving ball. Close up, we can see an incredible level of detail, Allowing us to thread a needle or read a small print,——detect a vast range of colours.——The eye acts as a highly sophisticated biological video camera".

An extract, with thanks, from
American College of Physicians,
'Complete Home Medical Guide,'
DK Publishing Inc, New York, 1999

BLACK EYE

A bruise caused by an injury makes the skin around the eye black because of coagulation of blood below the surface. The surrounding area is swollen.

Distinguishing symptoms of the patient	Medicine and potency
• Caused by an injury.	Arnica 200. Administer as early as possible.
• Because of blow or concussion. • Specific for an **injury to nerves**.	Ledum 200

BLEEDING

See *Haemorrhages* below.

BLEPHARITIS

An inflammation of the margins of the eyelids with irritation.

Symptoms: Redness. A feeling of grit. Swelling. Margins covered with greasy, soft scales which dry into crusts making the eyelashes stick together.
Hold a damp, warm, clean cloth against the eyelids for comfort.
In order to prevent Blepharitis, dandruff, if any, on the scalp of the patient, must be treated. For removal of dandruff, a shampoo with diluted Savlon is effective.

Distinguishing symptoms of the patient	Medicine and potency
• Eyelids **swollen. Red** eruptions. • Margins covered with **scales and crust**.	Graphites 200
• **Chronic** cases. Eyes dull, sunken, red, and itching. Inflamed	Antim Crud 200

- Canthi **fissured**.
- Throbbing, **needle pain** in the   Hepar Sulph 200
  inflamed lids.
- **Pus formed or** about to form.
- Worse by cold application.
- With acne of the face.   Pulsatilla 30
  Consumption of **heavy food**.
- **Tendency to form sties**.
- **Ulceration** of the eyelids. Severe   Merc Cor 30
  Blepharitis.
- Eyeballs **ache**.
- Sensitive to cold application.

BLINDNESS

A partial or total loss of vision that cannot be corrected by lenses. Day blindness or colour blindness is the lesser evil. The terms are self-explanatory.

Distinguishing symptoms of the patient	Medicine and potency
• **Day** blindness.	Bothrops 30
• **Haemorrhage** in conjunctiva, in retina.	
• **Colour** blindness.	Carbo Sulph 30
• Sensitivity to **red and green** colours lost. White visible.	
• Vision clouded.	
• Night blindness caused by **anaemic retina.**	China 200
• Black spot and pressure in eyes.	
• Eyes sunken. Weakness caused by **excessive discharges from body**, in cold, menstruation, haemorrhage etc.	
• While **reading**, lines **waver**, images move away, **words disappear**.	Cicuta 200
• **Spasm** in the eye caused by an **injury**.	

- Squint.
- **Night** blindness. Pupils contracted.   Physostigma 30
- Increasing myopia. **Paralysis** of the
  eye. Glaucoma. Photophobia.

BLISTERS

A local swelling of the skin containing watery fluid. Caused by irritation or burning.

Distinguishing symptoms of the patient	Medicine and potency
• Tiny blisters on cornea.	Euphrasia 200

BURNING

Distinguishing symptoms of the patient	Medicine and potency
• Smarting, burning sensation. **Bland discharge from eyes**, acrid from nose.	Allium Cepa 200
• Cannot tolerate light.	
• Better open air.	
• Acrid tears.	Arsenic Alb 200
• **Lids red, ulcerated, granulated. Swollen**.	
• Intense dislike of light. **Restlessness.**	
• Warm application helps. **Worse midnight**.	
• Eyes sore. **Intolerable** sensation of burning.	Merc Cor 30
• Lids swollen, red, skin surface torn.	
• Discharge acrid.	
• **Ulcers** on the margins of lids.	Sulphur 200
• Cornea **hurts like powdered glass.**	
• **Black floaters.**	
• **Chronic** inflammation [Ophthalmia].	

CANTHI

Plural of canthus, which are the angles formed by the meeting of the upper and the lower eyelids at either side of the eyes.

Distinguishing symptoms of the patient	Medicine and potency
• Raw and **fissured**.	Antim Crud 200
• **Inner** canthi swollen, red.	Arg Nit 200
• **Intense itching and soreness**. Inflammation.	Zincum Met 200
• Discharge **tears the skin** surface. Worse inner canthi.	

CATARACT

The lens of the eye gets clouded. There is loss of vision. It is a slow and painless process.

Symptoms: Misty veil over the eyes. Sees green halo around candle light. Star-shaped flickers of light visible at night while looking at bright lights.

As of today, a minor surgical procedure rectifies the defect and the sufferer can see and read comfortably with the aid of glasses.

Distinguishing symptoms of the patient	Medicine and potency
• **Chronic dilatation** of pupils.	Calcarea Carb 200
• Spots and **ulcers on** cornea.	
• Foggy vision. Watering eyes.	
• **In early stages**, one dose of 1000 potency every week.	Causticum 1000
• Severe myopia.	
• Misty veil over eyes. **Black spots**.	Phosphorus 200
• Printed words appear **red**.	
• A **green halo** is seen around candlelight.	

CHALAZION

Swollen pockets on the eyelids looking more like a sty. Do not form on the edges.

Distinguishing symptoms of the patient	Medicine and potency
• Fatty deposits under the skin of the eyelids, forming **heads on the outside**. • **Recurring styes**.	Staphysagria 200

COLOUR

Distinguishing symptoms of the patient	Medicine and potency
• **Dirty yellow** in the whites of the eye. • **Liver malfunction.** • Neuralgia over right eye.	Chelidonium 30
• Conjunctiva yellow. • **Liver, spleen enlarged.** • Diabetic patients. Restless and apathetic.	Chionanthus 30
• Sees countless **stars in flickering colours**. • Digestive upset. • Vision dims on waking up. Worse open air, evening.	Cyclamen 30
• Objects appear **green and yellow**. • **Black** floaters. • Detached retina.	Digitalis 30
• Iris **muddy** in colour. Neither contracts, nor dilates. • Lids swollen, **skin peeling off**, red, burning.	Merc Cor 30
• Sees **green halo** around candle light. • **Letters** appear **red**. Black floaters. • **Thrombosis** in retinal vessels. • Orbital pain.	Phosphorus 200

COLOUR BLINDNESS

An inherited problem in which the patient is unable to distinguish certain colours, most commonly red and green.

For medicines, refer '*Blindness*' above.

CONJUNCTIVITIS

Inflammation of the conjunctiva, the membrane covering the white of the eye and the inner surface of the eyelids. Very common. Rarely serious.

Symptoms: Feeling of sand. Redness of the white areas. When severe, eyelids swollen. Itching. Intense aversion to light. Profuse watering. Eyelids cannot be opened when pus has formed.

Distinguishing symptoms of the patient	Medicine and potency
• Conjunctiva **swollen**. Lids **red**. Piercing **pain**.	Apis 1000. Use as a **first medicine**.
• Hot discharge.	**Great results**.
• Chronic feeling of **sand**.	
• Better on cold application.	
• **Acute** cases. Swelling. Inflammation.	Arg Nit 200
• **Granular** sensation.	
• **Copious** discharge that hurts.	
• **Chronic ulcers** on margins of the eyelids.	
• Conjunctiva red, **dry, burning**.	Belladonna 200
• Sudden onset.	
• Eyelids swollen. **Eyes protruding, fiery**.	
• Intense **pain in orbits**.	
• Intense **dislike of light**.	
• Worse on movement.	
• **Non-stop, unpleasantly sharp, bitter** discharge from the conjunctiva. Bland discharge from the nose.	Euphrasia 200

- **Sticky mucous** on cornea.
- **Blisters** on the cornea.
- Pressure in the eyes.
- **Pus** formation. Copious flow.   Hepar Sulph 200
- **Shooting pain** in the **upper orbits.**
- Ulcers on cornea.
- Pus in iris. Iritis.

CORNEAL ULCERS

Infected pits in the cornea caused by an injury or viral infection, by herpes simplex. Sometimes, by wearing contact lenses.

Symptoms: Stabbing pain. Ophthalmia. Redness. Watering. Photophobia.

Distinguishing symptoms of the patient	Medicine and potency
• Acute cases. **Piercing pain**.	Hepar Sulph 200
• Ulcers with pus on the cornea. Eyelids inflamed.	
• Sensitive to touch and cold air.	
• Inflammation and ulceration of the cornea.	Silicea 200
• Discharge of **pus**, **thick and yellow**. Sometimes **blood-tinged** or thin but copious.	
• Most inveterate and **chronic** cases.	
• Intense photophobia.	
• Sensation of **foreign matter** in the eye.	

DACRYOCYSTITIS

A minor inflammation and infection of the tear duct.

Symptoms: Copious watering of the eyes. Redness, pain, and swelling near the tear duct. Discharge of pus in some cases.

For medicines, refer '*Discharge*' below.

DAY BLINDNESS

Defective vision in bright light.
For medicines, refer '*Blindness*' above.

DETACHED RETINA

Light sensitive retina at the **back of the eye gets detached** from the tissue underneath which supports it. This is not to be taken lightly. **Requires urgent medical attention**.

Symptoms: Sudden, painless loss of vision preceded, at times, by flashing lights in the corners. Dark spots in the field of vision.

Distinguishing symptoms of the patient	Medicine and potency
• Inflammation and **opacity** of the retina. A **curtain** across the field of vision.	Aurum Met 200
• **Upper half** of the vision **curtained**. Lower half clear.	
• Yellow, crescent shaped bodies floating obliquely upwards in the field of vision.	
• Occasional **showers of light, star-like bodies in upper dark section**.	
• Detachment due to **injury**.	Arnica 200

DISCHARGE

Copious flow of water, acrid or otherwise from the eyes. For different reasons. Apparent symptoms will help you select the correct remedy.

Wash with clean, cool water as often as you feel like. Do not rub.

Distinguishing symptoms of the patient	Medicine and potency
• **Bland** from the eyes. Acrid from the nose.	Allium Cepa 200
• Eyes burn and smart.	
• Full of **pus**. Copious.	Arg Nit 200
• **Acute** conjunctivitis.	
• Inflammation in the **canthi**.	
• Acrid with **granulated, ulcerated** lids.	Arsenic Alb 200
• Lids swollen.	
• **Restlessness**.	
• **Yellow**, thick, **lumpy**. **Chronic** cases.	Calc. Sulph 30
• Smoky cornea.	
• Yellowish, full of **pus**, mucous **flowing inwards** through the nose, quite often tinged with **blood**.	
• From **exposure to damp, cold** weather.	Dulcamara 200
• Thick, yellow discharge, granulated lids.	
• **Acrid** from the eyes and bland from the nose. Copious.	Euphrasia 200
• Inflamed conjunctiva, running **non-stop**.	
• Profuse, burning, with **inflammation of cornea.**	Merc Sol 200
• **Iritis**.	
• Unpleasantly bitter with **skin peeling** off the inside of the lids.	Merc Cor 30
• Lids swollen, red.	
• Profuse, yellow, thick, bland.	Pulsatilla 30
• Lids inflamed, **glued together**.	
• Tear ducts swollen and watering.	Silicea 200.
• **Abscess** in the eye. Chronic cases.	May have to be used for
• Dislikes daylight. **Sunlight hurts** the eyes.	quite sometime.

DOUBLE VISION

A defect in the muscles that coordinate the eye movement, causes double vision. It is also known as 'Diplopia'.

Distinguishing symptoms of the patient	Medicine and potency
• Caused by **myopia**, **by chill**, by congestive **headache**.	Gelsemium 200
• Sees double **with both eyes**, normal with one eye.	Plumbum Met 30
• **Squint**.	Hyoscymus 200
• Objects seen with **double border.**	
• Pupils dilated, shining, fixed.	

ECTROPION

A turning out of the eyelid. Causes considerable discomfort and inconvenience. Tears cannot be drained down the tear ducts into the nose. Eyes continue watering.

For medicines, refer '*Eyelashes*' below.

ECZEMA

Dermatitis. Blistering patches on the skin. Red, watering, and itching. Crusts form when discharge has dried.

Symptoms vary.

Main entry in the chapter, '*The Skin*'.

Distinguishing symptoms of the patient	Medicine and potency
• On the eyelids, with **fissures**. Eyelids red and swollen.	Graphites 200

ENTROPION

Turning in of the eyelids. Tears flow. Eyes are red and sore. For medicines, refer '*Eyelashes*' below.

EYELASHES

Distinguishing symptoms of the patient	Medicine and potency
• Turned **outwards**.	Apis 200
• Turned **inwards**.	Borax 200
• **Drooping**. Intense dislike of light.	Conium 200
• **Loss of eyelashes**.	Petroleum 30
• Blepharitis in the margins.	
• **Fissures in canthi**.	

FISTULA OF THE LACHRYMAL DUCT

An abnormality in the tear duct.

Distinguishing symptoms of the patient	Medicine and potency
• Watering. **Worse in open** air and early morning.	Calcarea Carb 200
• Sensation as if a **wind is blowing through** the eyes.	Fluoric Acid 200
• **Swelling in the bone** above the nose and between the eyes.	
• Violent itching in the inner canthi.	
• Chronic cases.	

FOREIGN BODY IN THE EYE

A speck of dust can cause irritation and discomfort. The eyes water and smart.

Do not rub. Clear the foreign body gently with soft, wet cotton or the wet corner of a clean handkerchief.

In an accident caused in a factory, or by a spray of chemical into the eye, **seek urgent medical help**.

First aid consists of washing the eye with running, clean water or by dipping the head, with lids forcibly open, into a bucket of water.

Distinguishing symptoms of the patient	Medicine and potency
• Takes care of the injury and consequent pain and pus formation.	Arnica 200
• Looks after **injury to the nerves** of the eye.	Hypericum 200. Continue until the pain disappears.

GLAUCOMA

Progressive loss of vision with increased pressure inside the eyeball. Mostly affects persons above forty. If no recovery takes place in the initial stages, the damage is irreversible. **Seek medical help as early as possible**.

Symptoms: Severe pressure inside the eye. Acute pain. Blurred vision. Rapid deterioration of the vision. Nausea. Vomit due to severe pain. Seen at night: colourful halos around a source of light. Eyes red, watering. Mild attacks precede a severe attack.

Distinguishing symptoms of the patient	Medicine and potency
• With iridescent vision. **Rainbow-like halos** around light. Green halo.	Osmium 30
• **Violent** supra orbital and infra-orbital **neuralgia**.	
• Objects look **red, often blue** in the field of vision.	Phosphorus 200
• Momentary **blindness** as if from fainting.	

GOUT

Painful inflammation of the joints, sometimes spreading to the eyes.

Distinguishing symptoms of the patient	Medicine and potency
• **Violent pain** in the eyeball **preceding glaucoma**. • Better on pressure.	Colocynthis 200

HAEMORRHAGES

Rupture of a blood vessel in the retina or anywhere else in the eye. **Consult an ophthalmic surgeon immediately.** Don't take it easy. Use the following medicines as palliatives only.

Symptoms: Floaters in the eye in minor episodes. Sudden loss of vision in major episodes.

Distinguishing symptoms of the patient	Medicine and potency
• Conjunctival haemorrhage into **retina**, resulting in **day blindness**.	Bothrops 30
• **Retinal**, non-inflammatory. Below the conjunctiva.	Crotalus 30
• **Ciliary neuralgia**. Dislikes **light**.	

INFLAMMATION

Localised protective reaction of tissue to irritation, injury or infection.

Symptoms: Redness, heat, swelling and pain. At times, loss of function.

Distinguishing symptoms of the patient	Medicine and potency
• **Sudden. Bright red** inflammation. On exposure to dry cold air.	Aconite Nap 30
• Lids swollen. Sensation of a foreign body.	
• Suppurating. Burning. Stinging pain.	Apis 200, 1000
• **Chronic conjunctivitis**.	
• With profuse purulent **discharge**.	Arg Nit 200
• Severe inflammation.	
• **Sudden, violent** inflammation in the optic nerve and in retina.	Belladonna 200
• Eyes **throbbing**, **red**, **protruding**, painful.	
• Worse motion, light, cold air exposure.	
• **Piercing pain** in the upper orbits.	Hepar Sulph 200
• Pus formation.	
• Inflammation of **cornea**. Effects of exposure to glare of fire.	Merc Sol 200
• Burning pain. Black floaters. Burning flow.	
• Marginal Blepharitis.	Petroleum 200
• Canthi **fissured**. Eyelids inflamed.	
• Of lids, with **thick**, **profuse, easy** flowing, bland, **yellow** or green discharge.	Pulsatilla 30
• In **chronic** and **recurrent** inflammation of cornea. Succession of abscesses.	Syphilinum 200. Once a day.
• Intense pain at night. Worse at night in summer.	
• Dislikes light.	
• Copious discharge.	
• Of **inner canthi** with severe itching.	Zincum Met 200
• **Skin peeling off**.	

IRITIS

An inflammation of the iris. Also known as 'anterior uveitis'. Symptoms develop slowly. In posterior uveitis, symptoms develop with speed. **Consult a doctor**.

Symptoms: Redness. Copious watering. Blurred vision. Pain in the eyeball. Pupil becomes small and irregular in shape.

Distinguishing symptoms of the patient	Medicine and potency
• **Pus and shooting pain** in anterior chamber.	Hepar Sulph 200
• Eyes red, inflamed. Worse on touch.	
• Iris **muddy** in colour.	Merc Cor 30
• **Thick**. Neither dilates, nor contracts.	
• **Syphilitic** iritis.	
• Tearing, shooting, burning pain. Worse at night.	

ITCHING

Distinguishing symptoms of the patient	Medicine and potency
• **Intolerable** itching of the eyeballs.	Ambrosia 200
• In **hay fever**. With watery flow from the nose, sneezing, wheezing, and coughing.	
• Eyes smart, burn, and water.	
• Severe itching in inner **angles**. Eyes sore.	Zincum Met 200
• Discharge excoriating.	

OPACITY

Distinguishing symptoms of the patient	Medicine and potency
• Of cornea. Night blindness.	Cadmium Sulph 30
• **In cataract**.	Calcarea Carb 200
• **Chronic dilation** of the pupils.	
• Foggy vision.	
• Fistula in tear duct. **Duct closed on exposure** to cold air.	

- Spots and **ulcers** on the cornea.
- Worse open air, in the morning.
- **Detachment of retina**.   Naphthalene 30

OPHTHALMIA

Severe inflammation of the eye.
For medicines, refer '*Inflammation*', above and '*Red*' and '*Swelling*'
below in this chapter.

PAIN

Distinguishing symptoms of the patient	Medicine and potency
• Piercing, burning pain in trachoma, in **chronic granular** lids.	Apis 200, 1000 **Most effective**. Quick.
• **Injury**.	Arnica 200
• **Bruised**, sore after close, strenuous work.	
• **Weary** after sight seeing, after a movie.	
• **Throbbing, deep** in the eyes.	Belladonna 200
• **Sudden**. **Violent**.	
• Pupil dilated and **protruding**. Eyes staring, shining, **red**, swollen, **dry**.	
• In the **right** eye, right cheek, right ear.	Chelidonium 30
• **Pain in the liver** followed by profuse tears.	
• Intense pain in the eyeball, **running** into **head.**	Cimicifuga 200
• **Dislike of artificial light**.	
• Pain **travelling from tear ducts**, from canthi, into the temple, across the **brow into the ears.**	Cinnabaris 30
• Shooting pain in the orbital bones. Ciliary neuralgia.	
• Entire eye red, lids granulated.	

- With **onset of influenza.**   Gelsemium 200
- In detached retina.
- Orbital pain.
- Constriction and **twitching** of muscles.
- **Piercing** pain in the **upper bones**.   Hepar Sulph 200
- Conjunctivitis with **pus**.
- Trachoma with **pus**.
- Eyelids red. Sensitive to touch and air.
- Pain deep in orbits.   Kali Bich 200
- **Infected sinus**.
- Supra orbital pain with aching in the   Lycopus Virg 30
  scrotum.
- Severe ache beyond the eyeballs.   Merc Cor 30
  Eyes feel being **forced out.**
- Discharge peels off the skin.
- **Chronic trachoma.**
- Muddy, **atrophied iris**. Inflamed.
- Pain in the eyes of **anaemic persons**   Natrum Mur 200
  on looking down. Headache in
  schoolchildren.
- Reflex neuralgia of the eye because of   Plantago 30
  toothache or inflammation of the
  middle ear.
- Eyeball tender to touch.
- Eyestrain following minute work. Headache Ruta 200
  follows. Burning in eyes.
- Eyes feel **too large** for their sockets.   Spigelia 200
  Pain **on turning**, deep in the eyeball.
- Stabbing, throbbing pain, in temple, eye,
  zygoma, cheek, jaws, teeth. Worse on motion.

PHOTOPHOBIA

Abnormal visual intolerance to light.

Distinguishing symptoms of the patient	Medicine and potency
• **Bland discharge**. Burning. Cannot stand light.	Allium Cepa 200
• **Restlessness** for any reason and intolerance of sunlight.	Ars Alb 200
• Swelling. Burning.	
• **Upper half** of objects invisible. **Retina detached**.	Aurum Met 200
• Intense photophobia.	
• **Protruding** eyes. Painful.	Belladonna 200
• **Red, dry** conjunctiva.	
• Dislike of **artificial light**.	Cimicifuga 200

RED

Distinguishing symptoms of the patient	Medicine and potency
• On **exposure** to dry, cold air.	Aconite 30
• **Acute** trachoma. Lids red, swollen.	
• **Inner** angles red.	Agaricus 200
• Canthi red, **fissured** and raw.	Antim Crud 200
• Chronic cases.	
• **Inner canthi** red, swollen. **Pus**. **Copious** flow.	Arg Nit 200
• Eyelids red, burning. Acrid discharge.	Arsenic Alb 200
• **Restlessness**.	
• Conjunctiva **red**. Violent.	Belladonna 200
• **Protruding eyes**.	
• **Sudden** onset.	
• **Red spots afloat** in the field of vision.	Dubosia 30
• Acute or chronic conjunctivitis.	
• **Red**, swollen.	Graphites 200
• **Fissured** lids.	
• **Eczema** of the eyes.	

- In **chronic trachoma.**   Marc Cor 30
- Lids red, excoriating. Eyes sore.

RINGS AROUND THE EYES

Distinguishing symptoms of the patient	Medicine and potency
• **Blue rings** around eyes. Eyes dull.	Abrotanum 30
• Dark rings. Anaemia. Eyes **sunken**.	Acetic Acid 30
• Blue rings in cases of **excessive discharge** from any part of body leading to debility.	China 200
• Blue rings. Eyes look **glassy**.	Phosphoric Acid 30
• Eyeballs forcibly **pressed together inwards**.	

SAND

Distinguishing symptoms of the patient	Medicine and potency
• **Acute** sensation of sand.	Aconite 30
• On **exposure** to dry, cold air.	
• **Chronic** granular lids.	Apis 200, 1000
• Eyes swollen and watering.	

SQUINT

The patient sees two images. The eyes, particularly in children, appear to focus in different directions.

Distinguishing symptoms of the patient	Medicine and potency
• **Spasmodic**, periodic squint. Eyes staring.	Cicuta 200
• Result of an injury.	

- Sees double. **Objects recede, approach**.
- **Disturbed muscular functioning** of   Gelsemium 200
  the eye.
- Corrects **blurring and discomfort** even
  after prescription and use of correct lenses.

STARE

Distinguishing symptoms of the patient	Medicine and potency
• In epileptic attacks. • Quick rolling of eyeballs. Eyes fixed, **staring, sunken, glistening**.	Cuprum Met 200

STYE

Formation of pus in a gland of the eye, at the root of an eyelash.

Distinguishing symptoms of the patient	Medicine and potency
• With **swollen** eyelids.	Apis 200
• Near **inner canthi**.	Lycopodium 200
• Pus formed. **Stabbing pain**.	Hepar Sulph 200
• First medicine. Usually a **cure**.	Pulsatilla 200
• **Recurring** sties.	Staphysagria 200

SWELLING [OEDEMA]

Distinguishing symptoms of the patient	Medicine and potency
• Chronic granular eyelids. **Stinging** pain. • Conjunctiva bright red and puffy.	Apis 200

- **Acute** granular conjunctivitis.   Arg Nit 200
- Swelling around eyes.   Arsenic Alb 200
- Eyes **ulcerated**, red. **Acrid tears**.
- Swelling in **non-stop catarrhal**   Euphrasia 200
  conjunctivitis.
- In **fissured** eyes.   Graphites 200
- **Upper lids** swollen like bags.   Kali Carb 200
- Swelling of the **bone between** the eyes.
- Eyelids feel **stitched together** in the
  morning.
- Swelling with **excoriation** of the lids.   Merc Cor 30
- **Severe burning**.

TEAR DUCT BLOCKED

When eyes are watering copiously, the cause can be a blocking of the tear duct due to an infection. It is common in babies and old persons.

Distinguishing symptoms of the patient	Medicine and potency
• Copious flow. **Intolerable** itching.	Ambrosia 30
• Non-stop excoriating discharge.	Euphrasia 200
• Inflamed **lids glued** together.	Pulsatilla 200
• Bland, yellow, thick discharge.	

TRACHOMA

A serious infection of the eye, spread by contaminated hands or towels. It damages the cornea that lies transparent in front of the eye. Repeated attacks can be very harmful. **Can lead to blindness**.

Symptoms: Acute aversion to light. Conjunctiva inflamed. Pus formation. Thick discharge. Sensation of sand.

For medicines, refer '*Pain*', and '*Red*' above, according to symptoms.
However, Apis 1000 gives quick relief.

TWITCHING

Distinguishing symptoms of the patient	Medicine and potency
• Of eyelids, of eyeballs.	Agaricus 200

ULCERS

Distinguishing symptoms of the patient	Medicine and potency
• Ulcers on the eyelids.**Restlessness**.	Arsenic Alb 200
• On **cornea**. Pus formed. **Needling** pain.	Hepar Sulph 200
• **Deep ulcers** on cornea.	Merc Cor 30
• Acrid lachrymation.Excessive photophobia. Lids swollen. Iris muddy in colour, thick, **neither contracts nor dilates**.	

THE NOSE

The nose is the part of the human face that contains the nostrils and the organs of smell. It forms the beginning of the respiratory tract which, besides the nose, includes the mouth, nasal sinuses, nasopharynx, left and right bronchi, and the lungs.

Functionally, the nose traps infection and prevents it, not always successfully, from reaching the lungs. The trapped infection leads to cold, running nose and sore throat.

The nasal cavity, lined with mucous membranes, is a narrow chamber going up high. Its floor is the roof of the mouth and its ceiling, the brain case. In its roof are located olfactory bulbs and sensory epithelia. The inhaled air passes over the latter and activates the bulbs to convey a sense of smell to the brain.

The lining in the nasal cavities provides moisture and warmth to the air entering the nose. Their walls secrete mucous which in turn blocks any foreign bodies like bacteria or dust trying to enter the respiratory system.

Infection often sets in the nasal sinuses which are hollows in the bone and connect the nasal cavity with the skull. This infection becomes chronic because it is difficult to clear. In such cases, homoeopathic remedies such as Pulsatilla, Kali Bichrome, Silicia and Hepar Sulph come in handy, with remarkable results.

Congested and blocked sinuses cause pain in the entire region. Infection leads to flow of green/yellow/grey mucous into the throat or outwards. In severe cases this mucous smells foul. The patient can hardly breathe. He has to breathe through an open mouth. His sleep is disturbed.

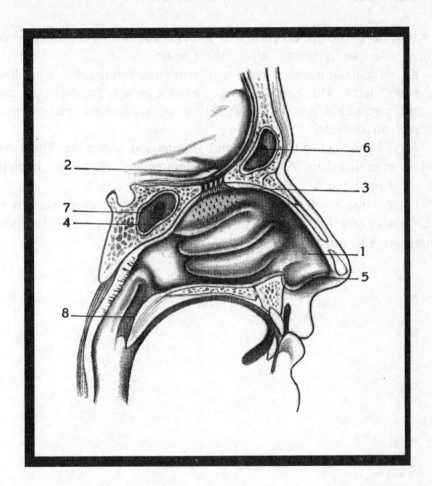

1. Nasal cavity. 2. Olfactory bulb. 3. Sensory epithelium. 4. Olfactory nerve. 5. Inlet for air. 6. Frontal sinuses. 7. Sphenoid sinus. 8. Eustachian tube.

The opening behind the nasal cavities leads to the Eustachian tubes. There is a connection to the middle ear at this junction. Infection travels into these tubes and causes severe pain.

None can avoid a common cold. Grin and bear it. However, the remedies indicated in the following sub-chapters will help in alleviating your distress and provide cure in most cases without any side effects. Antibiotics do not destroy viruses that cause common cold.

Once the symptoms appear, take rest, and use warm and moist inhalation. Drink a lot of warm water repeatedly, holding the sip for a few seconds in the throat. Have fruit juices at room temperature. Sneeze into a tissue so as not to infect others nearby.

Keep the nasal passages clean with water and soft tissue. Never blow your nose hard. This can injure the delicate lining. Similarly, do not forcefully scratch dry scabs. Moisten them with water, coconut oil, and clean them delicately.

A cold can lead to bronchitis and an infection of the ear. These are serious complications. Attend to them immediately. Refer to chapters on '*the Lungs*' and '*the Ears*', for appropriate remedies.

Do not use nasal drops to clear a stuffed nose except when it is unavoidable and that too for a short duration and under medical advice. These are harmful in the end.

BLEEDING

Distinguishing symptoms of the patient	Medicine and potency
• Nosebleed. Epistaxis. • **Sneezing**.	Ambrosia. Mother Tincture, 10 drops in water during attack. Every 15 minutes until bleeding stops.
• **Mucous with blood** blown out of nose. • **Persistent** nosebleed.	Ammonia Carb 30 Camphor, Mother Tincture to smell. Plus 10 drops on sugar dose every 15 minutes until bleeding is under control.
• Nosebleed. **Daily attacks. Face pale**. Weak. • **Dark, stringy**, and clotted bleeding. • **Small haemorrhage** in coryza. Handkerchief always stained. • **Hard crusts** in the nose. Bleed on loosening. • Nasal bones sensitive. **Chronic cases**.	Carbo Veg 200 Crocus 30 Phosphorus 200 Silicea 200

BURNING

Distinguishing symptoms of the patient	Medicine and potency
• Acute burning with nose **dripping like a tap.** • Incessant sneezing • Restless. Better hot application, worse cold.	Arsenic Alb 200

CARIES

Decay of a bone.

Distinguishing symptoms of the patient	Medicine and potency
• Decay of the **nasal bone**, of the **palate.** • **Fetid discharge**. • Nose obstructed, painful, ulcerated, and swollen.	Aurum met 200
• Caries in nasal bones with **swelling**.	Merc Sol 200

CATARRH

Excessive discharge accompanied by inflammation of the mucous membrane of the nose, of air passages in the nose or the throat.

Choose medicine according to symptoms as suggested in this chapter, such as the type of discharge, inflammation, swelling, and pain.

CHRONIC COLD

Symptoms: Refer '*Common Cold*' below.

Distinguishing symptoms of the patient	Medicine and potency
• Discharge inside as **well as outside.** • Sneezing.	Arsenic Iod 30
• Chronic, lingering cases of nasal catarrh. Thick, yellow, rusty mucous. • Large **blood stained lumps** thrown out in the morning.	Calcarea Carb 30
• Fetid odour, **greenish** crusts. • Nose stuffed. **Pain** from nose into the ear.	Elaps Cor 30
• **Chronic** inflammation of frontal sinuses. • Acute **pain in the orbits**, at the root of the nose, in the bones, in sinuses. • Thick, greenish, **stringy** discharge, glued to the throat, **not coming out.**	Kali Bich 200

- Nose blocked, smell lost, violent sneezing.
- **Dry catarrh**. No flow. Nose blocked.   Lycopodium 200
- **Chronic**.   Pulsatilla 30, 200
- Yellow, greenish, bland, fetid mucous **coming out easily**.
- Sense of smell lost.
- No thirst.
- Cold which **fails to yield**.   Silicea 200
- Sputum full of fetid, thick, yellow mucous.
- **Violent cough** when lying down.

COMMON COLD

Viral infection that covers the whole of the upper respiratory tract.

Symptoms: Lining of the nose inflamed, swollen. Inflammation in the throat, in the sinuses and the larynx. Dry cough. A sensation of tickling in the palate, gums and the nose. At times, congestion in the head. Breathing difficult.

For medicines, refer to the sub-chapters according to symptoms, in this chapter.

A few doses of Arundo 200 at the beginning taken at 30 minutes interval considerably alleviate the suffering. Hot fomentation eases discomfort.

DISCHARGE

Distinguishing symptoms of the patient	Medicine and potency
• Nose waters; eyes water. **Acrid** discharge.	Allium Cepa 200
• Violent sneezing.	
• **Intolerable itching** of the eyelids. Copious flow of water from the eyes.	Ambrosia 30
• **Acute, violent cold**.	
• **Trachea, bronchial tubes irritated**.	

- Nose **bleeding.**   Arsenic Alb 200
- **Excoriating**, thin flow in hay fever.
- Restlessness.
- **Chronic** nasal inflammation of the   Arsenic Iod 30
  mucous membrane with **free discharge
  inwards and outwards.**
- Discharge thick, yellow with sneezing.
  Excoriates.
- **Ulcers** in the nose.
- Fetid pus in **nasal decay.**   Aurum Met 200
- **Pain deep** in the nose.
- Fetid, thick, **ropy**, yellow, or greenish   Kali Bich 200
  discharge **inwards**.
- Mucous **difficult to take out**.
- Chronic sinusitis.
- Violent, **fluent, changing to stoppage** of   Nat Mur 200
  the nose.
- Loss of smell and taste.
- Chronic with **small haemorrhages.**   Phosphorus 200
- Green, yellow, or grey, **flowing outwards**   Pulsatilla 30, 200
  and **easy**.
- **Smell lost**. Nostrils blocked.
- Large, green, fetid scabs in the nose.
  Can be smelled fetid from a distance.
- Chronic cases.

DRY COLD

Distinguishing symptoms of the patient	Medicine and potency
• **Dry, stuffed** coryza, acute or chronic.	Ammonium Carb 30
• Has to **breathe through mouth**.	
• Chronically dry, stuffed nose.	Lycopodium 200
• Fan like motion of cartilaginous flaps on the outer side of the either nostril.	
• No discharge, yet **needs to blow** constantly.	Sticta 30

- Pain in frontal sinuses. Heavy **pain** and pressure at the **root of the nose**, in the forehead.
- **Discharge** provides **relief**.
- **Chronic inflammation** of the mucous membrane. Dry scabs.
- **Bleeding easily on scratching.**
- Polyps and adenoids.

Sulphur 200

ECZEMA

Distinguishing symptoms of the patient	Medicine and potency
• Of the nose. Sore, **crusty**, scruffy.	Antim Crud 200

EYE, COLD SETTLING IN

Distinguishing symptoms of the patient	Medicine and potency
• **Every cold** settles in the eye. • Worse in cold, damp weather.	Dulcamara 200

ITCHING

Distinguishing symptoms of the patient	Medicine and potency
• **Severe, unbearable itching** in the eyes, palate, gums, nose, ears with sneezing at the onset of cold.	Arundo 200
• Itching of the nose at **all times**. Picks until bleeds. • Worms in the abdomen. • The child grits his teeth while sleeping,	Cina 200

jerks, coughs, and chokes. Stretches out
his feet spasmodically.
- Itching in the soft palate, in the throat.   Gelsemium 200
- Onset of cold, influenza. **Body pain**.

PAIN

Distinguishing symptoms of the patient	Medicine and potency
- Nose red, swollen. **Stinging pain**.	Apis 200
- Caries in nasal bones. Nose **ulcerated**, swollen, obstructed. **Fetid pus**.	Aurum Met 200
- In influenza, severe pain in the **bones**. Bursting head.	Eupatorium Perf 200
- **Muscular soreness** in influenza, in coryza.	Gelsemium 200
- Feeling of a **band tightening around the skull.**	
- **Chill up the spine**. Sluggishness. Face besotted, stupefied.	
- Chronic sinusitis. Pressure at **the root of the nose. On stooping**, bending head forward.	Kali Bich 200
- In bones above the eyes, **deep in the eye sockets**.	
- Ulcerated septum. **Ropy, green mucous inwards**.	
- With swelling of the nasal bones. Caries.	Merc Sol 200
- Thick, yellow **mucous outwards**.	
- In **dry cold**, with heavy pressure at the root of the nose.	Sticta 30
- **Relieved by discharge**.	

POLYPS, NASAL

A growth protruding from the mucous membrane of the nose.

Distinguishing symptoms of the patient	Medicine and potency
• Foul smell. Caries. Ulcers in the nose.	Cadmium Sulph 30
• With acute coryza, **body pain**, **sneezing**.	Gelsemium 200
• Easy **bleeding** in bits. Chronic catarrh.	Phosphorus 200
• Nose full of mucous. **Irregular clinkers** blown out.	Teucrium Marum 30. Dry powder for local
• **Crawling sensation** in blocked nostrils	application.
• Foul breath.	

POST-NASAL DRIP

Distinguishing symptoms of the patient	Medicine and potency
• Thick, **ropy** mucous flowing **inwards**. Difficult to take out.	Kali Bichrome 200 **Remarkable results**.
• Chronic sinusitis with **pain deep in the eye** sockets and behind ears.	
• Wants **desperately to clear** the throat early morning.	

RHINITIS

An inflammation of the nasal lining which blocks the nose, running or stuffed. Acute rhinitis is called common cold.

For medicines, look according to symptoms in this chapter.

SEPTUM PERFORATED

Distinguishing symptoms of the patient	Medicine and potency
• Green, **ropy mucous inwards.**	Kali Bichrome 200
• Severe **pain, deep** in bones of the face, in sinuses and in eye sockets.	
• Foul smell.	

- Perforated septum in **old** sinusitis.   Kali Iodide 30
- Putrid smell.
- Perforated septum with **fetid discharge**.   Merc Cor 30
  Decay in the nose.

SINUSITIS/ACUTE OR CHRONIC

Sinuses are air-filled cavities in the bones leading from the skull to the nose. An infection of sinuses is painful. The situation is worse when the cold becomes chronic.

Symptoms: Pain, deep in bones around sinuses and eye sockets. Headache. Worse when stooping down. Foul nasal discharge inwards or outwards. Pain in the teeth and the jaws. Difficulty in breathing. Sense of smell and taste diminished or totally lost.

Distinguishing symptoms of the patient	Medicine and potency
• Infected sinus with **pus** formation.	Hepar Sulph 200
• Green, **sticky** mucous **inwards**.	Kali Bichrome 200
Difficult to take out.	**Great results.**
• **Pain** in sinuses, **deep** in eye sockets.	
Worse stooping.	
• Nose stuffy but **no discharge**.	Kali Iodide 30
• Perforated septum.	
• Putrid smell.	
• Bland, green mucous **easily coming out**.	Pulsatilla 30
• Chronic cold.	**Remarkable results.**
• Smell and taste diminished.	

SMELL

Distinguishing symptoms of the patient	Medicine and potency
• **Acute.**	Carbolic Acid 30
• After influenza, weakness.	

• Lost in chronic sinusitis.	Kali Bich 200
• Mucous **difficult to take out**.	
• Lost. Chronic cold.	Pulsatilla 30
• Bland, green mucous that **flows easy outwards**.	

SNEEZING

Sneezing is caused involuntarily by an irritation in the nasal passages.

Distinguishing symptoms of the patient	Medicine and potency
• On **exposure to dry, cold** air.	Aconite 30
• Without relief with **excoriating discharge.**	Arsenic Alb 200
• Burning sensation. Restlessness.	
• Acute, **unbearable itching** in the palate, gums, nose, and throat with sneezing.	Arundo 200
• With **congestion** in the skull bones. The skull feels tied with a **band of steel.**	Gelsemium 200
• **Chill up the spine**, in the shoulders.	
• Influenza cases.	
• Cold **starts with sneezing.**	Natrum Mur 200
• Violent, fluent flow from the nose.	
• In between, nose stuffed.	

STUFFED/SNUFFLES

Distinguishing symptoms of the patient	Medicine and potency
• Nose stuffed **at night**. Snuffles of **children.**	Ammonia Carb 30
• Old coryza.	
• Must breathe through mouth.	Aurum Triph 30
• **Bleeds on picking**. Blood streaked mucous. **Ulcers.**	

• Stuffed on exposure to **wet weather.**	Dulcamara 200
• Stuffed. **Old cheese smell**.	Hepar Sulph 200
• No discharge.	
• Highly sensitive to cold weather.	
• Sinusitis. Pain **deep in eye** sockets.	Kali Bich 200
• Ropy, green mucous **dripping inwards.**	
• Chronic cases.	
• Nose stuffed **at night**.	Nux Vomica 200
• Chronic cold.	Pulsatilla 30
• **Bland, green**/yellow mucous **flowing outwards**.	
• **Stuffed nose**. Take in addition to other chosen remedy. Once early morning for a few days.	Sulphur 200

SWELLING

Distinguishing symptoms of the patient	Medicine and potency
• **Stinging** pain. Nose red.	Apis 200
• Painful **ulceration** and swelling.	Aurum met 30
• Caries of nasal bones.	
• Of **nose and upper lip** with discharge of thick, yellow mucous.	Baryta Carb 200
• **Polyps** swelling at the root of the nose.	Calcarea Carb 30
• **Decay** in the nasal bones. Pain.	Merc Sol 200
• Greenish, **fetid discharge**.	

TENDENCY TO CATCH COLD

Distinguishing symptoms of the patient	Medicine and potency
• Every cold settles in **the throat**. **Tonsils enlarged and hardened**.	Alumen 30
• **One cold ends, another begins**.	Nitric Acid 200

- Offensive smell. Nasal catarrh
- Splinter pain in the nose.
- **Green crusts** flowing out every morning.

• Catches cold from a bath, from overheating, in a cold room, from exertion, from change of weather	Sulphur 200 In chronic cases, one dose early morning, once a week, for
• **Frequent sore throat.**	three months.

TICKLING

Distinguishing symptoms of the patient	Medicine and potency
• Annoying itching and tickling in the nostrils, palate, eyes with violent sneezing. • Unpleasant onset of cold.	Arundo 200

THE EARS
With ears, we hear music and bird song

The human ear performs two functions: hearing and maintaining equilibrium. The loss of the former leads to deafness and a disturbance of the latter to dizziness.

The visible outer ear consists of a flap known as the pinna and the outer ear canal. These collect and regulate sound waves from any source into a funnel.

The middle ear consisting of the eardrum, hammer, anvil, stirrup, and the Eustachian tube, receives the sound waves and transmits them to the inner ear.

The sound waves at first meet the eardrum known as tympanic membrane.

The Eustachian tube is a link between the middle ear and the nasopharynx lying behind the nasal cavity. It regulates the air pressure within the middle ear. Any disturbance of this balance leads to acute discomfort.

The hammer, anvil, and the stirrup are three small bones connected with each other.

The inner ear consists of the cochlea and the labyrinth. The cochlea that looks like a shell, converts the sound waves into nerve impulses for transmission into the brain via the auditory nerve.

The labyrinth in the inner ear monitors the movements of our head and body so that we can keep our balance. This sense of balance is an unconscious understanding of the orientation of the body in space. It

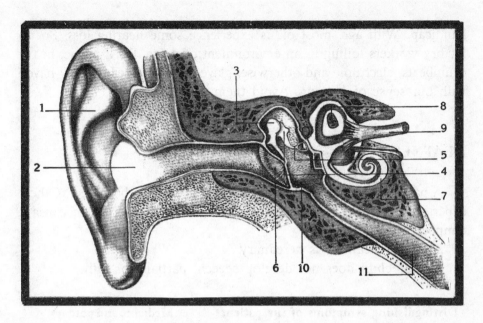

1. Pinna. 2. Ear canal [external ear]. [3-5. Middle ear bones.]
3. Hammer. 4. Anvil. 5. Stirrup. 6. Ear drum [tympanic membrane.]
7. Cochlea [internal ear or labyrinth.] 8. Semicircular canals.
9. Auditory nerves. 10. Tympanic cavity. 11. Eustachian tube.

allows us to maintain an upright posture and move without stumbling. A disturbance of this balance causes vertigo.

Hearing any sound, even if it is music, at very high volumes, is a threat to the health of our hearing system. It causes irreversible damage in the end. The power of the sound waves is measured in units called decibels. For every increase of ten decibel in power, our ears hear double the loudness. We converse at around 60 decibels. Normal traffic produces around 80 decibels. Noises above 120 decibels can cause serious damage to our hearing. In India, strict laws are in place to control noise pollution. Unfortunately, it is considered fashionable to hear music at 150 decibel and above. The enforcement is slack.

Persistent ear ache indicates an infection. This must be taken care of without any loss of time. Such an infection, if left untreated, can damage other parts of the body.

Problems relating to loss of the hearing faculty require attention. This loss is a social embarrassment. However, it is, largely, a reparable handicap. With age, most of us experience some hearing loss. So do factory workers toiling in an environment of noise. Rock music, heavy drumbeats, electronic and otherwise, played at high decibels play havoc with our sense of hearing. Avoid them.

DEAFNESS

A partial or total loss of hearing. Some people are born deaf. Others experience deafness because of age. Certain ear problems can cause a temporary deafness.

At times, deafness is hereditary.

A deaf child does not develop speech, partially or fully.

Distinguishing symptoms of the patient	Medicine and potency
• **Pus** with pain and **swelling**. From **working in water**.	Calcarea Carb 200
• With eczema.	Calendula, mother tincture,
• Worse in damp surroundings.	only for local application.
• **Roaring** and humming noise.	Causticum 200
• **Tinkling** sound.	
• **Fissures** in the ears.	Graphites 200
• Inner ear dry.	
• Hissing. Booming of guns.	
• **Hears better in noise**.	
• Fetid **pus** in ears. **Shooting pain**.	Hepar Sulph 200
• Whizzing, throbbing sound.	
• **Pus in Eustachian tubes**.	Hydrastis 30
• Roaring noises.	
• Eustachian tubes **obstructed.**	Iodum 30
• Due to **chronic coryza.**	Kali Mur 200
• External ear red, **swollen**.	Pulsatilla 30
• Diminished hearing.	

DISCHARGE

Distinguishing symptoms of the patient	Medicine and potency
• **Burning**, thin, offensive.	Arsenic Alb 200
• Inside **skin raw, peeling off**.	
∘ Spasmodic pain. Roaring noises.	
• Mucous flowing. **Glands enlarged**.	Calcarea Carb 200
Pulsating pain. Bleeding polyps.	
• Something pressing out.	
• Better dry weather, worse, cold air.	
• Fetid **pus in auditory canal**. Throbbing.	Hepar Sulph 200
• **Shooting pain.**	
• Better head wrapped up, warmth. Worse lying on painful side, cold air.	
• Pain with thick, green, **offensive discharge**. Chronic catarrh.	Pulsatilla 30
• **Red swelling** in the external ear.	
• Hearing quality diminished.	
• **Old, chronic catarrh of the ear.**	Silicea 200
• **Offensive** discharge.	Goes beyond Pulsatilla.
• **Roaring**, hissing sounds.	

DRYNESS

Distinguishing symptoms of the patient	Medicine and potency
• **Fissures** inside and outside the ears.	Graphites 200
• Hissing sounds.	

EARACHE/PAIN/OTALGIA

Distinguishing symptoms of the patient	Medicine and potency
• From **exposure to dry cold air,** throbbing, cutting pain.	Aconite 30

• Shooting pain in **Eustachian tube.**	Allium Cepa 200
• Eyes and nose **running**.	
• **External** ear red, **swollen**, sore.	Apis 200
• In **glands** around ears which are painful and swollen.	Baryta Carb 200
• **Unbearable**, tearing pain in the external and middle ear.	Belladonna 200, 1000
• Pain with **numbness.**	Chamomilla 200, 1000
• Soreness, heat, intolerable, stitching pain.	
• **Makes the person frantic**. Foul temper.	
• In the left ear with pain deep in **eye sockets.**	Kali Bichrome 200
• Green, **sticky mucous** flowing inwards.	
• With foul smelling, yellow, corrosive **discharge from external ear**.	Merc Sol 200
• **Inflammation** of the **middle ear** when pus formation has started.	Myristica 200 Hastens formation, release of pus and shortens its course.
• **With toothache**. Decaying teeth	Plantago 30.
• Pain travels from ear to ear.	Apply Mother Tincture locally.

EAR INJURY

An injury to the ear can be direct, or it can be caused by an injury to the head or by loud noise. It can be serious. **Seek medical counsel**.

Symptoms: An injury to the ear can damage the hearing nerves, resulting in total or partial hearing loss. Bleeding. Severe pain. Suppuration of the wound.

Distinguishing symptoms of the patient	Medicine and potency
• **Concussion or a direct hit** on the ear with bleeding or otherwise.	Arnica 200. First aid.
• **Severe pain** persisting even after Arnica has been administered.	Belladonna 200, 1000
• **Redness and swelling**.	

• Wound **suppurates**. Foul, green pus.	Hepar Sulph 200
• Shooting, **needling pain**.	
• A wound caused by a **pointed article** such as a hair clip, or a matchstick being inserted into the ear.	Ledum 200
• Injury to the **nerves**, to the **bones.**	Ruta 200
• A bruise above the ear.	

EARWAX

Earwax, though it looks messy and obstructs the ear, is produced by glands to moisten and clean the ears. It protects the ears from infection. It is an auto clean product. Yet, it sometimes accumulates and clogs the ear canal. Too much of this happening can lead to deafness in some cases.

If the earwax has been there for sometime and has hardened, get it cleaned by a doctor. In anticipation of this procedure, soften it by putting a few drops of olive or some other non-irritating oil into the ear. Lie down on the side other than the one on which the ear has to be cleaned. Do not clear the wax on your own. It is risky. You will merely push it inwards.

Distinguishing symptoms of the patient	Medicine and potency
• Helps in elimination of wax in the ears.	Conium 200

ECZEMA

Distinguishing symptoms of the patient	Medicine and potency
• Behind the ears, moisture and eruption.	Graphites 200
• **Fissures**.	
• Behind the ears.	Tellurium 30
• With catarrh of the middle ear.	
• Acrid discharge.	

EUSTACHIAN TUBE, OBSTRUCTION OF

Eustachian tube is a narrow canal that joins the middle of the ear to the back of the nose and throat. It controls air pressure in the middle ear.

Symptoms: The obstruction of Eustachian tube, for any reason, can cause acute, unbearable pain and temporary deafness.

The problem is caused by change of pressure while driving, diving, or during the landing of a flight. It can also be caused by common cold.

The patient should move his jaw in a chewing and swallowing motion and try to force breath out through the ears with the mouth and the nostrils closed. It helps in most cases. In chronic cases, the medicines noted under are of great help.

Before undertaking an activity wherein the blockage can occur, take a dose of Kali Bichrome 200. Repeat a few minutes before the descent of a flight. Take Belladonna in case nothing helps and the pain persists.

Distinguishing symptoms of the patient	Medicine and potency
Unbearable pain.	Belladonna 1000, 10000
Chronic sinusitis cases.	Kali Bichrome 200
Inward drip of mucous that is **tough to take out**.	
Severe pain in the frontal sinuses and **eye sockets**.	
Chronic cold but the mucous **flows outwards easily**.	Pulsatilla 30, 200

HAEMORRHAGE

Distinguishing symptoms of the patient	Medicine and potency
• Bleeding from **injury** to the ear.	Arnica 200
• Dullness of hearing after a **concussion**.	
• **Polyps** bleeding easily.	Calcarea Carb 200
• Black, **offensive** blood that does not **coagulate**.	Crotalus H 200

HERPES

Inflammation of the skin or of the mucous membrane, characterized by clusters of vesicles that tend to spread.

Distinguishing symptoms of the patient	Medicine and potency
• Herpes behind the ears. On nape of neck. • **Ulceration. Swelling**. Further, see '*Cold sores*' under '*The Skin*'.	Sepia 200

MENIERE'S DISEASE

An acute though rare condition, in which the fluid in the inner ear increases suddenly. The balancing mechanism swells. The condition recurs. Hearing worsens with successive attacks. The loss of hearing can be permanent in course of time.

Symptoms: Pain that causes incapacitating dizziness. Nausea, vomiting. Sensation of the room spinning around. The victim falls to the ground. Simultaneous deafness and a ringing noise in the affected ear. Abnormal, jerky movement of the eye.

Consult a doctor. It is urgent.

Distinguishing symptoms of the patient	Medicine and potency
• **Buzzing and ringing** in ears. Defective hearing. • Better in open air. Worse in warm, damp weather.	Carbo Sulph 30
• **Sudden vertigo**. Giddiness starting in the ears. • While deaf to voices, **sensitive to high-pitched sound. Buzzing in the ears.**	Chenopodium 30
• Loud **pistol like sound**. Buzzing. Roaring • Caries of mastoid, a bone behind the ears. Fetid pus.	Silicea 200

MOTION SICKNESS

Nausea, vomiting, caused by sensitivity to motion by sea, rail, road or air. It is caused by a disturbance in the balancing mechanism of the inner ear.

Symptoms: Headache. Nausea. Vomit. Fatigue.

Do not drive a vehicle on your own if you suffer from motion sickness. Take a dose of Cocculus 200 before embarking on your journey. Repeat as often as required. It is of great help.

Distinguishing symptoms of the patient	Medicine and potency
• Nausea **while travelling** by road, sea, air, or rail. Aversion to food, drink.	Cocculus 200
• Oesophagus dry. **Deglutition** muscles partially **paralysed**	
• **Flatulence. Diarrhoea.**	
• Pain in the eyes as if they are being pulled out.	

NOISES/TINNITUS

Tinnitus has been defined as a sound in one or both ears, such as buzzing, ringing, or whistling, occurring without an external stimulus. It is usually caused by a specific condition, such as an ear infection, the use of certain drugs, a blocked auditory tube or canal, or a concussion on the head. Age is an important factor.

Tinnitus may also be an indication of an imminent attack of epilepsy, or of fainting.

If the underlying cause is treated, improvement can occur. **Your doctor will be your best guide in handling this condition** because a number of alternatives, besides remedies, are available to reduce the distressing nuisance. In specific symptoms, the following remedies help.

Distinguishing symptoms of the patient	Medicine and potency
• When chewing, swallowing.	Baryta Mur 200
• **Buzzing and singing** noises. Hearing diminished.	Carbo Sulph 30
• Hears his **own echo**.	Causticum 200
• While climbing mountains.	Coca 30
• Caused by catarrh, by **inflammation of the middle ear.** Chronic cases.	Kali Mur 30
• During **menstruation**.	Kreosote 200
• Like ringing of bells.	Ledum 200
• Of a **windstorm**.	
• **Humming and rolling sounds**. Hardness of hearing.	Lycopodium 200
• Hears his own echo.	
• Crackling noise when **chewing**.	Nitric Acid 200
• Rolling noises. **Pus** in the ears. Chronic cases.	Silicea 200
• **Preceding menses**.	Veratrum Alb 200

OTITIS EXTERNA

The outer ear canal is infected by fungal, viral, or bacterial infection.

Symptoms: Discharge of pus. Earache and rash at the site.
Refer '*Discharge*' and '*Earache*' above.

OTITIS MEDIA

Inflammation of the middle ear caused by viral or bacterial infection.

Symptoms: Severe pain and inflammation of the middle ear. Often accompanied by high fever, diarrhoea, and irritability.
Refer '*Discharge*' and '*Earache*' above.

PAIN

Refer '*Ear ache*' above.

PERFORATED EARDRUM

A hole in the eardrum. Usually caused by an acute bacterial infection of the middle ear, by poking cotton swabs or pins, and sometimes by imbalance of pressure inside the ear and outside.

Symptoms: Deafness, ringing in the ears, discharge of pus and blood. Shooting pain.

Consult your doctor immediately if you suspect a rupture. The prognosis is good. However, the remedies indicated below are of great help.

Distinguishing symptoms of the patient	Medicine and potency
• **Shooting pain**. Fetid pus.	Hepar Sulph 200
• Sensation of **throbbing** in the ears.	
• Worse dry, cold winds.	
• **Chronic catarrhal** earache.	Pulsatilla 30, 200
• **Offensive, thick, green pus flows out easily**.	
• **Chronic** cases of thick, green discharge	Silicea 200
• **Roaring, hissing sounds** in the affected ear.	

PUS

Distinguishing symptoms of the patient	Medicine and potency
• Foul smelling pus in auditory canal. At times, bloody.	Hepar Sulph 200
• **Shooting pain.**	

- Rupture in the eardrum.
- Fetid, **corrosive**, green, and thick pus from   Merc Sol 200
  the ruptured eardrum.
- Heavy flow.
- Severe, **incorrigible** suppuration of the   Myristica 200
  middle ear.
- Thick, green, bland, and offensive pus   Pulsatilla 200
  flowing out easily.
- Hearing diminished.
- **Chronic** cases of **pus formation**.   Silicea 200

SWELLING

Distinguishing symptoms of the patient	Medicine and potency
Glands around ears swollen. **Severe pain**.	Baryta Carb 200
Glands **hardened**, inflamed.	Merc Sol 200

THE MOUTH, THE LIPS, THE TONGUE, AND THE PALATE

The mouth is a part of the digestive system. Here food is chewed by the teeth and mixed with saliva by the tongue. Infections in the mouth are caused by bacteria, viruses, or fungi.

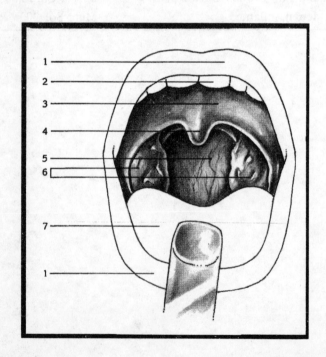

1. Lips. 2. Teeth. 3. Soft palate. 4. Uvula. 5. Tonsils. 7. Tongue.

The lips are mucous surfaces, fleshy parts, or folds that form the margins of the mouth. They play a vital role in word formation and speech.

Dry winter or cold can inflame the lips.

Cancer of the lips is a serious problem.

The teeth and the jaws have a separate chapter devoted to them.

The tongue, besides doing the mixing job, is the centre of our sense of taste. It detects the chemicals in the mouth. The sense of taste goes hand in hand with the sense of smell centred in the nose. A fetid odour can cause a nasty taste in the mouth. Our enjoyment of a meal depends on a complicated interaction between the sensations from the tongue, the palate, and the nose. A coryza patient loses his smell as well as taste temporarily.

Microscopic nerve endings called taste buds are located in the mouth and on the tongue. The upper surface of the tongue is covered by papillae, tiny, hair like projections with taste buds scattered in between. Different tastes are detected by different parts of the tongue.

The taste buds are activated by certain chemicals in the food. They, in turn, send messages to the brain. The latter sorts out the signals and gives us a feeling of taste.

Chewing tobacco has a pernicious effect on the tongue and the jaws. It causes cancer. Give up the use of tobacco in any form.

Sick persons, particularly those running a temperature, have a tongue which has a white, or yellow, furry coat on its surface. Ordinarily this is not a cause for worry. A sick person talks less, eats less. His mouth is dry. Secretion of saliva has been reduced. That is why his tongue is less active and collects white or yellow layers of bacteria. I recommend proper oral hygiene. With one's health improving, the tongue returns to its normal condition.

The roof of the mouth consists of an anterior bony portion called the hard palate and a posterior muscular portion known as the soft palate. These separate the oral cavity from the nasal cavity. The palate is connected with the respiratory system. That is why when the respiratory system is under attack by cold viruses, the palate experiences an intolerable itching.

BAD BREATH

If we do not clean the mouth and the teeth properly and regularly, food particles stagnate and a foul odour emanates with our exhalation. Injured teeth can become septic. Pus has an unpleasant odour. Bleeding gums are another source of foul breath.

Consumption of certain foods which in themselves have strong odours, sometimes, leads to bad breath. In such cases, proper oral hygiene is the only remedy.

Distinguishing symptoms of the patient	Medicine and potency
• Fetid breath. Bitter taste.	Arnica 200
• Because of **injury caused to the teeth**, gums, and resultant **septic**.	
• Foul breath pervades the entire room.	Merc Sol 200
• **Gums** spongy, **bleeding**, receding.	
• Excessive flow of saliva.	
• **Pyorrhoea**. Gum boils.	Silicea 200
• **Abscess** at the root of the teeth.	
• Teeth sensitive to cold air, to cold water.	

BLISTERS/ULCERS

Painful sores in the lining of the mouth, on the tongue, on the gums.

Symptoms: Formation of pits which are shallow, grey-white and have a red border. Pain on chewing spicy or hot food. Pus under raised skin blisters.

Distinguishing symptoms of the patient	Medicine and potency
• In the mouth. On the tongue. **Painful**.	Borax 200 Suck a few pills by placing these near the blisters.

• **Foul breath**, painful ulcers.	Merc Sol 200
• Blisters filled with **pus**.	Suck a few pills, placing
• **Ulcers on gums, lips, inside the cheeks.**	these near the blisters.
• **Teeth** leave an **imprint on the tongue.**	**Extremely effective.**
• Great desire for cold drinks.	
• On tip of tongue, on **palate**. Full of **pus.**	Nat Phos 30
• Roof of the mouth, the tongue at the **back coated yellow**. Swallowing difficult.	
• Stinging **pain in the evening**.	
• Ulcers on **soft palate**, in the mouth, on the tongue.	Nitric Acid 200 **Great remedy.**
• **Splinter pain**.	

CRACKS

Distinguishing symptoms of the patient	Medicine and potency
• In the corners of the mouth.	Antim Crud 200
• Digestion upset. **Foul belching**.	
• Corners of the mouth **sore, cracked.**	Aurum Triph 30
• Lips cracked, **burning**. Lips **bleed** on picking.	
• The palate feels **rough**.	

ITCHING

Distinguishing symptoms of the patient	Medicine and potency
• **Unbearable** itching at the roof of the mouth, in the gums, in nostrils, in eyes.	Arundo 200
• **Sudden onset of cold**.	

LIPS CRACKED, SWOLLEN, HOT

Dry winter or cold can inflame the lips and cause cracks. An application of any cooking oil will help.

At other times, cracked or swollen lips indicate a serious problem. The villain could be cancer or just cold sores.

Vitamin B or riboflavin deficiency can cause rawness, redness and swelling at the lip joints.

Distinguishing symptoms of the patient	Medicine and potency
• **Swelling** of lips. Any reason.	Apis 200
• **Insect** bites.	
• **Shooting pain**.	
• Sunken face. **Lips hot**.	Arnica 200
• Lips **black**, livid.	Ars Alb 200
• **Debility. Restlessness**. Exhaustion.	
• **Blue** lips. **Cancer.**	Aurum Ars 30
• Red spots. **Coppery** eruptions.	
• Parched, dry, cracked.	Bryonia 200
• Mouth, tongue **dry**.	
• Cancer of the lips. **Ulcerative** stage.	Condurango 30
• **Painful** cracks in corners of the mouth.	
• **Pus** formed. **Shooting pain.**	Hepar Sulph 200
• **Swollen**. Tender to touch.	
• Cracks worse **every winter**. Painful.	Petroleum 200
• **Skin rough and leathery**.	

Refer 'Cold sores' in the chapter, 'The Skin', and 'Cracks' above.

LIP TUMOURS

Distinguishing symptoms of the patient	Medicine and potency
• Tumour on the lip. **Cheeks hot** and flushed.	Acetic Acid 30
• Lips **black, blue**. Ashen.	Arsenic Alb 200
• Exhaustion. **Debility. Restlessness**.	

PARALYSIS OF THE TONGUE

Refer '*Tongue, problems of*' below.

SALIVA

Distinguishing symptoms of the patient	Medicine and potency
• Saliva runs excessively and out **of the mouth during sleep**. • Increased saliva formation. • Mouth **smells foul**.	Syphilinum 200 Once a day for a few days. Merc Sol 200
• Copious flow although salivary **glands congested**.	Trifolium Mother tincture, 5 drops, four times in a day.

STOMATITIS

An inflammation of the mouth that is caused by bacteria, virus, or fungi, by neglected dental care or oral hygiene.

Symptoms: Bad breath, sore mouth, ulcers. Fever, sometimes. Refer '*Blisters/ulcers*' above.

TASTE

Distinguishing symptoms of the patient	Medicine and potency
• Foul breath. Taste of rotten **eggs**.	Arnica 200
• **Sour** taste. Mouth full of sour water.	Calcarea Carb 200
• Strong **metallic** taste in the mouth.	Cuprum Met 200
• Saliva flows copious.	
• **Varying** taste, salty, bitter, and foul. Sense of smell diminished.	Pulsatilla 30
• **Excessive intake** of heavy food.	

THIRSTLESSNESS

Distinguishing symptoms of the patient	Medicine and potency
• No thirst. Tongue and uvula **swollen**.	Apis 200
• **Mouth dry** but no thirst.	Pulsatilla 30

TONGUE—PROBLEMS OF, COATINGS, BLACK AND BLUE, CANCER OF

Cancerous tumours form on the lips, tongue, or on the lining of the mouth, mainly on the lower lip or the tongue.

Symptoms: Swelling anywhere inside the mouth or on lips. An ulcer that does not heal and enlarges slowly.

Consult a doctor so that a proper diagnosis can be done. Use the medicines below as palliatives. Cancer in this area is not a pleasant prospect.

Distinguishing symptoms of the patient	Medicine and potency
• **Pale, red** papillae.	Allium Sativum 30
• Voracious appetite. Or, constipated.	
• Indigestion from **gluttony**. Foul eructation.	Antim Crud 200
• **Milky white**, thick coating.	
• Tongue **fiery red**, scalded.	Apis 200
• Uvula swollen.	
• **Cancer** of the tongue. It **swells** to fill the mouth.	
• Ulcers. **Blue** colour.	Arsenic Alb 200
• Food poisoning cases. Alcoholism. caused by chewing **tobacco**. Sting bites.	
• **Paralysis** of the tongue. The **tip burns** and smarts.	Baryta Carb 200
• Excessive thirst. Mouth **always dry**.	Bryonia 200
• Lips dry, cracked.	

- Yellowish or **dark brown** coating.
- Taste bitter. Digestion upset.
  Tongue coated thick white.
- **Blisters** on the tongue.   Carbo Veg 200
- **Acidity**. Debility.
- **Series of unending illnesses**.
- Constant **protrusion and retraction** of the   Cuprum Met 200
  tongue like that of a snake.
- Tongue **paralysed**.
- **Epileptic** stroke. Saliva flows out.
  Stammering.
- Thick, yellow, indented.   Merc Sol 200
- **Teeth leave a mark**.
- **Ulcers** on the tongue.
- Tongue **black, paralysed.**   Opium 200
- **Frothing** at the mouth.
- **White blisters** on the backside of the   Thuja 200
  tongue.
- Tip painful, sore.

THE TEETH AND THE GUMS

The teeth are a part of the digestive system. They chew the food when taken into the mouth so that it can be mixed with saliva and enzymes for the first stage of digestion.

The gums are the firm, fleshy tissue covering the alveolar parts of either jaw and surrounding the necks of the teeth. Healthy gums are essential to protect the roots of the teeth from bacterial infection and corrosion.

A tooth is a living structure and the pulp in its middle receives a large supply of blood vessels. It has nerves which are sensitive to heat, cold, pain and pressure.

The pulp is surrounded by dentine, a hard substance. Enamel, an even harder substance, covers the dentine.

Shock absorbing tissue lines the bony socket of every tooth. This saves the skull and the jawbone from shock during biting and chewing.

Enamel is the hardest substance in the human body. Yet the acids produced in the mouth by bacterial action on sugar rub the enamel off and lead to tooth decay.

Food particles with mucous and bacteria gather on the surface of the teeth, to form plaque. This combined with sugar harm the teeth and the gums, more so if not cleaned within a few hours.

If dental plaque is not removed frequently, rough tartar is formed on the surfaces. This inflames the gums and leads to acute discomfort and foul breath.

Most disorders of the gums, and quite a few of the teeth, can be prevented by careful and regular oral hygiene. Brush after every meal

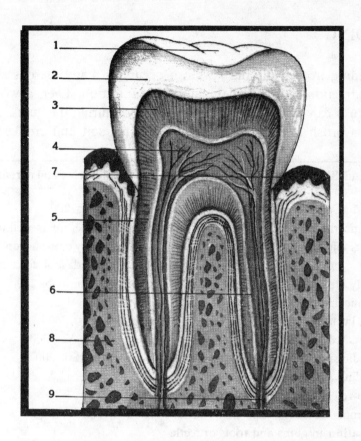

1. Crown. 2. Enamel. 3. Dentine. 4. Pulp. 5. Cement. 6. F ot.
7. Gum. 8. Bone. 9. Nerve and blood supply.

even if you do not use toothpaste each time. Develop this good habit in the children very early.

The bristles of the brush ought to be soft or medium soft, and not hard. Discard the brush as soon as the bristles begin to warp. Brushing with a toothbrush should be directional to clean all the recesses between the teeth and the margins where the teeth and the gums meet. Use of floss is desirable if food particles are not totally removed by a brush.

Consumption of sugar and fat should be limited. After having such food, clean your teeth immediately.

Keep your teeth healthy and sparkling clean. They enhance beauty as well as personality. You can say 'cheese' with confidence.

If taken proper care of, your teeth will last a lifetime.

BLEEDING

Bleeding from teeth and jaws can occur for many reasons such as tooth extraction, injury, inflammation, or infection. Even a worn out tooth brush can do more harm than good by injuring the gums. Hence, discard a brush as soon as its bristles become soft and crooked.

Distinguishing symptoms of the patient	Medicine and potency
• Bleeding and soreness **after extraction**.	Arnica 200
• Haemorrhage. **Swelling**.	Use before as well after
• Gums injured by a worn out brush.	surgery or extraction. Use for a few days, 4 doses in a day.
• Easily bleeding gums.	Arsenic Alb. 200
• Sceptic infections. **Ulcers.**	
• Dry, burning **heat**.	
• **Retracted**, easily bleeding gums. **Pyorrhoea**.	Carbo Veg 200
• Bleeding gums, **spongy, swollen**, and **receding.**	Merc Sol 200
• **Blue-red** margins on gums. Abscess in the roots.	
• **Pulsation** in gums and roots of teeth. Severe **itching**.	
• Gums ulcerated. Sensitive to touch.	
• **Teeth loose**, black, and dirty.	
• **Persistent** bleeding after tooth extraction.	Phosphorus 200

BLUE, BLACK

Discolouring of the teeth and the gums is a sign of plaque, infection, of tooth decay and of poor oral hygiene.

Distinguishing symptoms of the patient	Medicine and potency
• Purple, **swollen**, spongy, **bleeding** gums.	Lachesis 200 When Merc has failed.

- **Loose, black teeth.**
- Blue-red margins. Abscess. **Pulsating**.   Merc Sol 200

CARIES/DENTAL CAVITIES/DECAY

Formation of caries, cavities in the teeth, is the end-result of a process of decay. It is a slow process. To begin with, a small cavity forms in the enamel, the hard, protective covering on the teeth. If not checked in time, the cavity extends deep into the affected tooth. Ultimately, the nerves and blood vessels at the root are injured and infected.

Such teeth become sensitive to sweets and to cold or hot liquids. They loosen and fall in due course.

Caries are a site of severe pain.

Excellent dental care is available today. Have a regular dental check up to forestall the formation of caries. If the process has started, it can be arrested.

Good, daily oral care from childhood almost ensures that caries do not form.

Distinguishing symptoms of the patient	Medicine and potency
• Caries of teeth in **obese** children.	Calcarea Carb 200
• Teeth growing **crooked**.	
• Ugly, **black crowns** on **teeth**.	
• Necrosis of teeth. **Loss of enamel.**	Calcarea Fluorica 200
• Teeth **loosen** in their sockets.	
• Caries with **facial neuralgia**.	Hekla Lava 30
• Abscess in gums. Toothache.	
• **Upper jawbone enlarged**.	
• Decay **starting in childhood** and proceeding fast.	Kreosote 30
• **Teeth dark and crumbling.**	
• Swollen, bleeding. **Putrid odour**.	
• **Pulsation** in gums and roots of crumbling teeth. Abscess. Bleeding. **Severe itching**.	Merc Sol 200

GINGIVITIS

Gingivitis is an inflammation of the gums caused by accumulation of dental plaque at the junction of the tooth and the gums. Poor oral hygiene is responsible for this formation.

Symptoms: Gums swollen, purple, red, spongy. Bleed when brushed.

Refer '*Bleeding*', '*Pain/Inflammation*' and other symptoms in this chapter.

GRINDING

Distinguishing symptoms of the patient	Medicine and potency
• **Throbbing pain** in grinding teeth.	Belladonna 200
• Tongue swollen, painful. **Mouth dry**.	
• Intense desire to **press gums together**.	Podophyllum 200
• In **gastric** problems, in cholera.	

THE JAWS, PROBLEMS OF

Distinguishing symptoms of the patient	Medicine and potency
• **Protruding tongue** in epileptic fits.	Absinthium 30
• Jaws **fixed**.	
• Spasmodic facial **twitching**.	
• Face blue.	
• **Foaming** mouth in an epileptic fit.	Cuprum Met 200
• Jaws **contracted**.	
• **Hanging down** of lower jaw.	Opium 200

PAIN/INFLAMMATION

Distinguishing symptoms of the patient	Medicine and potency
• Gums inflamed. Terrible toothache. • Numbness. • On **exposure to dry, cold air**.	Aconite Nap 30
• Pain in **hollow** teeth.	Antim Crud 200
• Soreness after extraction or pain after **injury**.	Arnica 200
• **Throbbing** pain in gums which are red, hot. • **Red gum boils**.	Belladonna 200, 1000
• Boils with **hard swelling** on the jaw. • Teeth loose. • Pain **when chewing** food.	Calcarea Fluorica 200
• **Unbearable** pain after tooth extraction. • **Dentition** diarrhoea.	Chamomilla 200
• Worse from use of **tobacco**.	Clematis Erecta 30
• Dental neuralgia, radiating towards **ears and eyes**.	Ferrum Picrium 30
• Facial neuralgia because of caries. Abscess. • **Upper jaw feels enlarged**.	Hekla Lava 30
• **Pus** formed. **Shooting pain**.	Hepar Sulph 200
• Pain because of **decayed teeth.** • Gums spongy, purple.	Kreosote 200
• **Pulsating** pain in the roots. Receding, bleeding, and spongy gums. • **Foul smelling pus**.	Merc Sol 200
• **Tearing** pain. **Pulsation**. • Aggravated by cold as well as warm food.	Nitric Acid 200
• With **neuralgia of eyeballs**, and swollen cheeks. • Tooth decay. Worse on cold air contact.	Plantago Major 30
• Facial neuralgia on the **left side**. • Pain in teeth, jaws, eyes, and temple.	Spigelia 200

PYORRHOEA

Copious discharge of pus, generally from the gums, frequently accompanied by severe pain and loosening of the teeth. Usually develops as a complication of dental cavities.

Distinguishing symptoms of the patient	Medicine and potency
• **Easily bleeding** and retracted gums.	Carbo Veg 200
• Of gums **separating** from teeth.	Kali Carb 200
• **Ulcers** on the gums, in the mouth	Merc Sol 200
• **Foul smell**.	
• **Pulsating**, receding gums. Severe itching.	
• Abscess **deep in the roots**. Gumboils.	Silicea 200
• Sensitive to cold air and cold water.	
• Teeth **black and crumbling**.	Staphysagria 200
• Spongy, bleeding gums.	

THE THROAT

The throat is a part of the respiratory system as well as the digestive system. Shaped like a tube, it connects the back of the nose and the mouth to trachea [the windpipe] and the oesophagus [the food pipe].

The air we breathe in passes through the throat into the windpipe, on its way into the lungs.

Food shredded by the teeth, mixed with saliva, glides down the throat into the oesophagus on its journey to the stomach.

Larynx, the voice box, lies next to the throat. In larynx lie the vocal cords that produce sound when air passes over them.

On either side of the throat are glands known as tonsils. These provide a trap for harmful bacteria.

The entry of food into the windpipe is prevented by a tiny flap called the epiglottis.

Whenever your throat is affected and you are uncomfortable, you are running temperature, your voice is hoarse, and the throat is painful, take rest and stay in bed. Gargle with warm salt water frequently. Take hot liquids. Use medicines as indicated in the following sub-chapters.

Abstain from smoking. Better, give it up.

Continuous hoarseness over a long period is ominous. **Go for a check up. It could be cancer of the larynx or of the nasopharynx.** The symptoms are difficult and painful swallowing, difficult and loud breathing, repeated nosebleeds, earache, and loss of hearing, loss of the sense of smell, facial pain and swelling, change in voice, facial paralysis.

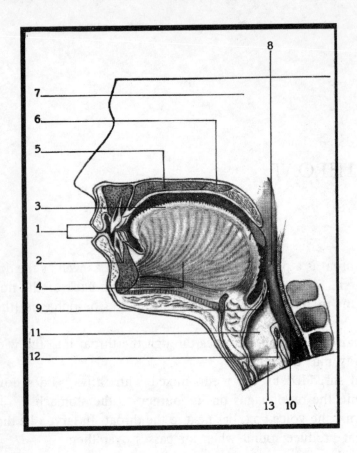

1. Lips. 2. Teeth. 3. Tongue. 4. Muscles of tongue. 5. Hard plate. 6. Soft palate.
7. Adenoids. 8. Throat. 9. Epiglottis. 10. Oesophagus. 11. Larynx. 12. Larynx.
12. Vocal cords. 13. Wind pipe [trachea.]

Do not take cold water immediately after taking greasy food. This can lead to hoarseness and wheezing. If such a situation develops, take Ipecac 200 a few times.

ADENOIDS, ENLARGED

Adenoid is a pad of lymphoid tissue that lies at the back of the nose and close to the mouth cavity. Its function is to help the body to fight infection. Its enlargement blocks the opening of the Eustachian tube and can lead to infection and pain of the middle ear.

Symptoms: As the airflow from the nose into the throat is obstructed, the child breathes through the mouth. Snores during sleep. Frequent pain in the middle ear. Constantly blocked or runny nose.

The problem does not last beyond childhood.

Distinguishing symptoms of the patient	Medicine and potency
• Adenoids with **pain in the middle ear**. Tonsils enlarged.	Agraphis Nutans 30
• To start the treatment with. No other medicine to be administered on that day, on the days before and after.	Bacillinum 200 One dose every fortnight.
• In pale and overweight children.	Calcarea Carb 30
• The child **perspires on the head at night**.	
• Tonsils swollen and painful.	

BURNING

Distinguishing symptoms of the patient	Medicine and potency
• Throat **numb, yet burning**. Red, hot.	Aconite 30
• Constriction. Tonsils swollen and dry. Tender to touch.	
• **Sudden** inflammation. On **exposure** to dry, cold air.	
• Throat feels as if **on fire. Scalding**.	Cantharis 200
• Burnt taking hot food	
• **Difficulty in swallowing fluids**.	

CANCER/GROWTH IN LARYNX, IN PHARYNX

Refer under *'Cancer'*.

DIPHTHERIA

A rare but serious infection of the throat.

Symptoms: Throat sore, swollen. Thick membrane forms on the tonsils, in the nose, on the windpipe. Difficult breathing. Fever. Swollen lymph nodes in the neck.

If not taken care of in time, diphtheria can lead to weakness, paralysis, heart failure, and death.

Today, diphtheria can be **prevented by immunization**. Children are immunized in early infancy. They receive three antitoxin injections in the first year and a booster dose later. Adults too can take booster doses.

Get immediate medical advice if diphtheria is suspected.

Distinguishing symptoms of the patient	Medicine and potency
• **Membrane** in throat **extending** towards larynx.	Kali Bichrome 200
• Thick, **yellow-brown** fur-like **coating** on the tongue.	
• Uvula relaxed.	
• **Greyish yellow** and curd like membrane.	Lac Caninum 30.
• **Silvery ulcers**.	Every two hours.
• **Paralysis** of the throat. Fluids return by nose.	
• Swelling from left to right.	
• **Sudden** attack. Left side.	Lachesis 200.
• Membrane **dusky**.	Every two hours.
• Thick, **white, ropy** mucous in the throat.	
• **Glands** around nose **swollen**.	
• Throat **malignant. Blackish** membrane at the back of throat.	Merc Cyanatus, 1000, 10000 One dose per day.

- Necrotic destruction of soft palate and fauces.
- Sudden. **Collapse imminent**.
- **Dark red**, blue, or **ash coloured** membrane.   Phytolacca 1000
- Burning as if a red-hot iron has been inserted into the throat.
- **Hands trembling**.
- Worse hot fluids.

DISCHARGE

Distinguishing symptoms of the patient	Medicine and potency
• **Stringy**, green, sticky mucous from nose, pharynx, larynx, trachea, bronchia, **flowing down into throat**. • All the time trying to clear the throat without much success.	Kali Bichrome 200

DRY

Distinguishing symptoms of the patient	Medicine and potency
• Throat **dry, red, tickling, burning**, stinging, constricted. **Larynx inflamed**. • Tonsils swollen, dry. • **Violent cough**. • On **exposure** to dry, cold air.	Aconite 30
• **Lips parched**. Tongue dry. **Throat dry**.	Bryonia 200

HOARSENESS

Distinguishing symptoms of the patient	Medicine and potency
• Hoarse due to **over-use**.	Arnica 200
• Larynx **inflamed. Squeaky** voice. Spasm in larynx.	Belladonna 200
• **Sudden loss** of voice. Constriction. Violent hoarseness.	
• Scraping, dry cough. **Result of having a cold drink after greasy food.**	
• On taking **oily** food, **followed by cold drinks** cold drinks.	Bryonia 200
• **Heaviness** in the throat. Congestion. Dry cough.	Ipecac 200 **Start with Ipecac.**
• **Wheezing**.	**Noticeable results**.
• Of public speakers, singers.	Wyethia 200
• Itching in posterior nares.	
• **Uvula swollen**.	
• Dry, hacking cough.	

Refer '*Laryngitis*' below as well as '*Voice lost*' in the chapter titled, '*The Respiratory System*.'

LARYNGITIS

It is an infection of the larynx [voice box], caused by environmental factors like smoke, chemical fumes and dust.

Symptoms: Hoarseness. At times, loss of voice. Pain in the throat when speaking.

Distinguishing symptoms of the patient	Medicine and potency
• **Acute** inflammation of the larynx. **Fever**.	Aconite 20
• On **exposure** to dry cold air.	

- **Total loss of voice**.
- **Suffocating cough**.
- Pain, like ulcers in the larynx.   Carbo Veg 200
- **Chronic catarrh of the aged**.
- Foul sputum. Debilitated.
- **Hoarse cough**. Toneless voice.   Drosera 200
- Sensation as if a **feather tickling** the larynx.
- Worse at night, lying down, drinking, singing, laughing.
- **Rough barking cough**.   Hepar Sulph 200
- Tenacious **pus** formation.
- Stitching **pain from ear to ear** while swallowing or turning head.
- Worse morning and indoors.
- **Chronic** laryngitis   Kali Bichrome 200
- Congestion. Swelling. **Sticky mucous** dripping inwards.
- Worse mornings when tough mucous nearly **strangles** the patient.
- **Violent tickling** in larynx while speaking. Phosphorus 200
- **Night cough**. Stitching pain. **Chilliness**.
- Larynx so **swollen** as to make a **second chin**. Tender neck.   Spongia 200
- Swollen sub-maxillary glands.
- On exposure to dry cold air. When Aconite fails.

MUMPS

Highly contagious swelling of the salivary glands, caused by a mild viral infection. These glands are located in the cheeks, just in front of the ears.

Symptoms: Pain in the ears. Swelling on both or one side of the face. These days, a routine immunization takes care of mumps.

At times, other glands such as testicles in men, ovaries in women, or pancreas can get inflamed.

Distinguishing symptoms of the patient	Medicine and potency
• Affecting **testes or breasts**. When Pulsatilla fails.	Abrotanum 30
• **Violent, acute, painful**.	Belladonna 200
• Alternate with Merc Iod Rub every half an hour until the acute stage is past. Later continue with Belladonna four times a day.	
• **Stiffness** of the muscles of the throat and of neck.	Merc Iod Rub 30
• Mumps with severe **pain in the ear**.	Pulsatilla 30
• Inflammation in **breasts or testicles**.	

PAIN

Distinguishing symptoms of the patient	Medicine and potency
• Stitching pain in tonsils **even if no pus** has formed.	Baryta Carb 200
• Pain in swallowing.	
• **Throbbing** pain in tonsils which are inflamed **red, hot, burning**.	Belladonna 200
• **Acute**, violent attack.	
• **Splinter pain** extending into ears. Pain as if someone is **piercing the tonsils** when **swallowing empty**.	Hepar Sulph 200
• **White patches** on the tonsils.	
• Pus formed or about to be formed.	
• **Chronic purple**, sore throat. Starts **left**.	Lachesis 200
• Deep **red or grey ulcers**. Mucous can neither be thrown out nor gulped.	
• Pain into the ear.	
• Worse on the slightest pressure.	
• **Uvula swollen**. Burning.	Merc Cor 30
• Throat red, sore.	
• **Post-nasal pain**, sharp into the ears.	

PARALYSIS

Distinguishing symptoms of the patient	Medicine and potency
Of oesophagus and throat, **after diphtheria**. Of vocal cords. Loss of voice.	Causticum 200
Larynx constricted. **Throat purple**. Vocal cords paralysed. Voice lost.	Lachesis 200

RED/ROUGH/SORE/PHARYNGITIS

An inflammation of the throat or of pharynx. Acute or chronic.

Symptoms: Rise in temperature, chill, and headache. Red, rough, sore throat. Dry cough. Pain in the ear, worse on swallowing. Heaviness in the throat. Enlarged and painful lymph nodes in the neck.

Gargle with warm salt water or with one soluble aspirin dissolved in warm water. Take plenty of hot liquids or very cold drinks. Take ice cream.

Distinguishing symptoms of the patient	Medicine and potency
• Throat is red, **burning, and numb**. Constricted. Sudden problem.	Aconite 30
• **Exposure** to dry, cold air.	
• **Uvula swollen**.	Apis 200
• **Deep red** congestion. Turning **dusky**. Worse on right side.	Belladonna 200
• Hot like **coals on fire**.	
• **Shining, swollen tonsils choking the throat**. Painful.	
• Sudden, violent.	
• Sore throat. A feeling of **heaviness**. Congestion of mucous. **Wheezing**. **Effect of oily food intake.**	Ipecac 200
• **Uvula swollen**.	Merc Cor 30

• Intense inflammation. Throat **red, painful, burning**.	
• Painful swallowing. Pain from ear to ear.	
• Sore with pus. Burning, raw. Pain into the ear.	Merc Sol 200
• Bluish, red swelling.	
• Rough, scraping in the throat. **Tickling sensation**.	Nux Vomica 200
• Stitches into the ear.	

SMOKER'S THROAT

Distinguishing symptoms of the patient	Medicine and potency
• Sore throat of smokers.	Capsicum 200

STAMMER/STUTTER/LOSS OF VOICE

To speak with involuntary pauses or repetitions.

Distinguishing symptoms of the patient	Medicine and potency
• Stammers. Awkward. **Things fall from hand**.	Bovista 30
• **Spasmodic repetition** of sounds, especially of initial components. Hesitation to begin.	Cannabis Sativa 30
• Loss of voice from **partial paralysis of vocal cords**.	Causticum 200
• Stammering	
• Rawness caused by **catarrh** in respiratory tract.	
• Stammering in patients of **epilepsy**.	Cuprum Met 200
• **Protrudes and retracts tongue** constantly.	
• **Paralysis of vocal cords** leading to loss of voice.	Kali Phos 30

SWELLING

Distinguishing symptoms of the patient	Medicine and potency
• **Swollen uvula** hangs like a water bag.	Apis 200
• Tongue swells and fills the mouth to **suffocation**.	
• **Sudden diphtheria**.	
• Uvula swollen like a bladder.	Kali Bichrome 200
• Ropy green **mucous, difficult** to take out.	
• **Inflammation** with swelling of uvula and **burning pain**.	Merc Cor 30
• **Pus** on tonsils. **Bluish red** swelling.	Merc Sol 200
• Loss of voice. **Excessive saliva**.	
• Throat swollen. Sensation of heaviness.	Wyethia 200
• **Itching** in posterior nares	
• Problems of **singers and public speakers**.	

TETANUS/LOCKJAW

Bacterial infection in a wound that results in acute contraction of the muscles of the jaw and of the neck.

Symptoms: Muscle stiffness in the arms, jaws, and neck. Fever, sweating, and headache. When the muscles of the throat and chest are affected, it leads to difficult breathing, suffocation, even death.

Tetanus takes time to develop. **Get immediate medical help** as soon as you notice the symptoms above or those indicated below.

Take an anti tetanus injection as soon as possible after suffering an injury with an open wound.

Distinguishing symptoms of the patient	Medicine and potency
• Convulsions with loss of consciousness.	Cicuta 200
• Face dark red. **Frothing**.	
• **Spasm of chewing muscles**.	

• High temperature, headache, and sweating.	
• From **injury** inflicted on **head or spinal column**.	
• Oppressed breathing.	
• Fear of tetanus after a **punctured wound**.	Hypericum 200.
• **Pain** in the wound and **nerves**.	To follow Ledum in early stages. Later use Hypericum alone.
• **First remedy when tetanus is feared**. As soon as a wound has been inflicted.	Ledum 200
• **Convulsions in the entire body**. Limbs rigid	Nux Vomica 200
• **Eyes distorted. Face red**.	
• Difficult breathing. Chest drawn in.	
• Spasm preceded by **violent chill**.	

TICKLING

Distinguishing symptoms of the patient	Medicine and potency
• Unbearable, intense, unpleasant **tickling in throat, jaws, eyes, ears.**	Arundo 200
• Sudden onset of cold.	

TONSILLITIS

Tonsils are located at the back of the throat and form part of the body's defence system. Their inflammation is called tonsillitis. It is a result of respiratory infections.

Symptoms: High temperature. White pus patches on the tonsils. Swollen Purple tonsils and throat. Discomfort on empty swallowing. Dry cough, headache, vomit, abdominal pain. Sometimes diarrhoea.

Tonsils provide a protective shield. Avoid their removal. Sulphur 200 taken once a week, for three months, eliminates the tendency to repeated tonsillitis and sore throat.

Distinguishing symptoms of the patient	Medicine and potency
• Tonsils swollen, red, hot on **exposure** to dry, cold air. **Acute** case.	Aconite 30
• Violent dry cough.	
• Tonsils **enlarged. Hard**.	Alumen 30
• Constriction in the oesophagus.	
• **Tendency to catch cold**, leading to tonsillitis.	
• Tonsils swollen, **suffocating** the throat.	Apis 200
• **Red, hot**, and painful tonsils. Shining. Swollen.	Belladonna 200
• Abscess in tonsils. Tingling pain in tonsils and all around.	Baryta Carb 200
• **Tendency** to inflammation of tonsils.	
• **Visible pus** spots on tonsils.	Hepar Sulph 200
• **Stabbing pain on empty swallowing**. Pain into ears.	
• Chronic cases.	
• Tonsillitis **with sinusitis**.	Kali Bichrome 200
• **Sticky**, green **mucous into the throat**. Difficult to take out.	
• Unbearable earache.	
• Deep **purple swelling** on tonsils.	Lachesis 200
• Throat livid. Abscess.	
• Starting left side. Difficulty in swallowing hot drinks.	
• **Pus** in tonsils but no shooting pain yet.	Merc Sol 200
• Loss of voice.	
• **Fever with chill** and sweat.	
• Chronic infection.	Silicea 200
• Prickly pain. **Where Hepar Sulph has been ineffective**.	

THE HEART AND THE CIRCULATORY SYSTEM

The heart is a muscular organ, almost the size of a fist. It lies in the centre of the chest, slightly to the left.

The human body requires oxygen and food to survive. While food provides fuel, oxygen is needed to burn this fuel. Both these substances are required by every cell in the body. Blood performs the function of transporting fuel and oxygen to every part of the body. It carries away waste products from wherever these have accumulated. It helps maintaining the body temperature. The heart plays an important part in the circulation of blood.

The circulation of blood is maintained through a complicated system. It depends on pumping and pressurizing the blood around the body. At the centre of this system lies the heart. In sixty seconds, the heart, beating steadily, pushes five litres of blood through a complete cycle through the body. It achieves this through contractions of its muscles.

The heart's contraction expels blood through the right side into the lungs, and from the left side into the aorta, the largest artery in the body.

The lungs receive blood from the heart through the pulmonary arteries. Here the blood gives up carbon dioxide and absorbs oxygen.

The oxygenated blood returns to the heart on its left side, via the pulmonary veins and is distributed by the aorta throughout the body. Even the tiniest of capillaries receive this oxygenated blood.

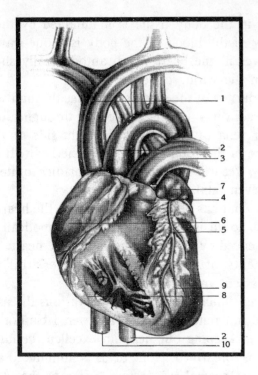

SECTION OF THE HEART
1. Superior vena cava. 2. Aorta. 3. Pulmonary artery. 4. Right coronary artery.
5. Left coronary artery. 6. Right atrium. 7. Left atrium. 8. Right ventricle.
9. Left ventricle. 10. Inferior vena cava.

The heart muscle itself requires abundant oxygen because it works non-stop from birth until death.

Oygen is carried by red blood cells. The blood plasma carries antibodies which protect the body from infection.

Oxygen is carried to the tissues in the body by capillaries.

Blood transports absorbed food from the intestines. It carries hormones which are produced by endocrine glands.

If the body is injured and the blood vessels are damaged, the clotting agents carried by the blood help in sealing the wound and in the formation of new skin.

Blood is the nectar in the body. Heat produced by metabolism in the body is circulated by the blood plasma. The blood carries waste products to the kidneys for excretion through urine.

Water level in the body tissue is maintained by the blood.

The journey of the blood in the body is a one-way street. This is ensured by valves in the heart which automatically shut if the blood tries to move in the wrong direction.

The return journey of the blood takes place through very small veins, then through larger veins. Ultimately flowing through superior vena cava and the inferior vena cava, it enters the right side of the heart.

At the centre of this vital activity beats the heart. It is the strongest part of the body. Yet it is prone to many maladies, quite a few of them debilitating or even fatal.

Contrary to what has been written by poets, the heart is not the seat of emotion. A beloved is a heartthrob only symbolically. The emotion of love is experienced by the brain and not in the heart. The heart beats faster in moments of love or fear. However, this is a result of communications sent from the brain.

The following sub-chapters discuss the various diseases of the heart in detail. I need not reiterate them. However, I cannot overemphasize the desirability of keeping our heart in excellent condition.

Forewarned is forearmed. None of us is immune to a possible heart sickness. There are several risk factors. Some or the other are present for each one of us. Nevertheless, awareness helps us to avoid the pitfalls.

The foremost risk factor is the high level of low density lipoprotein cholesterol in the blood stream. Its deposits inside the arteries make them hard, narrow and in course of time largely blocked. The process of plaque formation starts very early. However, it is only when the blockage chokes the supply of blood to the coronary arteries that the victim realizes the gravity of the situation.

Today the extent of deposits of cholesterol can be checked with a simple blood test. This ought to be done periodically. In case the levels of LDL, [the undesirable part of cholesterol], and the triglycerides are higher than permissible, medicine to reduce the same must be taken under proper medical advice. By reducing the level of the undesirable cholesterol, you have won half the battle in order to protect your heart.

Exercise helps in reducing LDL and increasing HDL [the healthy cholesterol]. The latter to a significant extent lowers the LDL by flushing it out of the arteries.

Lack of activity is a risk factor which can be easily tackled. Take regular exercise. Exercise speeds the flow of blood through the body and can increase it to an extent that that the blood goes round the body in ten seconds as compared to sixty seconds when the body is at rest.

Swimming is a complete exercise. Cycling is refreshing. It need not be strenuous. You can control your speed according to your capability. Climb a few steps several times during the day if possible.

Walk six kilometres, five to six times a week. Enjoy nature and its bounties. Stroll by the ocean looking at the rolling waves. These sights and sounds give you peace of mind and help you in relieving tension, stress, and anxiety. Your management of high blood pressure, if any, becomes easy when your mind is at peace.

For diabetics, exercise helps in controlling their blood sugar level. That in turn helps keep the heart stronger.

Smoking is an enemy of a healthy heart. It narrows the arteries and helps formation of plaque. If you are not a smoker, do not set on this course. If you are a smoker, give up as early as you can. Smokers have a two to three times greater chance of having a heart attack than non-smokers.

Hypertension or high blood pressure almost triples a man's chances of having a heart attack and more than doubles a woman's. The heart has to work harder when the arteries have narrowed. This wears the heart out. Further, the blood flow can loosen the plaque through friction. This leads to coronary thrombosis. Hence, control your blood pressure through proper medication and other measures recommended in the sub-chapter on 'Hypertension'.

The risk of a heart attack is more than doubled by abdominal obesity. Reduce and control your weight. Exercise. Control your diet. Consult a dietician.

Your diet plays a significant part in taking care of your heart. Seek guidance if you are not sure of what is a good diet for your constitution. However, as a rule avoid a diet rich in saturated fats. Increase the intake of fruit in your daily diet. Your meals should include a sufficient quantity of bran, fibre, cereals like oats, whole grains, and fresh vegetable (not overcooked). Avoid junk food which is high in calories. Cut down on coffee and colas.

Changes in lifestyle go a long way to keep our heart healthy. Anxiety, stress, overwork, mental tension for whatever reason, all contribute to damaging the heart by increasing the plaque formation, narrowing and hardening the arteries and raising blood pressure. Avoid late nights. Indulge in pleasant thoughts. Be nice to others. Learn to forgive. Take it easy. Find some time to 'stand and stare'.

It is in our interest to protect the heart which in a day pumps almost 8000 litres of blood through the body. It beats almost 1,00,000 times a day and almost three million times in a month. We live so long as the heart beats. Once the heart stops for good, 'the rest is silence'.

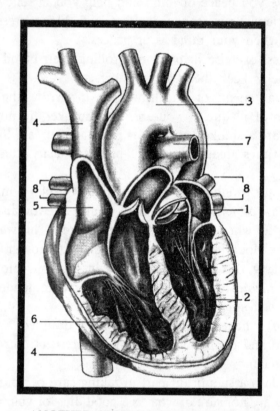

ANOTHER SECTION OF THE HEART
1. Left atrium. 2. Left ventricle. 3. Aorta. 4. Vena cava. 5. Right atrium. 6. Right ventricle. 7. Pulmonary arteries. 8. Pulmonary veins.
This section illustrates the complicated inner design of the heart. Blood is conducted from the left atrium via the left ventricle to various parts of the body via aorta. After a complete circuit of the body, impure blood running through the vena cava enters the heart through the right atrium. From there blood is carried into the right ventricle and thereafter by pulmonary arteries to the lungs for purification. Purified and oxygenated blood is carried by pulmonary veins from the lungs to the left atrium.

ANEURISM, AORTIC

The bulging section of an artery is known as 'aneurism'.

When the blood pressure is high and an artery is weak or diseased, the weaker part balloons outwards. Usually the main artery of the chest and abdomen, known as aorta is involved.

An aneurism must be taken care of as soon as detected. Seek medical advice.

If an aneurism bursts, **immediate surgical intervention is required**. A delay can be fatal.

Symptoms: For chest aneurism: pain in the chest, in the upper back between shoulders, wheezing, severe cough, and shortness of breath, hoarseness, and difficulty in swallowing.

For abdomen: throbbing, pulsation in the abdomen, pain spreading to the back.

A rupture leads to loss of consciousness, fast pulse, severe pain. **The following medicines are mainly palliative.**

Distinguishing symptoms of the patient	Medicine and potency
• Stitches in the chest, **worse inhaling**.	Baryta Carb 200
• Palpitation while lying on the **left side**.	
• Chronic loss of voice.	
• Dilated blood vessels. Chest **pain, shortness of breath**.	Calcarea Fluorica 200 One dose daily
• Palpitation worse at night.	Lycopodium 200

ANGINA PECTORIS

Pain in the chest, originating in the region of the heart, running mainly into the left arm and shoulders. It is caused by strain, fatigue, or excessive exercise. It is a result of an inadequate supply of blood to the heart muscle. It is relieved on rest.

Angina can occur in persons with coronary heart disease, hypertension, high levels of cholesterol, diabetes mellitus. Smokers are at great risk. So are persons who have high fat diet and do not exercise.

If a person is not already a heart patient, angina is the first warning shot. Worsening angina might indicate the formation of a clot of blood. Anyone who suffers angina must sit or lie still until the pain subsides. **Seek competent medical counsel. Do not take it lightly.**

Symptoms: Constriction. Dull and oppressive pain felt in the centre of the chest, spreading via throat to left arm and shoulder, sometimes to both the arms.

At times angina is felt as heartburn because of indigestion. **Let a doctor distinguish the two**.

Distinguishing symptoms of the patient	Medicine and potency
• Sudden, severe pain travelling **down elbow of the left arm**. • Stitches in the region of the heart. **Constriction**. Someone pressing on the chest.	Arnica 200, 1000 **First aid** remedy. **An angina patient better carry it all the time**.
• Heart feels tied down with an iron **band. Suffocation**. • Acute pain, violent, clutching. Travelling down left arm. • **Face blue, lips blue**. • **Left arm numb**.	Cactus, Mother Tincture. In emergency: 10 drops in water every thirty minutes until condition stabilises.
• Extreme **breathlessness on least exertion.** • Sudden pain in the left centre of the chest, extending into the left arm.	Crataegus 200 **A heart tonic**. Ought to be used for a long time: mother tincture, 15 drops in water, four times daily.
• Onset of pain while **going uphill**. Any rush of blood brings fainting spells. • Pulse small. Skin pale.	Glonoine 200 In a sudden attack, administer 15 drops of Mother Tincture on sugar every fifteen minutes.

AORTIC VALVE STENOSIS
AORTIC INCOMPETENCE

The aortic valve lies at the exit of the main pumping chamber of the heart. It becomes thick and does not close properly. As a result, the supply of blood to the coronary arteries and the brain is obstructed.

In aortic regurgitation, there is leakage of blood backwards. This leads to aortic incompetence.

Symptoms: Shortness of breath in cases of aortic incompetence, fatigue and an awareness of heart beating forcefully. Swollen ankles in later stages. In cases of stenosis: angina, shortness of breath, fainting on exertion, dizziness while standing up from a sitting position.

I advise medical consultation.

Distinguishing symptoms of the patient	Medicine and potency
• **Chronic aortitis**. Acute inflammation of the heart muscle.	Arsenic Iod 30 Twice daily, half an hour
• Pulse slow. Palpitation.	after a meal, along with
• Breathlessness on climbing stairs.	other indicated medicines.
• Pulmonary stenosis.	Aspidosperma
• **Thrombosis of the pulmonary artery**.	Mother Tincture to be
• Shortness of breath.	given, when attack comes,
• **Vertigo** while standing up from a sitting position.	in 10-drop dose, every hour until relief is obtained.
• Hardening of the walls in the case of **old persons**.	Aurum Met 30
• Angina pectoris in **chronic rheumatism** patients, where **pain wanders** from joint to joint.	

ATRIAL FIBRILLATION

Atria are the upper chambers of the heart. Their rapid, uncoordinated contractions are known as atrial fibrillation.

Symptoms: Sometime none. In acute cases sudden palpitation, shortness of breath. Slight dizziness.

Distinguishing symptoms of the patient	Medicine and potency
• Chronic irregular heart beat. **Feeble** action. • Extreme weakness. • Extreme breathlessness on least exertion. • Heart is **dilated, tired. Irregular** in beats.	Crataegus Mother tincture, 15 drop dose, four times daily, for a few months. Digitalis 30

ARTERIAL THROMBOSIS AND EMBOLISM

Formation of a blood clot in an artery of the brain, the heart, or a leg. Other arteries can be involved. **It is potentially a serious complication and requires immediate medical intervention**.

A blood clot can form at one place and travel to another choking the supply at that spot. This latter happening is known as embolism.

Risk factors: High cholesterol levels. High fat diet. Smoking. Obesity. Lack of exercise.

Symptoms: Pain in the limb even at rest. Numbness. Lack of colour in the skin. Cold feet. In abdominal thrombosis: fever, vomit, severe pain in the abdomen.

Distinguishing symptoms of the patient	Medicine and potency
• Blood clot in the middle or end of a **thigh**. Thick, sensitive stirring all along the inner side of a thigh or in a leg.	Apis 200
• Thrombosis in a **cardiac artery**.	Bothrops 200
• **Skin swollen, cold**.	
• Thrombosis with **high blood pressure**.	Lachesis 200
• Worse on left side, on pressure. Constriction.	

ARTERIO-SCLEROSIS [ATHEROMA]

Inelasticity, hardening and narrowing of arteries because of accumulation of cholesterol and other fatty substances. Food rich in cholesterol and saturated fats is the villain.

Symptoms: No symptoms in the beginning. Later, hypertension, angina pectoris, headaches, pain, and cramps in the legs, disturbance of balance, vision, speech and difficulty in the use of arms and legs. Some complications like a massive heart attack can be fatal.

Change your dietary habits a. the earliest. Go in for low or no cholesterol food, fibre, fruit, vegetables, fatless milk. No saturated fats Take regular and well-directed exercise. Walk briskly for a minimum of forty-five minutes six times a week.

Reduce weight if you are overweight.

Give up smoking.

Get your cholesterol checked regularly. Cholesterol is a killer. **Take medication to reduce the same under medical guidance**. Today statins are available for this purpose.

All these steps are essential. There is no way out.

Consult your cardiac physician regularly.

If you take the above precautions, you can add years to your life. Remember that healthy living is happy living.

Distinguishing symptoms of the patient	Medicine and potency
• **Cerebral** Arterio-sclerosis.	Arnica 200
• **Vertigo** of the **aged**.	
• **Sudden**, excruciating **pain** in the affected limb.	Bothrops 200
• The limb goes **cold** and turns **pale**.	
• Fat deposits on the arterial walls.	Crataegus
• Extreme **shortness of breath** on least exertion.	An excellent tonic for the heart.
• **Fingers, toes blue.**	Mother Tincture, 15-drop dose, four times daily for quite some time.

• Of the **lungs. Asthma** in old persons.	Baryta Mur 30
• Surging of blood to the brain and the heart. Pulsating pain.	Glonoine 200
• Cannot recognize localities. **Confusion, dizziness.**	
• **Faints on exertion**. Limbs go numb. Throbbing in the entire body.	
• **Loss of consciousness** on exertion. Pain in the chest.	Opium 200

BLOOD PRESSURE, HIGH. HYPERTENSION

Blood pressure higher than normal, that is higher than 120/80. It damages the arteries and the heart.

Symptoms: Usually none. At very high levels: headache, blurred vision, dizziness, throbbing in temple arteries, a feeling of heaviness. Change lifestyle.

Seek and follow medical advice. You must lower blood pressure with proper medication. (Refer box)

Distinguishing symptoms of the patient	Medicine and potency
• **Violent headache**. Congestion in the head.	Aurum Met 200
• **Double vision**.	
• Sleeplessness.	
• Tumultuous **rebounding** of heart after a momentary stop.	
• Irregular pulse.	
• Surging of blood to **head**. Sensation of **heaviness**. Confusion. Dizziness.	Glonoine 200
• **Violent irregularity** of blood circulation. Sudden. **Throbbing pulsation** in the entire body.	

- Breathlessness on exertion or climbing steps.
- High blood pressure at the **climacteric**.   Lachesis 200
- Rush of blood to the heart with **coldness of feet**.
- Suffocation. Constriction.
- With **rheumatoid pain**.   Lycopus Virg 30
- **Cardiac asthma**.
- **Hardening of the arteries** with high   Plumbum Met 30
  blood pressure.
- **Burning of palms and soles**.   Sanguinaria 30
- Climacteric. Flushes of heat
- Distension of temporal veins. Pain in occiput.
- Congestion at the base of brain.   Veratrum Viride 30
  Congestion of the lungs. **Giddiness**.
  Bloodshot eyes. **Double vision**. Bloated face.
- **Both** systolic and diastolic pressure **high**.
- **Rheumatic heart**.
- Nausea. Vomiting
- **Pulse throbbing throughout** the body, particularly **the right thigh**.
- Burning pain in chest near the heart.

BLOOD PRESSURE, LOW

Low blood pressure can be debilitating. It is undesirable. Its causes are varied. Treat according to symptoms. Do not neglect. **Seek medical advice.**

Distinguishing symptoms of the patient	Medicine and potency
• **Irregular, feeble** pulse.	Cactus 30
• Violent palpitation with **vertigo**.	Mother Tincture, 10-drop
• Flatulence. Loss of breath	dose in water every half an
• **Face blue**. Cardiac incompetence. **Constriction**. Stitching pain.	hour in emergency.

• Stimulates the **feeble heart muscle** in threatened failure. **Low pulse rate**.	Caffeine 200
• Blood pressure low because of **imperfect oxygenation**.	Carbo Veg 200
• **Face blue, body icy cold**.	
• **Chronic acidity**. Weak digestion.	
• Caused by **exhausting discharges** from any part of the body. **Severe debility**.	China 200
• Anaemia. Dropsy.	
• Heart beat irregular, **weak**, and rapid, **alternating** with **strong** heartbeats.	
• In **chronic** heart disease. Dilated heart.	Crataegus
• **Heartbeat** distinctly felt in chest, throat, and head.	Mother Tincture, 15-drop dose, four times a day for a long time.

HYPERTENSION

Blood pressure is the pressure exerted by the blood against the walls of the blood vessels, especially the arteries. It varies with the strength of the heartbeat, the volume, and viscosity of the blood, and the elasticity of the walls of the arteries. It also depends on a person's age, health, and physical condition.

Heart rate is different from blood pressure in that the former is regulated by electrical impulses from the sinoatrial node, the heart's pacemaker, which is a small area of nervous tissue in the wall of the right atrium. Each one of these impulses causes a rapid sequence of contractions, first in the atria and then in the ventricles, that corresponds to one heartbeat.

Both heartbeat and blood pressure are controlled by the nervous system in the short term and by hormones over a longer period.

A healthy adult heart beats up to 60-80 beats per minute while at rest. During strenuous exercise, it can beat up to 200 beats per minute. Reverse flow of blood or flow in the wrong direction is prevented by one-way valves inside the heart. When these valves shut tightly, we hear the well-known rhythmic sound, 'dub-dub'.

When the heart beats, the blood flows and exerts pressure against the arterial walls. As the heart contracts in its cycle of pumping blood, blood pressure reaches its highest level. This is called systolic blood pressure.

The blood pressure reaches its lowest point when the heart is at rest and is relaxed. This is called diastolic blood pressure.

Normal blood pressure is 120/80 mm of mercury for a healthy person. There is no safe limit beyond normal.

A human being is said to have high blood pressure if continuously, the systolic and the diastolic pressures exceed the limit of 140/90. Medical advice is necessary. Values higher than 160/95 are placed in the danger zone.

If the blood pressure is too low, not enough oxygen reaches the body tissues. This results in debility, light-headedness. If untreated, its consequences are grave.

Blood pressure level varies depending on the following factors:

- The arteries are narrowed by cholesterol and plaque deposits. As the movement of blood through arteries builds up pressure, this pressure increases according to the resistance offered by the narrowing inner circumference of the arteries.
- The amount of blood which the heart has to pump out in a given period and the total volume of blood in the body. The amount of blood pumped out with each heartbeat is affected by mental tension, physical needs of the body due to exercise, and a number of other factors.
- Cardio vascular changes produced by constriction of blood vessels and increase in blood volume caused by hormones produced by glands and enzymes produced by the kidneys.
- The age and weight of an individual.

The following groups are more affected by blood pressure than others are:

1. More men below forty-five years of age than women in that age group.

2. Obese persons. The heart has to pump a greater volume of blood in proportion to the body weight and size than in the case of a person with normal body weight.
3. Children of parents either of whom might have suffered from hypertension.
4. Persons who use excessive quantities of table salt, pickles, processed meat, canned soup, processed cheese, seasonings like tomato ketchup, soya sauce, chilli sauce and so on. Sodium in salt leads to excessive fluid retention in the body and thus increases the overall volume of blood which the heart has to pump.
5. Some users of birth control pills.
6. Smokers. Nicotine narrows and constricts arteries, thereby boosting the blood pressure.
7. Persons who consume large amounts of alcohol.
8. Persons leading a stressful lifestyle. Persons who are competing all the time with others and with themselves. Unreasonably ambitious persons. Mentally discontented. Unforgiving. Angry for no reason.

Usually hypertension has no symptoms. A periodical check is, therefore, necessary.

However, in case the blood pressure is very high, the patient may suffer from headaches, blurry vision, or dizziness. There are other consequences, such as partial or total blindness, swollen ankles, mental and body debility and fatigue. Left unchecked and untreated, hypertension leads to many undesirable consequences.

First, the arterial walls become thick and hardened. There is no going back once the process has started and has reached an advanced stage. The smooth flow of blood is affected by narrow and inflexible arteries. The heart muscle comes under strain. It may give way and fail. Further, the supply of oxygen to the heart and the brain is reduced. Medically this condition is known as atherosclerosis.

Hypertension can lead to congestive heart failure. If a substantial part of the heart muscle has been damaged, blood collects in the extremities and in the lungs. It is not pumped efficiently. The heart is forced to pump against increasing resistance and perforce it fails.

A serious consequence of hypertension is 'Stroke', which damages the brain, sometimes for good. High blood pressure makes it difficult for delicate blood vessels to function effectively. The brain does not get proper nourishment by way of blood and oxygen. Blood rushing with greater pressure than normal, physically hurts the sensitive inner walls of the arteries. A deposit of plaque forms more rapidly than in normal circumstances. The blood vessels lose their elasticity. As the plumbing becomes rotten, defective, inelastic, a sudden choking occurs. The patient suffers a stroke which is sometimes fatal.

A stroke may not always kill. Nevertheless, once it has affected a person, his ability to walk, think, read, write, or speak is greatly reduced.

Congestion in the lungs caused by hypertension makes the patient short of breath. He develops a cough.

High blood pressure slows down the functioning of the kidneys. As a result, the blood retains more salt and water. This in turn increases blood pressure. It is a vicious cycle.

Hypertension cannot normally be cured. It can, however, be controlled with treatment. Seek medical advice and follow it faithfully.

A number of powerful drugs are available to reduce high blood pressure. These have side effects. However, it is better to treat hypertension with drugs than to live with it with all its unpleasant consequences.

Homoeopathic treatment according to symptoms is useful. There are no side effects.

Nevertheless, changes in one's lifestyle help deal with hypertension quite well. I suggest the following:

- Stop smoking. No medicine can help you if you persist with smoking.
- Reduce alcohol intake. Preferably, give it up.
- Cut down salt intake. Reduce having papadam, sauces, pickles, and canned food.
- Reduce weight.
- Reduce cholesterol with or without medication. Seek expert guidance. You just cannot ignore unhealthy cholesterol levels.
- Do not consume saturated fats.
- Control your diet. A voracious appetite paves the way to a never-ending cycle of sickness.
- Exercise regularly. Swim. Cycle. Do stretching exercises. Seek an expert's guidance on what to do and what to avoid in a gym.
- Join a support group or a circle of friends who meet regularly and care for each other.
- Be happy.
- Relax. Relaxation has a positive effect in reducing hypertension.
- Meditate. It lowers blood pressure considerably.
- Use visualization for mental concentration.
- Practice yoga and *pranayamma*.
- Give up anger, jealousy, hatred, and negative feelings towards fellow human beings. The milk of human kindness is a tonic for the heart.
- Read. It does wonders to your mind.
- Avoid movies and TV serials which show violence, horror, and scheming villains.
- Listen to Indian classical music, particularly, the slow movements called 'aalaap.'

BRADYCARDIA

Slowness of heart rate, usually fewer than sixty beats per minute in an adult person. On aggravation it can cause fainting or death. Generally, athletes or older persons suffer from Bradycardia.

Symptoms: Awareness of an irregular heartbeat, chest pain, shortness of breath, light-headedness, and unconsciousness in an extreme situation. **Any weak pulse requires expert intervention.**

Distinguishing symptoms of the patient	Medicine and potency
• Weak pulse. • Violent palpitation by the least movement. • Sudden sensation as if the heart stood still. Digitalis stimulates the heart, increases the force of systole, and lengthens its duration.	Digitalis 30. Mother Tincture for cardiac stimulation. 15-drops dose, every 30 minutes. Reduce dose as soon as the pulse rate has been raised to 80 beats a minute and the normal rhythm has been restored.

BURNING

Burning sensation in the heart region can be deceptive. It can be due to acidity or ulcers. It can also be a warning of a heart attack. Rule out an attack. **Seek medical advice immediately**.

Meanwhile, start taking Arnica 200 and Carbo Veg 200 at once. The former thins the blood and helps in angina. The latter looks after acidity.

If you are experiencing nausea, retching and cold sweat, take Veratrum Alb 1000 as well.

However, **consult a doctor immediately**.

Distinguishing symptoms of the patient	Medicine and potency
• **Violent burning pain** in the chest and stomach. Burning as in an ulcer.	Acetic Acid 30

- **Coldness** of **skin**. Cold **sweat** on forehead.
- With constrictive, burning pain extending to chest.   Carbo Veg 200
- **Acidity**. Burning ulcers.
- **Hyperacidity** with **pain radiating** from the centre of the ribs in all **directions**.   Argentum Nit 200

CHEST PAIN

Chest pain should always be taken seriously. **Seek medical advice immediately**.

Refer '*Angina' Pectoris*', '*Burning*', '*constriction*' and '*Coronary Thrombosis*', in this chapter, and '*Indigestion*' under '*The Digestive System.*'

CONSTRICTION

You feel as if some outside force is trying to crush your chest, your heart. You experience a heavy weight lying on your chest and pressing downwards. You are short of breath. You feel like vomiting but nothing comes out. You sweat. You experience pain originating in the heart region and spreading in various directions, particularly towards and down the left shoulder and arm. You fear death.

This sensation indicates a probable heart attack. **Get medical help immediately. Call an ambulance. Shift to a hospital**. In the meantime, administer the indicated medicine.

Constriction is present in Angina Pectoris as well. However, here the pain passes off if the patient is immobile. If the pain persists, the situation is as above.

A feeling of constriction of the heart is experienced in several situations discussed in this chapter. Never take it lightly.

Distinguishing symptoms of the patient	Medicine and potency
• The heart feels as if being **constricted by an iron band**.	Cactus 30 Mother Tincture, 10-drop

- Suffocation. Cold sweat. Nausea.

- Pain shoots down left arm.
- Pain in shoulders and neck.

dose in water every half an hour

until condition stabilizes.

CORONARY THROMBOSIS
[MYOCARDIAL INFARCTION]
HEART ATTACK

A blockage of blood in a coronary artery reduces or stops the blood supply to the heart muscle. It is called 'heart attack'.

While the angina pain subsides on rest, the Myocardial Infarction pain persists. Rather it goes on increasing. **Do not lose time. Contact a doctor. Call an ambulance. Rush the patient to the nearest Intensive Care Unit**.

The following medicines are of great help, in the meanwhile.

Symptoms: Constriction of heart as if squeezed by an iron band. Sudden, heavy, severe pain in the region of the heart spreading to the left shoulder, down into the left arm. Sensation of hyperacidity, at times. Nausea. Pallor. Cold sweat on the face and the body. Irregular heartbeat. Anxiety. Fear of death. Restlessness.

Distinguishing symptoms of the patient	Medicine and potency
• Tightness, **constriction after over-exertion or fatigue**.	Arnica 200 Use as a first aid remedy.
• **Helps in the dissolution** of a blood clot.	Bothrops 30
• Constriction of the heart as if squeezed by **an iron band**.	Cactus 30 In emergency, Mother
• Suffocation. **Cold sweat. Nausea.**	Tincture, 10-drop dose in
• Pain shoots down left arm.	water every half an hour
• Obstructed breathing. **Face blue**. Cannot lie on the left side	until condition stabilizes.
• Pain in shoulders and neck.	
• Acute coronary thrombosis	Lachesis 200
• Terrible **constriction** in the chest	
• **Numbness** in the left arm.	

• The heart feels **grasped in a vice**.	Lilium Tigrinum 200
• Sensation as if the heart has stopped for a while, followed by rush of blood and **violent palpitation**.	
• **Cold hands, cold feet, cold sweat**.	
• Pain travelling from left nipple through chest to back.	

ENDOCARDITIS

A bacterial infection of the lining of the heart cavity and of the heart valves. It can be acute or chronic.

Symptoms: Sudden rise in temperature. Night sweats. Signs of heart failure. Fatigue. In chronic cases, a general ache in the body. Poor appetite and weight loss. Low grade fevers.

It is a serious problem. Seek medical advice.

Distinguishing symptoms of the patient	Medicine and potency
• **High fever**. Congestion of the heart and of the lungs.	Aconite 30
• Palpitation. **Cardiac oppression**.	
• **Brief loss of consciousness** in transient cerebral anaemia or heart attack or a sudden lowering of blood pressure.	
• Severe **constriction**.	Cactus 30
• **Obstructed breathing. Face blue**.	
• Pulse **throbbing**, quick, **hard**.	
• With **rheumatism** of joints. Shifting pain.	Kalmia Lat 30
• Severe pain in the chest running into shoulder blades.	
• Heart beats **tumultuously**.	
• **Threatened paralysis** of the heart. **Body cold**. Weak pulse.	Naja Tripudians 30
• Palpitation. **Gasping for breath**.	

- Stitching pain in the heart region,
  extending to the nape of the neck,
  left shoulder, and left arm
- Anxiety. Fear of death.
- **Damaged** heart after infectious **diseases**.

HEART FAILURE

Inability of the heart to fulfil the pumping demands and thus to maintain circulation of blood sufficient to meet the needs of the body. Can be acute or chronic. It can be caused by the weakness of the heart muscle or by reduction in the supply of blood to the heart for any reason.

Symptoms: In acute cases, extreme shortness of breath, pale skin, sweating, and wheezing. Pink, frothy sputum with cough. In case of a heart attack, symptoms as indicated in '*Heart Attack*' above.

In chronic cases, general fatigue, loss of appetite, nausea, swollen feet and ankles, breathing difficulty when exerting or lying flat. Possibility of acute heart failure with dire consequences.

Seek medical advice. Symptomatic medicines as indicated help.

INFLAMMATION/MYOCARDITIS

An acute inflammation of the heart muscle, usually due to an infection.

Symptoms: Pain in the chest, fever, fatigue, awareness of the abnormally rapid heartbeat. In later stages, breathlessness and swelling of the legs and ankles. Numbness.

Even though the problem is considered a minor one in the initial stages, **consultation with a doctor is advisable** because, if not treated in time, it can lead to severe heart failure.

Distinguishing symptoms of the patient	Medicine and potency
• Inflammation of the middle and the thickest layers of the heart.	Arsenic Iod 30

- Fatty deposits. High cholesterol.
- Heart chronically weak. **Flutters irregularly. Tendency to faint**.
- Severe pain in cardiac region travelling to the back.
- Breathlessness on climbing steps.
- Myocardium weak and dilated. **Inflamed**.   Digitalis 30
- **Sudden**.   Mother Tincture in acute
- **Pulse abnormally low** but quickened by   cases to stabilize the least movement.   patient. 15-drop dose on
- Sensation as if the heart **would stop**   sugar every 30 minutes. **beating** if the patient moved.   Reduce dose as soon as
- Heavy breathing. Worse lying.   the pulse stabilises at 80
- **Faintness and exhaustion** like during a   beats per minute. No mild illness such as cold or influenza.   liquid to be taken for 20
- **Dropsy** of internal and external parts.   minutes before or after the dose.
- **Swelling on left foot, left leg, and**   Cactus **left hand**.   Mother Tincture, 10-drop
- Acute or chronic inflammation of the   dose in water four times heart.   daily.

PAIN

Any pain in the region of the heart is a cause for concern. **Consult a doctor**.

Distinguishing symptoms of the patient	Medicine and potency
• Violent, **burning pain** in chest and stomach followed by **coldness of skin**, cold sweat on forehead.	Acetic Acid 30
• Face swollen, waxen, **emaciated**. Eyes sunken. Anaemia.	
• Cases of weak heart, of angina pectoris.	
• **Angina pectoris**. Pain is **reduced** on complete **immobility**.	Arnica 200, 1000

- Severe pain in the left arm.
- **Angina** pectoris with constriction as of an iron band tightening.
- **Cold sweat, face blue**. Left arm numb.

Cactus, Mother Tincture, 10-drop dose in water every thirty minutes until condition stabilises.

- **Rheumatic pain** in cardiac region.
- Sudden shock to the heart.
- Pain in heart region before menstruation. **Pain in bladder** and while passing urine.

Lithium Crab 30

- Angina pectoris with **loss of voice**.
- Sharp, **lacerating** pain coming **suddenly** in the **left lung**, leaving the patient **breathless**.

Oxalic Acid 30

- Pain in the **right side of** the chest. Stabbing pain in the sternum, extending to back and near shoulders.
- **Cough** with profuse, **foul expectoration**.

Phellandrium 30

- Inflammation of the sac covering the heart. Stitching pain.
- **Frequent violent palpitations**.

Spigelia 200

PALPITATION

A disagreeable awareness of the heart-beat to the patient.

Distinguishing symptoms of the patient	Medicine and potency
• Palpitation with **distension of stomach**.	Abies Can 30
• Violent, **reverberating in the head**.	Belladonna 200
• Palpitation from the least exertion.	
• **Low** blood pressure. Weak heart. Pulse feeble.	Cactus, mother tincture
• **Violent** palpitation, **irregular, quick**.	
• With **breathlessness** while **climbing** a mountain.	Coca 30

- From **nervous irritation**.   Lycopus Virg 30
- Heart action tumultuous and forceful.
- **Hypertension**.
- With **coldness** of feet and heart constriction.   Natrum Mur 200
- Rapid heart beat in **anaemic** persons.
- Acute, **violent**, visible through clothes.   Spigelia 200
  Sound audible. The whole chest shakes.
- With **irregular and rapid pulse**. An   Veratrum Alb 200
  excellent heart stimulant.

PERICARDITIS

Inflammation of the pericardium, the double-layered sac surrounding the heart. Usually an acute infection.

Symptoms: Like those of the *'coronary thrombosis'*. [See above]. Constricting pain in the chest spreading into neck, into the left shoulder, the left arm, breathlessness, sweat, nausea, fear of death. Fever. Swelling in abdomen and in ankles.

Distinguishing symptoms of the patient	Medicine and potency
• Constrictive pericarditis with **tenderness in the abdomen**.	Bryonia 200
• **Ankles swollen**.	
• **Stitching pain in the chest**. Worse on motion.	
• Acute **rheumatic cases**.	Colchicum 30
• **Vertigo**. At times **loss of consciousness** on sitting upright.	
• Difficult breathing. Chest pain. Tightness in chest.	
• Pulse **imperceptible**.	
• For symptoms, see *'Inflammation'* above.	Digitalis 30
• For symptoms, see *'Endocarditis'* above.	Kalmia Lat 30
• **Rheumatic** cases.	Spigelia 200

- Piercing pain.
- Violent palpitations.
- Acute heart attack.
- Worse by leaning forward.

PULSE RAPID, SLOW/TACHYCARDIA

Refer '*Atrial Fibrillation*' above as well.

Distinguishing symptoms of the patient	Medicine and potency
• Abnormally rapid pulse.	Abies Nigra 200
• Indigestion. **Blockage in oesophagus**.	
• Abnormally rapid pulse.	Aconite Nap 30
• Full of **fear**, anxiety.	
• **Numbness and crawling in fingers**.	
• Irregular pulse, violent and rapid.	Cactus 30
• Infection of the lining of the heart.	
• **Numbness** in left arm. **Swelling** in left arm, leg, and feet.	
• **Very slow** pulse. Tired heart. Dilated heart.	Digitalis Mother Tincture, 15-drop
• Cardiac failure following **cardiac dropsy**.	dose on sugar or bread
• Skin, lips, and tongue **blue**.	every thirty minutes.
• At times, the pulse quickens.	Reduce dose as the pulse rate becomes normal.
• Abnormally rapid heart beat.	Natrum Mur 200
• **Anaemia**.	
• Constriction. **Coldness**.	
• Pulse **irregular, but rapid.** Great stimulant for the heart.	Veratrum Alb 200

THE RESPIRATORY SYSTEM
THE LUNGS

The respiratory system performs the functions of intake of air rich in oxygen and the exhalation of carbon dioxide.

The nose and the throat are a part of this system. For the sake of convenience, these have been dealt with separately.

The human body cannot survive without a sufficient supply of oxygen required by every living cell. Oxygen helps produce energy for various activities of the body. Absorbed by blood, it is carried to every nook and corner of the body. Carbon dioxide is produced as a waste product. It has to be got rid of. The lungs assisted by the heart, perform both these functions with the help of blood, the total volume of which passes through them every minute.

The surface area of the lungs plays a vital role in this exercise. It is forty times larger than the surface area of the human body.

The air we breathe is purified by the nose. The filtered air passes through the pharynx [throat] and moves into the larynx and onward into the trachea [windpipe].

The trachea divides into two bronchi, one going into each lung. The left bronchus and the right bronchus sub-divide into increasingly smaller bronchioles which end in small cavities shaped like balloons known as alveoli. In the thin walls of the alveoli occurs the exchange of oxygen for carbon dioxide with the help of tiny blood vessels. Each lung has 250 million alveoli.

Moist membranes known as pleura surround the lungs. They help the lungs to move freely to perform their job.

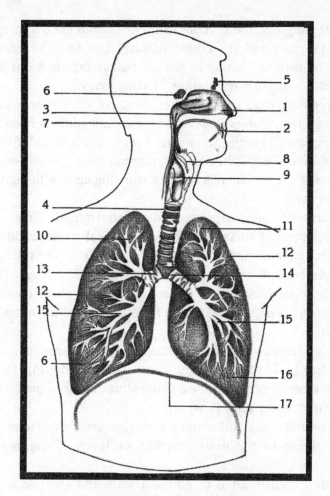

THE RESPIRATORY SYSTEM
1. Nasal cavity. 2. Mouth. 3. Pharynx. 4. Trachea. 5. Frontal sinus. 6. Sphenoid
sinus. 7. Tonsils. 8. Larynx. 9. Vocal cords. 10. Right lung. 11. Left lung.
12. Pleura. 13. Right principal bronchus. 14. Left principal bronchus. 15. Bronchi.
16. Respiratory bronchiole. 17. Diaphragm.

Just below the lungs lies the diaphragm, a partition wall separating
them from the stomach. When we breathe, the diaphragm contracts, the
space in the chest is increased and the lungs expand.

The stronger the action of the rib muscles and the diaphragm, the
greater is the air which enters the lungs. Further, the greater the quantity
of carbon dioxide which has to be expelled from the blood stream, the
faster is the rate of breathing in and out.

On breathing out, the muscles of the chest and the diaphragm relax. The rib cage sinks and the lungs contract. The air is squeezed out.

Traces of carbon dioxide in the air that is breathed out are useful in the mouth-to-mouth respiration in emergencies.

Hundreds of organisms, either bacteria or viruses, attack the respiratory system. Babies under six months can suffer serious disorders of the respiratory system. So do the very weak and elderly who can suffer from acute bronchitis or pneumonia.

Smokers run a serious risk because smoking chokes the lungs, in the end, irreversibly.

A respiratory illness saps the body of its strength. Such a patient, after recovery, ought to take up heavy, physical work gradually.

The common cold and sinusitis, although disorders of the respiratory system, have been discussed under the chapter, *The Nose.*' The throat problems have been discussed under the chapter of that name.

This chapter primarily deals with the afflictions of the lungs and their components.

Lifestyle changes can help us maintain our respiratory system in good condition. Do not smoke. Even passive smoking is harmful. Partying in closed rooms among a suffocating and drinking crowd is not conducive to a good lung function.

Factory smoke and automobile pollution are other factors vitiating the environment to the detriment of our lungs. These may not be avoidable.

The safest course out is to go for a walk and exercise regularly in open air. *Pranayama* and deep breathing exercises, besides giving us peace of mind, tone up the lungs. Swimming and running too are beneficial for health of the respiratory system. Laugh as often as you can, louder the better.

ASTHMA BRONCHIAL

Swelling and narrowing of the small bronchial passages resulting in breathing difficulty and wheezing.

Bronchial asthma is purely a respiratory problem. It is not to be confused with cardiac asthma which troubles patients with heart disease and is more serious.

Symptoms: Painless tightness in the chest, difficult cough, wheezing sound on breathing out. Panic. Sweating.

At times, the skin turns blue. The pulse beats fast.

Inflammation of the bronchi produces excess mucous that blocks the small airways further.

In babies and young children, difficulty in breathing results in the lower ribs being drawn inwards.

Usually worse at night. Worsens as the night progresses.

Distinguishing symptoms of the patient	Medicine and potency
• **Sudden, violent** attack. • **Stitches** through and constant **pressure** on the chest. • **Hoarse, dry**, croupy cough. • Restlessness, **fear of death**. Better in open air. Worse at midnight, in a warm room, lying on affected side, from dry cold wind, from tobacco smoke.	Aconite Nap 30 An excellent first remedy. Alternate with Ipecac 30, every 15 minutes, stirred in warm water, in an acute attack until it subsides.
• Lungs **choked** with mucous. **Unable to take it out**. Coarse rattling.	Antim Tart 200, 1000 Effective where nothing else expels mucous.
• Severe at **midnight. Chronic** lung problems. • **Burning** in the chest. • Terrible wheezing. Frothy expectoration. • Restlessness, moaning, agitation. Great exhaustion. **Cold perspiration**.	Arsenic Alb 200

When asthma follows pneumonia.

- Lungs of **old persons**. Chronic catarrh.   Bacillinum 200
  Reduced pulmonary circulation.
- Humid asthma. **Bubbling rales.**
  Oppressed breathing.
- Expectoration full of **pus**.
- **Sudden, violent spasm** with breathing   Belladonna 200
  attended by constriction of chest and
  throat. A feeling of suffocation.
- **Loss of voice**. Larynx painful.
- Uneven, oppressed, quick respiration.
- Asthma of **old age**. No strength in   Carbo Veg 200
  the body.
- **Skin blue**. Imperfect oxygenation.
- Appetite lost. Acidity. Indigestion.
- **Spasmodic** asthma alternating with   Cuprum Met 200
  spasmodic vomiting. Chest constricted.
- **Face blue. Eyes turned up**. Loss of
  colour in fingers and nails. Cramped
  fingers as in **epilepsy**.
- Attack in **cold, wet** weather.   Dulcamara 200
                                          Combine with other
                                          remedies.

- Asthma acute or chronic.   Ipecac 200
- **Nausea** present all the time.   In acute attack use as
- Constriction, severe wheezing, incessant,   indicated above with
  violent cough. Loss of voice.   Aconite.
- At times lung **haemorrhage**.
- Phlegm does not yield while coughing.
- Threatened **paralysis of lungs**. Sudden   Lachesis 200
  flushes of heat, flooding of lungs.
- Wants to loosen clothes. Severe suffocation.
- Cold sweat.
- Asthma with **yellow expectoration**.   Kali Sulph 30
  Rattling in chest.
- Asthma incited by **anger or**   Lycopodium 200
  emotional upset.

- In nervous patients.
- **Always catching cold, easily tired**, exhausted.
- **Burning** in oesophagus.
- Aggravation in the evening.

ASTHMA CARDIAC

Older persons with a history of serious heart disease can get attacks of cardiac asthma at night.

Distinguishing symptoms of the patient	Medicine and potency
• Palpitation with anxiety. **High blood pressure.**	Aconite 30 Also as first aid as indicated under, '*Asthma bronchial*'.
• Irrational **fear of death**.	
• Numbness and tingling in the fingers.	
• Worse at midnight and after, worse in a warm room, and after a cold drink.	
• **Want of breath** during **exertion**.	Aspidosperma
• Specific for cardiac asthma. **Stimulates respiratory centres** and increases oxygen absorption in the blood.	Mother tincture 10 drops every hour until the patient is stable.
• **High blood pressure** patients. Pulse is full and hard.	Baryta Carb 200
• **Black spots** before eyes.	
• Deep sounding mucous in the chest.	
• Old asthmatic patients with **high blood pressure.**	Baryta Mur 200
• Unable to take out mucous.	
• Worse by every change in weather.	
• Asthma with **chronic bronchitis and a weak heart**.	Digitalis 200
• Short of breath. Wants to breathe deep all the time. **Sudden** sensation as if **heart stood still**. Quickened by least movement.	

BRONCHIOLITIS

A viral respiratory infection, affecting infants, mostly in winter.

Symptoms: Cough, cold, spreading to the small air tubes deep in the lungs. Congestion of mucous and pus in the lungs. Difficult, rapid breathing. Lower ribs and upper abdomen sucked in with each breath. Skin turns pale or yellow.

Distinguishing symptoms of the patient	Medicine and potency
• Acute, sudden, **violent** attack.	Aconite Nap 30
Violent cough.	First aid as indicated in
• **Lower ribs sucked in**. Oppressed breathing.	*'Asthma bronchial'*, above.
• Child restless, mentally and physically.	
• Worse at and after midnight.	
• **Pus** in the lungs.	Calcarea Sulph 30
• **Short and rapid breaths**.	Ipecac 200
• Wheezing. Constriction.	
• Face turns **pale or blue**.	
• Restlessness and irritability.	

BRONCHITIS ACUTE

A sudden viral inflammation of the bronchi, the larger airways leading to the lungs.

Symptoms: Dry, hacking cough with stitching pain in the centre of the rib cage. Clear mucous. Expectoration of green or yellow mucous as the infection spreads. Oppressive breathing. Wheezing. Fever.

Seek immediate medical counsel in case the patient has a history of heart or lung disease and throws up discoloured sputum.

Distinguishing symptoms of the patient	Medicine and potency
• **Rattling** of mucous, **audible** across the room.	Antim Tart 200, 1000

- **Difficult to take out mucous**.
- Weakening cough
- Impending paralysis of the lungs.
- **Stitching pain** in the chest, in the centre of the ribs. Severe pain on the least coughing.
- Infection of trachea and of lungs.
- Little expectoration.
- Worse on least movement. Worse after eating, drinking.
- Bronchitis **following influenza**.
- Debility caused by outflow of liquids, mucous etc
- Violent cough after every meal.

Bryonia 200.
First remedy. A dose of 10 pills dissolved in one-half of a teacup of lukewarm water, sipped slowly, repeated every four hours, gives relief.
China 200

- **Suffocative catarrh**.
- With **nausea** and terrible **wheezing**.
- Violent, difficult breathing. Weight on chest.
- **Bleeding** from lungs at times. Lungs full of mucous.
- Face pale. Sunken eyes with blue margins.
- **Acute bronchitis in infants**. Coarse rattling. Wheezing. Pain below the ribs. Bad cold ending in bronchitis.

Ipecac 200
Alternate with Antim Tart 1000 in case it is difficult to take out phlegm.

- Profuse expectoration which is **thick, ropy, and greenish**.
- Constant desire to take a deep, long breath.

Natrum Sulph 200

- Bronchitis with **thick, bland,** greenish, or yellowish discharge flowing easy.

Pulsatilla 200.
Alternate with Bryonia 200.

BRONCHITIS CHRONIC

Virtually, an irreversible process. The bronchi become narrow. The delicate air sacs of the lungs are destroyed. Oxygen supply to the blood is reduced.

Chronic bronchitis may lead to heart failure.
Seek medical advice at the earliest.

Distinguishing symptoms of the patient	Medicine and potency
• Chronic bronchitis. **Hard, croupy cough** with **wheezing**. • Inability to raise sputum. • Patient **aged** and weak. No strength. No appetite. • Pneumonia and bronchitis **together**. It is a serious condition. **Get medical help immediately**.	Antimony Jodat 200
• **Inability** to take out phlegm the sound of which can be heard across the room. • Sharp stitches in the **centre of the** ribs while coughing. • Worse on the slightest movement.	Antimony Tart 200, 1000 Combine it with Bryonia. Bryonia 200, 1000 **A must**. Combine with other indicated remedies.
• **Mucous white** and **frothy** or thick, ropy and greenish. • Increasing breathlessness and cough.	Natrum Sulph 200
• **Burning sensation** in the chest with pain in the ribs while coughing. • Feels oppressed. Wants windows open. • Expectoration full of **pus, is sweet**. Rattling sound. • Worse morning.	Sulphur 200 One dose, early morning, before having any food or drink, besides other indicated remedies.

COUGH

Cough is a natural response to infection or irritation of the respiratory tract. It helps clear blockages or irritants from the airways.

If a cough does not ease in a day or so, consult a doctor who will look into the underlying cause which can be serious at times.

Distinguishing symptoms of the patient	Medicine and potency
• **Dry**, hoarse cough. On **exposure** to dry, cold air.	Aconite Nap 30
• Sudden aggravation.	
• Worse at midnight and after midnight.	
• Whooping cough with **flatulence** and **vomit**.	Allium Cepa 200
• On taking in cold air. **Pain into ears**.	
• With **facial herpes**, violent, spasmodic cough.	Arnica 200
• **Face turns red**. Violent, sudden onset.	Belladonna 200
• **Larynx painful**.	
• Tickling, short cough, worse at night.	
• With **piercing pain in the chest,** in the centre of the rib cage. **Hacking pain.**	Bryonia 200
• **Bronchitis**. Almost no expectoration.	
• Cough arises from the upper trachea. Must sit up.	
• Loose cough, with expectoration of **large pieces like cast** of bronchial tube.	Calcarea Acetica 30
• Better bending backwards.	
• Whooping cough attack ending in **white tough mucous**.	Coccus Cacti 30
• **Chronic** bronchitis. Feels as if being **strangled**. Tickling in larynx.	
• Whooping cough attack **ending in catalepsy**.	Cuprum Met 200
• Face turns **blue**. Nails lose colour. **Clenched thumbs**. Cramped fingers.	
• **Whooping cough**, deep and hoarse. **Main remedy in whooping cough.**	Drosera 200
• Spasmodic, dry, irritating. **Paroxysms, one following the other rapidly**.	
• Yellow mucous. **Blood** from nose and mouth. **Retching**.	

- Worse after midnight.
- Sudden with **nausea**. **Any type of cough with nausea.**
- Vomits all food. Face red.
- Incessant and violent cough.
- Terrible **wheezing**. Phlegm does not easily yield.

Ipecac 200.
Use Antim Tart 1000 if Ipecac fails to take out the phlegm from the lungs.

- **Metallic**, hacking cough. Brassy sound in catarrhal cough in laryngitis.
- **Ropy, green mucous** going inwards. Very difficult to take out.

Kali Bichrome 200

- With thick, **green, bland mucous coming out easily**. Loose cough in the morning.
- Dry cough in the evening and at night. Must sit up for relief.

Pulsatilla 30

- **Chronic** cases. Cough fails to yield.
- Thick, **yellow lumps** thrown out.

Silicea 200

- Cough with **sneezing**.
- **Bronco-pneumonia**.

Squilla 30

CROUP

Viral infection leading to inflammation of trachea. Mostly children between six months and three years suffer from croup. It usually starts with the symptoms of a common cold.

Symptoms: Acute inflammation of larynx. Noisy breathing producing a croaking sound. Hoarseness. Barking cough. The chest wall drawn inwards with every breath. Fever.

If the skin turns blue, send for a doctor.

Distinguishing symptoms of the patient	Medicine and potency
• Sudden, dry, hoarse croup. • On **exposure** to dry, cold air • **High fever**. Dry skin.	Aconite 30. Provide mild steam inhalation covering the

- Child awakened from sleep by long, suffocating attacks.
- Fear of being choked to death. Anxiety, restlessness.
- Severe catarrhal croup.
- **Rattling mucous**. Lungs choked. **Cannot take it out**.
- Face cold, **bluish**, covered with **cold sweat**.
- Pulse rapid, weak. **Collapse**.
- Highest grade of croup. **Face blue, pulse weak**, slow, intermittent.
- **Complete insensibility**. No cough or muffled cough.
- Wheezing. Difficult breathing.
- Rattling, choking cough. The child **chokes with every spasm**, has to sit up and bend for comfort.
- **Profuse, sour sweat** before midnight.
- Cannot take out mucous but can breathe easy.
- Evening cough with **convulsions, nausea, wheezing**.
- Gradual onset of croup.
- Coarse, **metallic cough** with loud rales.
- **Tough, stringy mucous flowing inwards**.
- Aggravation towards 3 am.

child's head and the vessel of water with a towel spread like an umbrella.

Antim Tart 200, 1000

Carbo Veg 200

Hepar Sulph 200

Ipecac 200

Kali Bichrome 200

EMPHYSEMA
CHRONIC OBSTRUCTIVE PULMONARY DISEASE

Progressive loss of lung elasticity usually caused by smoking. A chronic disease. The tiny air sacs in the lungs are inflated and distended. Their walls become thin and rupture.

Symptoms: Difficulty in breathing, in exhalation. Wheezing. Severe, persistent cough. Chest shapes into a barrel. Loss of weight. Skin colour turns blue with exertion. Morning cough produces sputum. Production of yellow or green sputum as time passes. As the disease progresses, shortness of breath even while at rest.

Worse in cold weather or with other respiratory problems like influenza.

Consult a doctor at the earliest.

Distinguishing symptoms of the patient	Medicine and potency
• Stitching pain in the chest.	Ammonium Carb 30
• Bronchial tubes lack strength. **Breathing oppressive,** asthmatic, resulting in **fainting**.	
• Persistent cough. Worse 3 to 4 A. M.	
• **Pulmonary oedema**.	
• **Lungs choked with mucous**. Difficult to expectorate.	
• **Burning** in the chest.	Arsenic Alb 200
• **Face blue. Cold perspiration**.	
• Suffocates while breathing.	
• Chest tight as if **bound by a hoop**.	
• Great **anxiety. Restlessness**.	
• Better, from heat, warm drinks, head elevated.	
• Worse during wet weather, after midnight, from cold, cold drinks, cold food.	
• Often **follows Arsenic in chronic**, neglected cases of emphysema.	Carbo Veg 200
• Cough spasmodic, violent.	
• **Watery**, copious expectoration.	
• **Cold hands, cold feet, cold breath. Skin blue**.	
• **Wheezing, nausea**.	Ipecac 200
• Lungs full of mucous.	If mucous does not yield
• Dry, spasmodic cough in **old patients**.	use Antim Tart 1000.
• Difficult inhaling and exhaling.	

EXPECTORATION

Distinguishing symptoms of the patient	Medicine and potency
• Little **balls of mucous** with cough that ends in a **sneeze**.	Agaricus 200
• Bronchial tubes choked with **noisy mucous**. Very difficult to take out.	Antim Tart 200, 1000
• Expectoration full of **pus in humid asthma**.	Bacillinum 200
• Large pieces of **casts of bronchial tubes** thrown out while coughing.	Calcarea Acetica 30
• **Green mucous** with **high fever**. Pneumonia.	Calcarea Iod 30
• Chronic cough.	
• Thick, **lumpy secretions** from lungs. White or yellow.	Calcarea Sulph 30
• Pus in lungs.	
• Expectoration of **pure blood in pneumonia**.	Ferrum Phos 30
• Spitting of **pure blood while coughing**.	Millefolium 200
• Bleeding from lungs with **nausea and wheezing**. In bronchitis, in asthma.	Ipecac 200
• **Glutinous**, yellow, or green mucous flowing down the throat. **Difficult to take out**.	Kali Bichrome 200
• Expectoration thick, yellow, or green, bland, **easily coming out** with loose cough in the morning.	Pulsatilla 30
• Thick, yellow, **lumpy** with violent cough.	Silicea 200
• Thick but easy expectoration.	Tuberculinum 200
• Hard, hacking cough. Rales all over the chest.	
• Profuse sweating. **Loss of weight**. In **tuberculosis**.	

INFANTS/CHILDREN

Distinguishing symptoms of the patient	Medicine and potency
• **Croup. Dry cough**. • On **exposure** to dry, cold air. • **Frightened**, restless. • Sudden attack at midnight.	Aconite Nap 30
• Lungs do **not yield mucous**. • Terrible **rattling sound audible** across rooms.	Antim Tart 200
• Bronchitis. **Severe hacking pain** in the centre of the **rib cage.** • **First remedy in Bronchitis**.	Bryonia 200 Use with Antim Tart 200 if phlegm does not yield. Use Pulsatilla 30 as well, if the phlegm is green and comes out easily.
• Bronchitis. Severe pain in the centre of the rib cage. • **Rapid wheezing** and loss of breath. • Pneumonia. Chest loaded with **mucous. Nausea**, vomiting. • Face pale, turning blue.	Ipecac 200
• Snuffles. **Nose blocked**.	Nux Vomica 200
• **Bronco-pneumonia** in children. Further, refer '*Croup*' above.	Tuberculinum 200

LUNG CANCER

Malignant growth in one or both the lungs. Cigarette smoking is one of the major causes of lung cancer.

Symptoms: Terrible, persistent cough. Yellow/green sputum. Red or brown blood in sputum. Difficult breathing. Sharp chest pain, worse on inhaling. Wheezing. Abnormal curvature of the finger nails.

In some cases, no symptoms appear until the cancer has advanced.

Early detection helps. Give up smoking. **Follow your doctor's advice**.

Further, refer the chapter, '*Cancer*'.

Distinguishing symptoms of the patient	Medicine and potency
• Coughing up of **pure blood**.	Millefolium 200
• **Streaks of blood** in mucous from the lungs.	Phosphorus 200
• Thick, **yellow, lumpy mucous**. Violent cough.	Silicea 200

OLD PERSONS, PROBLEMS OF

Distinguishing symptoms of the patient	Medicine and potency
• **Inability** to take out noisy rattling mucous. Lungs' function weak.	Antim Tart 200
• **Chronic catarrh** of the lungs.	Bacillinum 200
• Enfeebled pulmonary circulation.	
• Bronchial affliction along with **cardiac dilation**.	Baryta Mur 30
• **Asthma** in aged persons. Extreme **debility**.	Carbo Veg 200
• Face blue. Imperfect oxygenation.	
• **Poor digestion. Acidity**.	
• Bronchitis in **old, exhausted** persons.	Hydrastis 200
• Thick, yellow, tenacious expectoration.	

PAIN

Distinguishing symptoms of the patient	Medicine and potency
• **Sudden** pain in the chest on **exposure** to dry, cold air. In **pleurisy**.	Aconite Nap 30

• Pain caused by **injury** to chest, bones, and cartilages.	Arnica 200
• Severe pain in the **upper right** lung.	Arsenic Alb 200
• Severe pain in **larynx**.	Belladonna 200
• Soreness of **muscles and bones** in influenza.	Eupatorium Perf 200
• **Left lung** sore.	Oxalic Acid 30
• **Loss of voice** with cardiac problems.	
• Larynx painful. **Cannot talk**.	Phosphorus 200
• Sharp stitches and heat in the chest.	

Refer '*Pleurisy*' and '*Pneumonia*' below.

PARALYSIS OF LUNGS

Distinguishing symptoms of the patient	Medicine and potency
• Inability to take out coarse, rattling, noisy mucous.	Antim Tart 200 Please refer Carbo Veg in '*Pneumonia*' below.

PLEURISY

An inflammation of the two-layered membrane which separates the lungs from the chest wall. It can be wet or dry.

Symptoms: Movement caused by breathing results in sharp, stabbing chest pain. Rise in temperature. Shallow, rapid breathing. Difficult breathing.

Distinguishing symptoms of the patient	Medicine and potency
• **High fever**. Fast pulse. • Stitching **pain in a fixed spot** in the chest.	Aconite 30

- Hot skin. Great thirst.
- **Superficial**, hurried, short respiration.
- Aggravation by breathing, coughing, sneezing.
- Because of an **injury** to the chest wall in an accident.　　Arnica 200
- Sharp hacking pain in the **centre of the chest**　　Bryonia 200 while coughing. No mucous expectoration.
- Persistent, **high fever**.
- Pain **worse on movement**, on coughing, even on breathing.
- Seat of pain **sensitive to pressure**.
- **High fever**. Accumulation of pus in the　　Hepar Sulph 200 pleura. **Chronic pus**.
- Repeated attacks of chilliness, fever, sweat. Extreme debility.
- Pleura-**pneumonia** of the **right side**.　　Kali Iod 30 Cannot lie on this side. Difficulty in breathing.
- Complications of the heart.
- **Acute** stabbing pain in the chest.　　Ranunculus B 30 Chest sore, tender to touch.
- Inflammation and **swelling** in pleura.
- Short and oppressed breathing.

PNEUMONIA

An acute inflammation of the alveoli [air sacs] of the lungs.

Symptoms: High fever, delirium, confusion, rapid breathing, dry, persistent cough, pain in the chest, rusty blood in sputum.

In infants, high fever is accompanied by rapid respiration in which the lower ribs are drawn inwards.

Seek medical advice.

Distinguishing symptoms of the patient	Medicine and potency
• Acute, sudden inflammation. Terrible shortness of breath. • Mucous streaked with **blood**. • **High fever**. • Dry, croupy cough • Fear of death, anxiety. **First remedy for Pneumonia**.	Aconite Nap 30 Repeat at 30 minutes interval in acute cases. As the patient stabilizes, shift to 200 potency, four times a day.
• **Inability to take out** noisy mucous lodged in the lungs.	Antim Tart 200, 1000 Use with other indicated remedies.
• **Chronic** pneumonia with **abscess** in the lungs. **High fever**.	Arsenic Iod 30
• **Last stage. Face blue**. Gasping for breath. • Foul smelling sputum. • Threatened paralysis of the lungs.	Carbo Veg 200 With Antim Tart 200 in case mucous does not yield.
• Pneumonia with expectoration of **pure blood**.	Ferrum Phos 30
• **Infantile** pneumonia.	Ipecac 200
• **Pulse weak, rapid, irregular**. • Heart failure apprehended.	Strophanthus 30

TICKLING

Distinguishing symptoms of the patient	Medicine and potency
• In larynx. **Hoarseness**. • Violent, rapid inflammation. **Hacking cough**.	Allium Cepa 200
• Extremely bothersome, unpleasant tickling in palate, nose, eyes. **Acute onset of cold**.	Arundo 200

TUBERCULOSIS

A destructive infectious disease affecting virtually every part of the body. However, the lungs are the most common site. Tuberculosis of the lungs is called pulmonary tuberculosis or consumption. There can be tuberculosis of the brain or of the bones or of the gastrointestinal tract.

Avail of the best medical help. Very effective treatments are available.

Symptoms: No symptoms to begin with except a dry cough and a feeling of unease. However, later, persistent cough producing green/ yellow mucous, at times streaked with blood, pain in the chest while inhaling, fever, shortness of breath, weight loss, poor appetite, fatigue, and excessive sweat at night.

Distinguishing symptoms of the patient	Medicine and potency
• Pulmonary tuberculosis with **constant rattling** of mucous in bronchi. • **Severe pain** in the chest. • Mucous difficult to take out.	Allium Sativum 30
• **Early stages** of pulmonary tuberculosis, caused by **influenza**. • Emaciation. • Intense thirst but **cold-water distresses**. Hot drinks preferred.	Arsenic Iod 30
• To clear congestion of lungs, to decrease sputum formation, and make it less purulent **before other medicines are administered**.	Bacillinum 200 Begin treatment with this remedy. One dose a day for 3 days.
• **Last stages** of pulmonary tuberculosis. • Cough shakes the head, **rattles the brain**, and is distressful. • Sputum full of **offensive pus**. • **Suffocating hoarseness**.	Carbo Animalis 30
• Tuberculosis of larynx. **Chronic hoarseness**.	Mag Aceticum 30

• Stitches in larynx, extending into ears.	
• Bloody, **rusty, sputum full of pus**.	Phosphorus 200
• Hoarse, violent, tickling cough. Chest oppressed.	Once a day until cured. **Primary drug for tuberculosis**.

VOICE LOST/HOARSENESS

Distinguishing symptoms of the patient	Medicine and potency
• Total loss of voice in professional **singers**.	Arg Nit 200
• **Chronic** laryngitis.	
• Due to **overuse** of voice.	Arnica 200
• Larynx raw, dry, tickling	Chamomilla 200
• Patient **irritable**.	
• In **whooping cough** patients.	Drosera 30
• Voice **deep** and hoarse.	
• Paralysis of larynx because of **hysteria**. **Nervous** hoarseness.	Gelsemium 200
• **Complete loss** of voice with **wheezing**, nausea. Acute cases.	Ipecac 200
• **Paralysis** of vocal cords.	Lachesis 200
• Nervous loss of voice with cardiac derangement.	Oxalic Acid 30
• **Left lung** painful.	
• **Inflammation of the larynx**. Terrible pain.	Phosphorus 200
• Accumulated mucous	
• Thirst for cold water.	
• **Capricious** hoarseness: comes and goes.	Pulsatilla 30
• Loose cough. **Bland, green mucous**. Refer '*Hoarseness*' under '*The Throat*' as well.	

WHEEZING

Distinguishing symptoms of the patient	Medicine and potency
• Wheezing **for any reason**. In bronchitis, in asthma. • Suffocative cough. Constant constriction in chest. • **Heaviness in the throat**. • Child stiff, **blue**.	Ipecac 200

WHOOPING COUGH

A bacterial infection which causes bouts of severe coughing. It affects infants and children who have not been immunized against it. At the end of a spasm, there is a sudden, noisy drawing in of breath. Cough is followed by vomit.

Symptoms: Severe, repeated bouts of cough as described above. Vomiting. Cold. Running nose. Large amount of sputum during the coughing fit.

Go in for immunization.

The medicines are indicated under *'Cough.'*

THE DIGESTIVE SYSTEM

"Other men live to eat, whereas I eat to live", wrote Socrates, the Greek philosopher, four hundred years before Christ. In this brief sentence, he described the functions of the digestive system and the precautions one ought to take to eat well in order to live healthy.

Our body needs a tremendous amount of energy to live, to function. The food we take, supplies us with this energy. However, the process of the release of energy by food is complicated and elaborate. The digestive tract performs this function with the help of enzymes, hormones, nervous impulses, and systematic muscular action.

The digestive tract consists of the mouth, the pharynx, the oesophagus, the small intestines and the large intestines. It ends in the rectal canal and the anus, each organ performing different tasks.

In its functioning, the digestive system is helped by the teeth, the tongue, the spleen, the liver, the gall bladder, and the pancreas.

Food consists of starches, proteins, vitamins, fats, water, and minerals. All these have to be broken down for absorption into the blood stream. As we eat, our teeth chew the food. Simultaneously saliva, supplying liquid and enzymes, is mixed into the mouthful in order to help digestion. Almost without a change, this mixture passes through the throat and the oesophagus into the stomach.

The function of oesophagus, a muscular tube linking the pharynx with the stomach is to propel the food, liquids, or solids, into the stomach. Any inflammation of oesophagus can obstruct this vital function.

A digestive enzyme contained in the saliva, converts starches into maltose, a form of sugar which is soluble. In the stomach, the food is

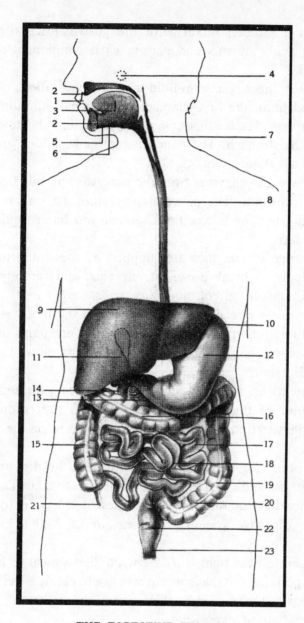

THE DIGESTIVE SYSTEM
1. Mouth. 2. Teeth. 3. Tongue. 4. Parotid gland. 5. Sub-lingual gland. 6. Sub maxillary gland. [Glands at 4, 5 and 6 produce saliva.] 7. Pharynx. 8. Oesophagus. 9. Liver. 10. Spleen. 11. Gall bladder. 12. Stomach. 13. Pancreas. 14. Duodenum. 15. Ascending colon. 16. Transverse colon. 17. Small intestine. 18. Ileum. 19. Descending colon. 20. Large intestine. 21. Appendix. 22. Rectum. 23. Anal canal.

mixed as in a kitchen mixer with the gastric juice consisting of hydrochloric acid, mucous and pepsin, each component assisting in different tasks.

From the stomach, the semi-fluid mass of food called chime, moves into the duodenum, the first chamber of the small intestine. Here the chime encounters alkaline digestive juices as against the acidic juices it had met in the stomach. The pancreas, the gall bladder, and the liver supply these alkaline juices.

At this stage, the enzymes from the pancreas and bile from the liver break down the food. The pancreatic enzymes act on carbohydrates, proteins, and fats. The bile, a thick, green, and bitter liquid, helps in emulsifying fats.

A vast range of enzymes are supplied by the lining in the small intestine helping to break down fat, proteins, and carbohydrates into amino acids, glucose, glycol, and fatty acids.

The food is now ready for absorption into the blood stream. This is done in the jejunum and the ileum, which are parts of the small intestine. Most of the nutrients are carried by the blood into the liver for further digestion.

The nutrients are absorbed into the blood stream through the veins. The remainder of the food moves down into the colon and after progressive dehydration, it is passed out of the body via the rectum and the anal canal.

It takes hours for the food to pass through the digestive tract. It is the oesophagus and the stomach that enable us to take in a substantial quantity of food at one time. It is then digested at leisure. In an average lifetime, the digestive system processes almost 30,000 kilograms of food.

Thus, Socrates was right when he wrote that we eat to live. He was also right in pointing out that some others live to eat. It is here that many human beings go wrong and suffer severe consequences of a wrong choice of food or of overeating.

The quality of life depends not only on the 'liver', the organ but also on the liver, the person who lives it. The 'liver' produces bile, stores fats, minerals and vitamins, filters blood, converts sugar into glycogen, and performs a host of other metabolic activities. It has the capacity to regenerate itself into its normal state only if the damage caused to its cells is limited. That is where the '*liver of life*', the human being, can save, survive, or destroy himself.

The quality of diet matters. Excessive consumption of alcohol can damage the liver irreversibly. Contaminated food can result in food poisoning and death. Tobacco can lead to lung cancer. Fried food can cause heartburn and indigestion. Overeating, besides causing flatulence and dyspepsia, converts into obesity which, in turn, can lead to heart and respiratory problems.

Regular eating habits go a long way in keeping us healthy and fit for the daily grind. Start your day with a light snack followed by regular, moderate, yet vigorous exercise according to your age. Walk briskly for at least forty-five minutes daily. Swim. Cycle. Play games. Go to the gym.

Make your breakfast the main meal of the day. Be sure to include a lot of fibre, fruit, and green vegetables, toned milk and curds, carbohydrates like oat bran, wheat flakes, and muesli. Add almonds and walnuts. Avoid white bread. Repeat fruit five or six times a day, each time a different one, if possible.

Lunch and dinner ought to be light. Have a light snack every three hours. Indulge in sweets but moderately unless you are a diabetic. Shun alcohol, tobacco, and cholesterol-rich food such as full cream dairy milk, yellow of the eggs, butter, cheese, and red meat.

Do not pile your plate in a buffet. Select a little at one time and relish its taste, aroma, and flavour. Try to stop eating while still hungry and unsatisfied. You do not have to eat all that is on the menu.

Ensure that your diet is well balanced. Besides carbohydrates, proteins and unsaturated fat, it should include vitamins and minerals like calcium and iron.

Besides the content, the hygienic quality of food matters. It must be cooked in the cleanest of utensils and surroundings and eaten in a pleasant environment.

Time your motions for regularity. Never suppress the urge. Take care of constipation in time.

Grief, worry, bad temper, or anger affects the digestion adversely. Peace of mind and happy surroundings help in the better functioning of the digestive process.

ABSCESS OF THE LIVER

Distinguishing symptoms of the patient	Medicine and potency
• **Piercing pain** in the region of the liver when walking, coughing, breathing, or touching it.	Hepar Sulph 200
• Abdomen distended.	
• Chronic cases.	Silicea 200
• **Hands yellow, nails blue**.	
• Colic. Bloated hard abdomen.	
• No appetite. Excessive thirst.	

ACHALASIA OF THE CARDIA

An uncommon disease in which the muscles of the oesophagus do not function properly because of lack of coordination between the muscles and the nerves involved in swallowing.

Symptoms: Difficulty in swallowing liquids or solids. Feels as if food sticks behind the breastbone. At times, severe pain in the chest.

Distinguishing symptoms of the patient	Medicine and potency
• As if a **hard-boiled egg** has been lodged in the oesophagus near the cardiac end.	Abies Nigra 200
• Pain after food intake.	
• The **simplest food distresses**. Digestion slow.	Carbo Veg 200 Take the medicine for a
• **Chronic cases** of difficulty in swallowing.	few weeks.

ACIDITY

The sensation of burning and hot contents of stomach rising behind the breastbone.

Symptoms: Acidic, hot liquid moves upwards in the oesophagus. In hyperacidity, severe pain radiates from the centre of the ribs.

Sitting with back resting against pillows and having cold milk alleviate the symptoms. Do not lie down immediately after a meal. Avoid fried food and spices such as chillies. Eat less and have small portions at two-hourly intervals.

Distinguishing symptoms of the patient	Medicine and potency
• **Shooting pain radiates from the centre point of the ribs in all directions**. Hiatus hernia.	Argentum Nitricum 200
• Hyperacidity. Ulceration in the stomach. **Burning. Constriction**.	
• Colic with distension.	
• Worse after having cold food, sweets, and at night. After a meal. From warmth in any form.	
• **Acidity without much pain**.	Carbo Veg 200
• Foul eructation.	
• Tense flatulence. **Ulceration. Burning sensation**.	
• Results of **overindulgence in food and drink**.	
• Contractive pain extending into chest.	
• Better belching.	
• Worse from fats, butter, coffee, wine, spices, fried food. In the evening.	
• Acute. Chronic.	

You can depend upon these two remedies in cases of acidity. Nothing else gives such speedy relief as these two.

APPENDICITIS

An inflammation of the appendix, a small structure rising from the beginning of the large intestine. Can be acute or chronic.

Comes suddenly and requires immediate medical attention lest it bursts. The appendix is removed surgically.

In chronic cases, attacks of pain occur in the right lower abdomen, quite often for a few months.

Symptoms: In acute appendicitis, the first symptom is intermittent pain on the right side of the abdomen or near the navel. The pain worsens and becomes continuous. It is worse on movement. There is nausea and vomiting. At times, constipation. Foul breath.

Distinguishing symptoms of the patient	Medicine and potency
• **Severe pain** in the right, lower abdomen.	Belladonna 200, 1000 Administer this if Iris
• Worse from shaking. Inability to bear the slightest touch.	Tenax fails or is not available. Similar
• **Vomiting. Throbbing headache**.	symptoms.
• Stitching, burning pain, worse on movement.	Bryonia 200 Give every half an hour
• **Thirst for large quantities of water**.	until pain subsides.
• Pain less when lying on the painful side and by pressure.	
• In case of **nervous patients** suffering in mind as well as body.	Ignatia 1000
• Symptoms similar to those indicated against Belladonna.	Iris Tenax 1000 Start treatment with this.
• Chronic appendicitis.	Lycopodium 1000 once a week to stop recurrence of attacks.

APPETITE—LOSS OF

Distinguishing symptoms of the patient	Medicine and potency
• **Tones up** appetite and digestion. Results in improved mental and physical vigour with weight gain. • Induces **mental exhilaration**, a feeling of general well being. • Helps in **depositing fat**, corrects tissue waste.	Alfa Alfa Mother Tincture, 10 drops five times a day. Continue until its tonic effects are apparent.
• Loss of appetite because of **indigestion**, because of **overeating**.	Antim Crud 200
• Loss of appetite in cases of **hyperacidity**.	Arg Nit 200
• When **overworked**.	Calc Carb 200
• The **simplest food distresses**. • **Slow digestion**. Aversion to milk, fats, and meat. • **Acidity**. Eructation after eating and drinking. • Distension in the stomach. Pain in the liver. • **Revives the entire digestive system**.	Carbo Veg 200
• In persons leading a fast life. Drinking, late nights.	Nux Vom 200

AVERSION TO FOOD

Distinguishing symptoms of the patient	Medicine and potency
Cannot bear the sight of food. **Restlessness**. Great thirst but drinks little at a time.	Arsenic Alb 200
The simplest of foods distresses. **Chronic indigestion and acidity**. Aversion to fats, meats, and milk.	Carbo Veg 200

Aversion to **milk**.	Nat Carb 30
Aversion to fats, warm foods, and drinks.	Pulsatilla 30
Dislike for butter.	

BOWEL—CANCER OF

If detected early, the prognosis is good.

Symptoms: A change in bowel habits. Pain in the abdomen with distension, after eating. Stool contains dark blood and mucous. Unexplained loss of weight, of appetite. Nausea, vomiting.

The patient feels generally sick.

Seek expert medical advice. Use the following medicines as palliatives.

Distinguishing symptoms of the patient	Medicine and potency
• Malignant symptoms. **Oesophagus choked. Nothing seems to pass**.	Arsenic Alb 200
• Gnawing, burning pain in the stomach.	
• Distension with pain.	
• **Ice-cold. Great exhaustion**. All prevailing debility.	
• Hates the sight and smell of food.	
• Unquenchable thirst.	
• Nightly aggravation.	
• **Burning and flatulence in the upper part of the stomach.**	Carbo Veg 200 4 times a day for months.
• As **a general medicine** in the cancer of the bowel with other chosen remedies.	
• Vomiting of **bloody, slimy mucous**. Black or coffee coloured **vomit**.	Crotalus H 200
• **Trembling, fluttering** sensation in the part of the abdomen lying above the stomach.	
• **A sinking sensation** in the stomach.	
• Worse lying on the right side. In spring. In open air. Onset of summer.	

• With this medicine, the patient starts vomiting a **black jelly-like substance** on the first dose and gets relief.	Ornithogalum Mother tincture. One drop in a teaspoonful of water.
• Second dose to be repeated after 48 hours if the reaction does not occur.	
• Ulceration has set in. **Sharp, cutting pain.**	Phosphorus 1000
• **Coffee-coloured vomit**.	Once a week.
• A gone sensation in the abdominal cavity.	
• **Carcinoma of the lower bowel.**	Ruta 200
• **Prolapse of anus** every time there is movement.	
• Tearing, stitching pain in the rectum.	

BURNING/ULCERS

An ulcer is a lesion of the skin or of mucous membrane lining the stomach or duodenum, the first part of the small intestine. It is a result of inflammation, of formation of pus and decay of the surrounding tissue.

Symptoms: Sharp, cutting pain. Loss of appetite. Weight loss. Nausea. Sometimes vomiting. Fullness in the abdomen.

Distinguishing symptoms of the patient	Medicine and potency
• Violent, burning pain in the stomach and chest.	Acetic Acid 30
• Coldness of the skin. **Cold sweat** on the forehead.	
• **Burning thirst. However, cold drinks distress.**	
• Vomits any food.	
• Hiatus hernia. **Hyper-acidity. Pain spreads from the centre of the ribs in all directions.**	Arg Nit 200
• **Ulcer pain. Shooting, gnawing**.	
• Severe distension.	

- **Live coals on fire inside**. Unbearable pain.   Arsenic Alb 200
- Tongue dry, brown, or black.
- Nausea, retching. Vomiting after eating or drinking. Vomit of bile.
- **Hot drinks relieve burning**. Cold drinks or foods do not agree.
- With **acidity** without pain in the   Carbo Veg 200 upper digestive tract.
- **Burning ulcers. Pain in the chest as if coals on fire.**
- Slow digestion
- Eructation. Heaviness. Flatulence.
- Burning in **alimentary canal throughout.**   Iris Veriscolour 200
- **Profuse flow of saliva**. Vomiting.
- Chronic intestinal ulceration.   Kali Bich 200

CHOLERA

An acute, intestinal infection. Often a fatal disease. It is caused by bacteria in contaminated food.

Symptoms: Profuse rice water diarrhoea, vomiting, cramps, dehydration.

Emergency. Call a doctor. Urgent hospital treatment is required to replace lost minerals and fluids.

Meanwhile administer *Veratrum Alb* 1000 immediately.

Give plenty of glucose water [boiled and cooled], with a pinch of salt added.

Complete rest is advised.

For medicines, refer '*Cholera*' under '*The Stool*'.

CIRRHOSIS OF THE LIVER

A chronic condition of the liver in which the damaged cells are replaced by scar tissues. The condition is more or less permanent.

Mostly, it is caused by excessive intake of alcohol. Eventually cirrhosis leads to liver failure and death.

Because there are no obvious symptoms, cirrhosis is not diagnosed early.

Symptoms: Any loss of weight, appetite, fatigue, weakness, disinterest in sex, shrinking testicles, a feeling of numbness in feet and fingers, anaemic, pale complexion, yellow in the whites of the eye, ought to sound a warning to persons fond of a drink too many.

You need medical advice at the earliest. Timely action can stall the progress of the disease.

Distinguishing symptoms of the patient	Medicine and potency
• Skin **yellow**, wilted, cold, clammy. Jaundice.	Chelidonium 30
• **Eyes** dirty **yellow**. **Tongue** yellow. Bitter taste. **Urine copious, yellow, and foamy**. Bright, pasty stool.	
• Enlarged liver	
• **Constant pain under the inferior angle of the right scapula.**	
• Preference for hot food and drinks. Temporary relief on eating.	
• **Chronic** swelling of the liver with jaundice.	Chionanthus 30
• **Constipation**. No appetite	
• Liver painful to touch	
• Skin, tongue, stool, yellow. **Urine dark. Bile in urine**.	
• Liver enlarged and tender.	Merc Sol 200
• **Profuse anaemia.**	
• **Skin ever moist and itching.**	
• Deficient bile secretion.	
• Cirrhosis caused by **excessive intake of liquor.**	Nux Vomica 200
• No thirst. Despondency.	
• Disseminated through blood.	Phosphorus 200
• Liver sore. **Degenerated with fat deposits. Congested**.	
• **Large yellow spots on the abdomen.**	
• **Stool greyish**, white.	

COLIC

An acute abdominal pain which comes in paroxysms. It is caused by spasm, obstruction, or distension of intestines and other hollow organs nearby. Often a condition of early infancy.

Symptoms: Severe pain. Chronic irritability and crying.

Distinguishing symptoms of the patient	Medicine and potency
• No relief from bending up double.	Chamomilla 200
• Pain with **numbness**.	
• Occasioned by anger. Uncivil behaviour. Irritable.	
• **In children**. Distension. **Child tosses in agony**.	
• **Terrible, tightening pain** made **slightly less by bending double** or pressing something hard against the stomach.	Colocynthis 200
• Neuralgic colic caused by anger, annoyance.	
• **Vomiting because of pain**.	
• Pain begins at the umbilicus and radiates all over the abdomen, chest, back, arms and legs.	Dioscorea 200
• Sharp pain from **liver to right nipple**. From **gall bladder to chest.**	
• Belches **offensive gas**. Too much flatus.	
• A sinking feeling in the pit of the stomach.	
• Pain aggravated by bending forward.	
• Relief on standing erect, in open air, by pressure.	
• Comes and goes **like lightning.**	Magnesia Phos 200
• **Uterine** colic. Painful menstruation.	
• Neuralgic pain in **extremities**, in face, stomach, pelvis, uterus.	
• **Cramps always present.**	

- Better by bending double, rubbing, pressure, and hot application.
- Abdominal wall feels **drawn to the spine with a string.** Plumbum 200
- Obstructed flatus. Intense colic.
- Colic alternates **with delirium.**
- Constant vomiting. **Constriction in oesophagus**. Difficulty in swallowing solids.
- In cholera. **Non-stop retching**. White rice-like **water stool**. Veratrum Alb 200, 1000
- **Cold sweat**. Collapse.

COLITIS

A chronic problem caused by inflammation of the lower bowel.

Symptoms: Severe pain like a cramp, in the abdomen. Constant pressure in the rectum. Watery diarrhoea, at times with mucous and blood.

Distinguishing symptoms of the patient	Medicine and potency
• Violent burning pain in stomach and chest. **Ulceration.**	Acetic Acid 30
• **Haemorrhage** from bowels.	
• Cold sweat.	
• Burning thirst but **cold drinks distress.**	
• Cannot retain any food.	
• With **offensive diarrhoea.**	Lachesis 200
• Haemorrhage from bowels **like charred straw.**	
• Bowels **perforated by ulcers**, severe pain.	
• Constant pressure in the rectum but no stool.	
• Paroxysmal hot **flushes**.	

- Chill in the back. **Feet cold**.
- Stool **bloody, slimy, hot, and offensive.**   Merc Cor 30
  Shreds of mucous membrane.
- Cutting pain.
- **Tenesmus**. Not relieved by stool.
- Fever and chill. Profuse perspiration.
- Burning, painful, **weight-like pressure**.   Sulphur 200
- Severe acidity.   Start the treatment with a
- Complete loss of appetite.   dose of Sulphur twice a
- Frequent **flushes of heat.**   day. Most effective.
- Feels weak around 11 a m.
- **Chronic diarrhoea of mucous and blood.**   Trillium 30
- **Faints. Feels dizzy.**

CONSTRICTION

Distinguishing symptoms of the patient	Medicine and potency
• Of oesophagus. As if, a **hard-boiled egg** is lodged at the cardiac end.	Abies Nigra 200 **Remarkable results.**
• Resistance to **any food going down** the oesophagus.	
• Can swallow **only liquids.**	Baptista 30
• **Vomiting** due to spasm in the oesophagus.	
• Inflammation in the stomach. **Ulcers.**	
• In cases with **heart problems.**	Cactus 30

Further, refer '*Oesophagitis*' and '*Paralysis of oesophagus*' below.

CRAMPS-ABDOMINAL

Spasmodic pain in the abdomen.
Refer '*Pain*' below.

DUODENAL ULCERS

Ulcers which develop where the stomach joins the duodenum, the first few inches of the small intestine. Ulcers in the duodenum.

Symptoms: Burning, gnawing pain below the ribs. Starts after a meal and continues between two meals. Relieved by milk and food.

For medicines, refer '*Acidity*' and '*Burning/Ulcers*' above and '*Pain*' below.

DYSPEPSIA

Discomfort and pain in the upper central part of the abdomen. Normally it occurs because of a wrong choice of food. It is accompanied by eructation and nausea.

For medicines, refer '*Indigestion*' and '*Pain*' below.

ERUCTATION

To eject gas spasmodically, noisily from the stomach through the mouth.

Distinguishing symptoms of the patient	Medicine and potency
• Eructation tasting of food recently taken. • **Constant belching** after a meal. • **Foul smell. Stinking flatus.** • Result of habitual overeating.	Antim Crud 200
• **Despite effort cannot belch.** • Loss of appetite. Feeble digestion.	Arg Nit 200
• Rancid, sour, putrid eructation. • **Acidity**. Indigestion. Slow appetite. Tense flatulence. • The **slightest of food distresses.**	Carbo Veg 200
• Indigestion due to intake of fermented food like cabbage.	Lycopodium 200

- **Passes wind all the time**. Gluttonous.
- **Burning eructation** near pharynx.
- After intake of **too much** greens,   Pulsatilla 30
  fruit and fat.
- **No thirst.**

FLATULENCE

Excessive formation of gas in the stomach or intestine. Caused by taking food fast and simultaneously swallowing air.

Symptoms: Abdomen bloated like a tent. A feeling of heaviness and discomfort.

Avoid foods which produce gas in the abdomen.

Distinguishing symptoms of the patient	Medicine and potency
• Distension with **palpitation of heart**.	Abies Can 30
• **Colic during stool**. Pain around navel.	Aloe 200
• Abdomen bloated. **Hot**, copious **flatus**. **Loud, rumbling**.	
• **Insecurity** of rectum.	
• **Upwards eructation**, sour and putrid.	Carbo Veg 200
• **Acidity all the time.**	
• No food agrees.	
• Abdomen **bloated like a tent**. Tense.	China 200
• **Belching gives no relief.**	
• No relief from eructation or passing of wind.	
• Distended like a drum. Food fermenting inside.	Lycopodium 200
• **Wind pressing and leaking downwards.**	
• Stomach full even after a light meal.	
• **Palpitation**.	
• Obstructed flatus with intense colic.	Plumbum Met 30
• **Post operative** flatulence.	Raphanus 30
• No flatus, upwards or downwards.	
• **Backache** due to flatulence.	Staphysagria 200

FOOD POISONING

Distinguishing symptoms of the patient	Medicine and potency
• Poisoning from **decayed food** or fruit or meat left in the open. • Unbearable pain. **Restlessness. Burning.** • **Black, bloody diarrhoea.**	Arsenic Alb 200

GALLSTONES

Formation of hard, stone like masses in the gall bladder. Result of chronic inflammation of the gall bladder. A common problem. **Consult a surgeon if the medicines below do not help.**

Symptoms: Severe or mild pain in upper abdomen. Often sets in the evening after a fatty meal. Nausea and vomiting.

Distinguishing symptoms of the patient	Medicine and potency
• Stitches **in gall bladder area.** • Worse pressure.	Berberis Vulgaris 200
• Prevents formation of gallstones. Helps in expulsion. • **Chronic** cases.	Chelidonium 30
• Pain in the region of the liver as from ulceration. Worse touch.	China 200

GASTRIC ULCERS

Ulcers in the lining of the stomach.

Symptoms: Burning, gnawing pain in the upper abdomen, below the ribs. It generally occurs in the early hours of the morning. Pain after a meal.

For medicines, refer *'Acidity'*, *'Burning/Ulcers'* and *'Pain'* in this chapter.

GASTRITIS

An acute or chronic inflammation of the lining of the stomach.

Symptoms: In acute gastritis, besides pain in the upper abdomen and nausea with vomiting, there is blood in the vomit. The attack comes because of intake of alcohol or infected food.

In chronic gastritis, the treatment is according to symptoms.

For medicines, refer *'Indigestion'*, *'Nausea'*, and *'Pain'* below.

GASTROENTERITIS

Inflammation of the lining of the stomach and the intestines due to infection.

Symptoms: Cramp-like abdominal pain. Nausea and vomiting. Diarrhoea. Fever, often with headache.

For medicines, refer *'Nausea'* and *'Pain'* below.

GIARDIASIS

An intestinal infection caused by a small parasite called *giardia lamblia*.

Symptoms: Diarrhoea with profuse and watery or bulky, loose, breezy stool. The patient feels restless and weak. Distension in the stomach.

Distinguishing symptoms of the patient	Medicine and potency
• Stomach hard and bloated. • **Twisting pain about navel.** • Stool preceded by colic. It has white **mucous formed like popcorn**. • Irritable, cross, hungry.	Cina 200

HEPATITIS

An inflammation of the liver. Can be acute or chronic.

Symptoms: Severe loss of appetite. Nausea and vomiting. Headache. Pain in the joints. A general feeling of being ill. Fever. As jaundice develops, the patient passes dark urine, and a light coloured stool.

Jaundice fades after two to four weeks. At times, it may take months.

Relapse occurs often in hepatitis. Complications can result in cirrhosis of the liver and scarring. Liver failure ultimately leads to death.

Seek medical advice as soon as hepatitis is detected.

The medicines below will help.

The patient must compulsorily rest in bed and take a diet high in calories, low in proteins and free of fats.

The patient's saliva, urine, and stool is infective. Take precautions if someone has to handle the patient's bedpans or clothes.

For medicines, refer '*Cirrhosis of the liver*' *above*, and '*Jaundice*', '*Pain*', '*Swelling*' and '*Yellow skin*' below.

HERNIA, FEMORAL

Common in women.

Symptoms: A cherry-size bulge grows below the middle of the groin crease.

Distinguishing symptoms of the patient	Medicine and potency
• Strangulated femoral hernia.	Plumbum Met 30

HERNIA, HIATUS

Protrusion of a portion of the stomach through a rupture in the diaphragm.

Symptoms: Severe, unbearable pain beyond the breastbone, often after a meal. Pain radiates in all directions from its centre. Worsened by tight clothing around the waist and sitting bending forward for any reason after having food. Cutting heartburn because acid and semi-digested food spill up into the oesophagus.

At times, these symptoms can be confused with a heart attack. **A proper diagnosis is essential. Talk to a doctor.**

The medicines given under *'Acidity'*, *'Burning/Ulcers'*, and *'Pain'* are of great help. Most of the time one dose of Arg Nit 200 relieves the pain. **Taken over a few days, it is almost a cure.**

However, the patient ought to change his eating habits. He has to cut down on fried food, alcohol, tobacco, or coffee. He must avoid bending forward while working at an office table or before a computer. An hour must pass before he lies down after a meal. He should avoid wearing tight clothes around his waist.

HERNIA, INGUINAL

Protrusion of intestines or other contents of the abdomen through a gap in the groin.

Symptoms: Swelling in the groin or scrotum.
Mostly, surgery is the only way out.

Distinguishing symptoms of the patient	Medicine and potency
• Inguinal hernia.	Calc Carb 30
• Hernia of the **right side.**	Lycopodium 1000
• **Distension** of the stomach. **Rumbling** sounds.	One dose every weak.
• **Left side.**	Nux Vomica 1000
	One dose every weak.

HERNIA, UMBILICAL

Babies suffer from umbilical hernia.

Symptoms: Round swelling near the navel.

Distinguishing symptoms of the patient	Medicine and potency
• Umbilical hernia in babies.	Aurum Met 200
• Umbilical hernia in babies.	Calc Carb 30

HICCUP

Involuntary and repetitive spasm of the diaphragm. Caused by an irritation of the nerve cells that control the contraction of the diaphragm.

By and large, hiccup is not a serious problem. Common in young infants. Need not cause any worry.

Distinguishing symptoms of the patient	Medicine and potency
• Hiccups.	Calc Fluor 30
• Violent, spasmodic.	Cicuta 200
• Followed by copious **vomiting.**	Jatropha 30
• **Violent.**	Ratanhia 200

INDIGESTION

A set of symptoms usually referred to as stomach upsets. It is caused by wrong eating habits like overeating, having rich or spicy food, eating in a hurry, by natural production of excessive acid in the stomach and weakness of the digestive system.

Tension, strain, and anxiety also cause indigestion and so does excessive fondness for alcohol or aerated waters.

Symptoms: A feeling of fullness in the stomach. Heart burn, acidity, nausea and/or vomiting. Accumulation of wind in the stomach. Distension. Cramps in the abdomen and the intestines. Constipation or diarrhoea. At times, lack of appetite.

Distinguishing symptoms of the patient	Medicine and potency
• From **overeating.**	Antimony Crud 200
• Nausea, fullness, and discomfort.	
• **Foul eructation** as soon as food is eaten.	
• Stomach distended though flat.	
• Milk coated tongue.	
• Hyperacidity. **Shooting pain in the centre of the ribs radiating all over.**	Arg Nit 200
• **Perforating ulcers in the stomach. Cutting pain.**	
• Vomiting of food.	
• Flatulence relieved by belching.	
• Longing for sweets although it aggravates and causes diarrhoea.	
• **Burning pain** in the stomach.	Arsenic Alb 200
• Results of **food poisoning.**	
• **Convulsive vomiting** of water, food, bile.	
• Slimy, bloody stool of **undigested food.**	
• Great prostration. Nightly aggravation.	
• **The slightest of food distresses.**	Carbo Veg 200
• **Acidity without much pain. Lack of appetite.**	
• **Ulcers** in the stomach. **Burning** in the stomach extending to spine.	
• Flatulence. Eructation.	
• Stomach **distended like a tent**. Colic caused by flatulence. No relief on passing wind or on belching.	China 200
• Gastritis pain, worse on left side, under the ribs, extending downwards.	
• Flatulence because of having food that	Lycopodium 200

ferments inside the system. **Foul wind
passing downwards.**
- **Burning eructation.**
- **Palpitation.**
- **Nausea** because of indigestion.   Ipecac 200
- **Vomit of undigested food.**
- Unyielding cases of gastritis where
  even a drop of water does not
  get digested.
- **Fermented stools**, foaming like
  yeast, with mucous.
- Sharp pain travelling from left to right
  in the stomach.
- Result of **irregular eating habits, of**   Nux Vom 200
  late nights, of liquor consumption.
- Constipation. Pain. Pressure and
  uneasiness in the rectum.
- Frequent desire to pass stool but can
  pass just a small quantity each time.
- Indigestion due to **excessive intake of**   Pulsatilla 30
  cakes, fruit, and creamy food.
- **Loss of taste. Loss of smell.**
- No thirst. Mouth dry
- Pain in the stomach an hour after a meal.
- Chronic constipation. Stool dry, hard,
  and difficult to expel.

JAUNDICE

Yellowish discolouration of the whites of the eye, skin, and mucous membranes caused by deposits of bile salts in these tissues. It occurs as a symptom of various diseases, such as hepatitis, that affect the processing of bile.

Old and damaged blood cells break down in the spleen to produce yellow pigment known as bilirubin. Normally this pigment is removed by the liver and discharged as bile into the intestines. When this process slows down, bilirubin collects in the blood and causes yellow discoloration all over the body. The skin and white of the eye take on a yellow colour. Urine becomes dark and the colour of the stool turns creamy.

The patient requires complete bed rest and treatment of the cause which might have led to jaundice.

For medicines, refer 'Cirrhosis of the liver', 'Hepatitis' above and 'Pain', 'Swelling' and 'Yellow skin' below.

MORNING SICKNESS

Pregnant women in the first few weeks of pregnancy experience nausea and vomiting.

Distinguishing symptoms of the patient	Medicine and potency
• **Persistent nausea**. No relief from vomit.	Ipecac 200

Please refer 'Nausea/Vomiting' below.

MUCOUS/DYSENTERY

Glutinous, sticky secretions of the mucous membranes.
The following remedies show remarkable results.

Distinguishing symptoms of the patient	Medicine and potency
• In large quantities in stool.	Aloe 200
• **Insecurity in the rectum.**	
• **Violent** tenesmus.	
• **Grass-green stool**. Amoebic dysentery.	Ipecac 200
• Griping pain.	
• **Blood and mucous in dysentery.**	Merc Cor 30
• **Persistent tenesmus**. Cutting pain.	

- Shreds of mucous membrane in stool.   Merc Sol 200
Start with this medicine.

- **Mucous dysentery**. No blood.
- Mucous dysentery with **pain in the thighs.**   Rhus Tox 200
- When Merc Sol or Cor fails.   Sulphur 200

NAUSEA/VOMITING

Symptoms: Feeling sick in the stomach with a desire to vomit. Accompanied by distaste, a loathing for food. The impulse to vomit is involuntary and uncontrollable.

Distinguishing symptoms of the patient	Medicine and potency
• Vomit of **bile, blood, green or brown-black mucous.**	Arsenic Alb 200
• **Food poisoning**. Nausea and retching after having a contaminated meal.	
• Intense nausea but **relief on retching.**	Antim Tart 200
• Body cold. **Cold sweat.**	
• Tongue thick, white. Has **red edges.**	
• Vomits **all fluids.**	Bismuth 30
• Nausea **when rising.**	Bryonia 200
• Pressure like that of a stone in stomach after a meal.	
• Vomit of **green, slimy mucous**. Vomit black.	Cadmium 30
• Vomit of **green, semi-digested food.**	Carbolic Acid 30
• Desire for stimulants and tobacco.	
• Fermentation inside the stomach.	
• In cases where **acidity is prominent.**	Carbo Veg 200
• In pregnancy, early morning.	
• Caused by **pressure on spine** and **cervical region.**	Cimicifuga 200
• During any kind of travel. **Travel sickness.**	Cocculus 200

- **Persistent** nausea, vomiting. **No relief**   Ipecac 200
  from vomiting.   **First remedy**.
- Vomits food, bile, blood or mucous.
- Cutting pain from left to right.
- Fermented, **foamy stool** full of mucous.
- Nausea in **pregnancy**. With **headache.**
  With **fever, chill,** heat and breathlessness.
- **Copious red haemorrhage** in nausea.
- Face pale, twitching.
- Child vomits **curdled milk in large lumps**   Valeriana
  after nursing. Screams violently.   Mother Tincture. 5 drops
      4 times a day.

- Nausea and retching during or   Veratrum Alb 1000
  without **cholera.**   Remarkable effect to stop
- Rice coloured, **watery stools.**   vomiting.
- Chronic vomiting of food.
- Cold sweat.

OESOPHAGITIS

Inflammation of the lower portion of the oesophagus, near the stomach. Caused by irritation by gastric juices.

Symptoms: Heartburn. Regurgitation of acid and food after a heavy meal. Pain on swallowing hot or cold food.

For medicines, refer *'Acidity'*, *'Constriction'* above, and *'Paralysis of oesophagus'* below.

OESOPHAGUS—STRICTURE OF

Spasmodic stricture of the oesophagus.

Symptoms: Vomiting of food immediately after swallowing
This problem requires immediate medical attention.

For medicines, refer *'Constriction'* above and *'Paralysis of the oesophagus'* below.

PAIN/COLIC

Distinguishing symptoms of the patient	Medicine and potency
• Painful spot over stomach, in the centre of the ribs. Piercing pain radiates in all directions. Hiatus hernia pain.	Arg Nit 200
• **Burning and constriction. Ulceration** of the stomach.	
• Hyperacidity.	
• Pain in **food poisoning**. Burning.	Ars Alb 200
• **Black, bloody diarrhoea.**	
• Pain because of enlargement of liver, spleen.	
• Hot food relieves. Cold food disagrees.	
• Spasmodic pain. Feels as if **clutched by a hand.**	Belladonna 200
• **Distension. Burning, cutting pain.**	
• Great thirst for cold water.	
• Stitches in the region of **gall bladder**, in the kidney area, extending to liver, **spleen, stomach, and groin.**	Berberis Vulgaris 30
• Ulcers in the stomach. **Sensation of burning coals.** Constrictive pain.	Carbo Veg 200
• Flatulent colic	
• **Acidity.**	
• From **enlargement of spleen.** Splenitis.	Ceanothus 30
• Pain on the left side.	
• Acute inflammation and pain of duodenum. Pain spreads from the **navel to the small of the back.**	Chamomilla 200
• Child peevish, in great agony.	
• Griping pain in **umbilical region.**	Chionanthus 30
• As if a string is tightened around intestines, then loosened.	
• Pain in enlarged liver, spleen. Jaundice.	

- **Gall stone colic.**
- Colic with **convulsions.**   Cicuta 200
- **Twisting about navel**. Because of   Cina 200
  worms of any type.
- **Severe cutting pain in the abdomen,**   Colocynthis 200
  compelling the patient to bend over.
- Dysenteric stool each time food is
  eaten. **Stool like jelly with foul odour.**
- As if stones are being ground together
  and that the stomach will burst.
- **Colic and cramp in calves.**
- Worse from indignation.
- In **abscess of the liver.**   Hepar Sulph 200
- Pain of amoebic **dysentery**. Worse   Ipecac 200
  around navel.
- **Nausea.**
- In **chronic liver** trouble. Swelling.   Lycopodium 200
- Brown spots on the abdomen.
- **Chronic appendicitis.**
- **Wind passing downwards.**
- Pain in cases of **irregular eating habits**,   Nux Vom 200
  leading a fast life, indulging in alcohol.
- Colic-like pressure from a stone a few
  hours after a meal.
- In gastroenteritis with **loose, yellow** stools,   Podophyllum 200
  gushing, fetid, and bilious vomiting.
- Following abdominal **surgery.**   Staphysagria 200
- In cholera with **nausea. Copious, rice**   Veratrum Alb 1000
  water, non-stop motions.
- **Cold sweat.** Collapse. Face pale.
  Skin blue.

Also, refer '*Peritonitis*' below.

PANCREATITIS-ACUTE

An acute inflammation of the pancreas, a gland near the stomach which produces hormones as well as digestive juices.

Symptoms: Severe abdominal pain, increasing with passage of time. In acute cases, rise in temperature, shock, low blood pressure, vomiting and clammy skin.

A life threatening condition that requires immediate medical attention. Hospitalization may be necessary.

Distinguishing symptoms of the patient	Medicine and potency
• **Haemorrhaging** pancreas. **High fever.**	Belladonna 200
• **Burning distress** in the region of the pancreas.	Iris Veriscolour 30
• Watery stool containing **undigested food.**	
• **Vomit of sweet water.** Saliva greasy.	

PARALYSIS OF THE OESOPHAGUS

Distinguishing symptoms of the patient	Medicine and potency
• As if **a hard-boiled egg is lodged** in oesophagus. Pain in swallowing.	Abies Nigra 200
• A **spasm**, as soon as food enters, causes **gagging and choking.**	Baryta Carb 200
• Can swallow **liquids only.**	Baptisia 30
• **Constriction** of oesophagus. Food does not go down because of a **spasm.**	Cactus 30
• **Paralysis** of oesophagus and of pharynx, at the end of diphtheria.	Causticum 200
• Spasm because of swallowing **sharp bone pieces.**	Cicuta 200

Please refer '*Constriction*' and '*Oesophagitis*' above.

PERITONITIS

An inflammation of the lining of the abdominal cavity due to various causes.

Symptoms: An acute situation. High fever. Darting, burning pain in bowels. Hard swelling in the stomach. Delirium. Stupor. Face puffed.

Seek medical advice.

Distinguishing symptoms of the patient	Medicine and potency
• High fever. Abdomen hot to touch.	Aconite 30
• Burning, cutting pain in the bowels.	
• **Restlessness. Agony. Fear of death.**	
• Aching soreness of the stomach.	Apis 200
Does not tolerate any pressure.	
• Sudden, knife like stabs through the abdomen.	
• **Face bloated.**	
• From an **injury**, a blow. From **confinement.**	Arnica 200
• Pain like a dagger going through a wound.	
• Stomach distended hard.	
• Worse right side.	
• Acute, violent pain. **Spasmodic**.	Belladonna 200
• High fever. **Delirium**. Stupor.	
• Abdomen distended, hot, and painful to touch.	

SWELLING

Medical consultation is advised.

Distinguishing symptoms of the patient	Medicine and potency
• Enlarged liver in **cardiac cases.**	Aurum Met 30
• Cirrhosis. Large quantity of **blood flooding** the liver. Jaundice.	Cardus Marianus 30

- Liver swollen. Hepatic and gall bladder obstruction.   Cheledonium 30
- **Jaundice**. Eyes, skin, yellow. Urine dark. Stool bright and pasty.
- Hard, swollen liver and spleen.   China 200
- **Chronic liver condition.**
- Pain on the right side.
- **Jaundice with constipation.**   Chionanthus 30
- Swollen liver.
- **Chronic liver swelling with flatulence.**   Lycopodium 200
- Brown spots on the abdomen.

TASTE DIMINISHED

Distinguishing symptoms of the patient	Medicine and potency
- In **chronic cold** or due to indigestion. - **Smell diminished**.	Pulsatilla 30

TYPHOID

Please refer under the chapter '*Fevers.*'

WORMS/ROUNDWORMS/TAPEWORMS/ THREADWORMS

Usually children suffer from worms. Many types grow in the abdomen. Harmful organisms in contaminated food or drink enter the body through the mouth.

Symptoms: Worms cause passing of abnormal stool. Sometimes bits of worms are passed in the stool with each motion.

Distinguishing symptoms of the patient	Medicine and potency
• Worms of **any type.** • Face pale, cold. Alternatively, red and hot. • Dark rings around eyes. • Loathing of food. Or, great hunger. • Nausea, vomiting. • Convulsions of head and limbs. • Rolling eyes in restless sleep. • Constant **rubbing of the nose**. • Grinding and **smashing of the teeth**. • Itching of anus.	Cina 200 4 times a day for a fortnight or more until all adverse symptoms have vanished.

YELLOW SKIN

Distinguishing symptoms of the patient	Medicine and potency
• Liver problems. Jaundice. **Foaming yellow urine.** • Tongue yellow. Taste bitter. • **Nausea.**	Cheledonium 30
• Liver enlarged with **constipation.** • **Urine dark**, full of bile and sugar.	Chionanthus 30
• **Cancer of the stomach**. Vomiting of bloody, slimy mucous. • Pain in the region of the liver.	Crotalus H 200
• **Bronze yellow skin.** • Complete jaundice.	Myrica 30
• **Large spots on the abdomen.** • Acute hepatitis. • Cirrhosis of the liver. • Pancreatic diseases.	Phosphorus 200

THE BACK AND THE NECK

The back is the rear part of the human body, extending from the neck to the end of the spine. The neck connects the head and the trunk.

From the neck to the lowermost part of the back, extends the vertebral column, the spine, which holds the body upright, and supports the head. It encircles the spinal cord. It is our backbone.

The vertebral column consists of thirty-three bones, or segments, known as vertebrae, consisting typically of a cylindrical body and an arch through which the spinal cord passes.

The vertebrae in the region of the neck, seven in number, are known as cervical vertebrae. The next twelve are known as thoracic [chest] vertebrae. These lie behind the ribs.

Just below but above the pelvis are five lumbar vertebrae.

The spinal column ends in the sacrum and the coccyx with five and four vertebrae each.

The spine is made flexible by joints and discs of fibrous tissue between most of the vertebrae. Ligaments and muscles stabilize it and control movement.

The discs vary in size according to the location. These consist of shock-absorbing fleshy material. The casing of the disc is made of tough fibres and contains a jelly like substance.

Spinal nerves come out of small holes placed in the side of the vertebral column.

Any dislocation of any part of the spine can lead to pain because the spinal cord is an important part of the central nervous system.

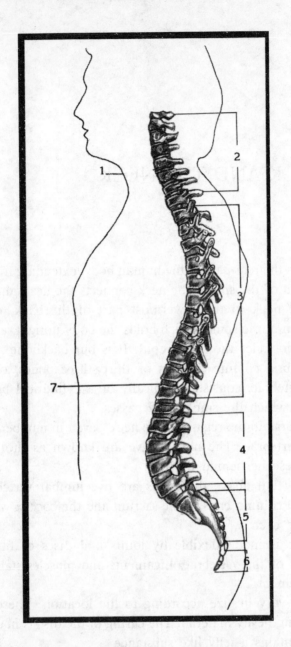

THE BACK AND THE NECK
1. Neck. 2. Cervical vertebrae, 7. 3. Thoracic [chest] vertebrae, 12.
4. Lumbar vertebrae, 5. 5. Sacrum, 5. 6. Coccyx, 4. 7. Intervertebral disc.
The spinal cord runs through the spinal canal of the spinal column.
Not shown here.

Women get a pain in the coccyx sometimes after childbirth. Coccyx pain also occurs after a concussion suffered in a fall.

Most of us have suffered from backache at one time or the other in our lives. Backache is seldom a sign of a serious disorder. Usually some minor strain or injury causes this pain. It can also be due to poor posture, or weak abdominal muscles. A muscular inflammation too can cause back pain.

The lower part of our spine has excellent manoeuvrability. It can bend in all directions. It can rotate. Even a small upset in these movements can cause backache.

The lower back is more often the area of pain because it is not supported by a strong bone formation as the rib cage above. The same is true of the neck.

The human spine is never at rest. It is involved in effort all the time. To this, we can add self-imposed burdens like excessive weight and the pleasant function of being pregnant for a woman.

In the cervical region, an irreversible degeneration leads to cervical spondylosis which is painful and leads to unpleasant giddiness.

A bulging of the discs puts pressure on the nerves next to the bulging disc and generates pain and weakness in muscles. A slipped disc in the lumber region can lead to sciatica or lumbago pain.

With age, we suffer from backache and cervical spondylosis. The bones become weak. Take it easy. Take the prescribed medicines. Take enough rest.

Strengthen your abdominal and back muscles with regular, gentle exercises. Reduce body weight if you are overweight.

Adoption of a correct posture while sitting, working, lifting weight, even while sleeping, helps avoiding backache. Sleep on a firm mattress.

Make sure that your spine is not bent beyond what it can bear. Be natural in your posture. Do not sit or stand in an awkward drooping posture. Do not walk carelessly.

Your working chair should support the small of your back.

Do not stoop to pick things, to lift heavy objects and do not carry heavy articles by yourself. Carry loads evenly balanced in both arms.

Seek guidance from a physiotherapist or get a good book on the subject and follow the directions.

Take calcium supplements under medical advice to strengthen your bones. Ask your dietician about your diet regime.

BACKACHE/LUMBAGO/PAIN

A common complaint but rarely a sign of serious disorder. Usually results from a wrong posture, wrong lifting of weight, from strain or injury.

Symptoms: Aching pain in the back and hips made worse by sitting and relieved by standing. Localized sharp pain in the small of the back. Stiffness. Difficulty in bending. Pain radiating to buttocks and legs. Tingling sensation and numbness.

Distinguishing symptoms of the patient	Medicine and potency
• Backache affecting **sacrum, hips.**	Aesculus 30
• Back and **legs give** way. Weak spine.	
• Pain in the **coccyx.**	
• Worse while walking or stooping.	
• **Cervical muscles twitch**.	Agaricus 200
• Pain in the lumbar region.	
• Severe pain in the back, as if **tightened in a vice.**	Ammonium Mur 30
• **Ice-coldness** between the shoulders.	
• **Violent** pain in sacro-lumbar region.	Antim Tart 200
• Sensation of **heavy weight** in the coccyx.	
• Slightest effort to move causes **retching, cold,** and clammy **perspiration.**	
• Pain caused by an **injury.**	Arnica 200
• Stitching pain in the back, in neck, in the **region of the kidneys**, around abdomen, **hips and groin.**	Berberis Vulgaris 30
• Kidney problems.	
• Pain with **stiffness in the neck, in the small of the back.**	Bryonia 200 First remedy in stiffness
• Worse on movement. Better on strong pressure.	and if pain is worse on movement.
• **Chronic** pain in the **lumbar** region.	Calcarea Fluorica 200
• In late menstruation with **dark blood**.	Calcarea Phos 30
• Unbearable pain in loins and hips.	Chamomilla 200, 1000

- **Numbness.**
- **Irascible** temper.
- **Stiff neck, head** drawn to the **left.**   Chelidonium 30
- Pain under the inner and lower angle
  of the right scapula.
- Sharp pain **across kidneys** as if **stabbed**   China 200
  with knives in the back.
- Worse at night, worse movement.
- Back bent backwards like an **arch.**   Cicuta 200
- Jerking, tearing in **coccyx** during
  menstruation.
- **Spasms and cramps** in the muscles of
  the nape of the neck.
- **Cervical spondylosis.**   Cimicifuga 200
- Rheumatic pain in back, neck,   **First remedy for cervical**
  lumbar, sacral region, down thighs   **spondylosis**. Combine
  and through hips. **All over.**   with Bryonia and Cicuta.
- Backache after **coitus.**   Cobalt 30
- **Small of the back** feels as if paralysed.   Cocculus 30
- Cervical vertebrae **crack** on movement
  of the head.
- From **incarcerated flatulence**, spreading   Cochleria 30
  from abdomen to back and into sacrum.
- **Suppressed** menses. **Prolapsed** uterus.   Helonias 30
- Painful weakness and **dragging** in lumbar.
- Spinal **concussion**. Severe pain.   Hypericum 200
- Injury to **nerves** in the spine.
- Pain in lumbar region, in the small of the   Rhus Tox 200
  back, caused by **exposure, by strain**, by
  getting **drenched** while doing a strenuous
  job or lying on damp sheets.
- Better for a short while on motion, or
  lying on hard surface.
- Pain in **coccyx, in lumbar vertebrae**, as   Ruta 200
  from a blow, from a fall.
- From **incarcerated flatus.**   Staphysagria 200
- Worse in the morning.

BURNING

A sensation caused by problems in parts of the body near the back.

Distinguishing symptoms of the patient	Medicine and potency
• Constant burning in the **kidney region**. Can trace outline.	Helonias 30
• Back tired. Pain running into legs.	
• In overworked women. A sensation of dragging **weight in sacrum and pelvis**.	

CEREBRO–SPINAL MENINGITIS

An acute inflammation of the meninges of the spinal cord and the brain.

Symptoms: High fever. Chronic jerking of the head.
Consult a doctor.

Distinguishing symptoms of the patient	Medicine and potency
• **Delirium**. Acute cerebral infection	Apis 200
• **Shrill cries** in sleep.	
• Chronic headache, **jerking** of the head.	
• Acute dropsy of the brain.	

Refer *'Meningitis'* under *'The Mind, Emotions, the Head, and the Brain'*.

CERVICAL SPONDYLOSIS

Irreversible degeneration of bones and cartilages in the neck leading to pain and stiffness.

Symptoms: Stiffness and aching pain in the neck and shoulders. Severe giddiness. Vertigo, very severe at times. A sensation of numbness and tingling in the fingers. Muscular weakness in the arms and the hands.

Distinguishing symptoms of the patient	Medicine and potency
• **Stiff** neck and shoulders with pain.	Bryonia 200, 1000
• **Numbness**. Tingling in fingers.	Cimicifuga 200,1000
• **Head spins** distressingly. Cannot stand or move erect. Severe vertigo.	
• Pain in **collarbones**.	
• **Spasms and cramps** in the muscles of the neck.	Cicuta 200

A mixture of the above medicines in equal measure gives early relief. If the problem is severe, use 1000 potency and reduce dosage to twice a day.

COCCYDYNIA

Pain develops at the base of the spine because of an injury to the spine. It is worse when the patient is sitting.

More women suffer from Coccydynia than men.

For medicines, refer '*Backache/Lumbago/Pain*' above.

CONCUSSION

Injury or shock to spinal cord, brain, from a fall, a blow.

Distinguishing symptoms of the patient	Medicine and potency
• On **injury** along with Hypericum.	Arnica 200
• **Concussion. Nerves damaged.**	Hypericum 200
• Injury to spine of women during **labour.**	
• Coccyx turns blue, **black. Abscess forms.**	
• Excruciating pain.	

CRACKING

Distinguishing symptoms of the patient	Medicine and potency
• Cracking of cervical **vertebrae** while moving head.	Cocculus 30

CURVED

Distinguishing symptoms of the patient	Medicine and potency
• Back bent backwards **like an arch.**	Cicuta 200

MALIGNANCY

Consult an oncologist.

Distinguishing symptoms of the patient	Medicine and potency
Malignancy in **glands of the neck**.	Cistus Can 30

MYELITIS

Inflammation of the spinal cord.

Distinguishing symptoms of the patient	Medicine and potency
• Inflammation, pain, and stiffness in the **small of the back.** • Pain and stiffness in the nape of the neck. • **Better motion for a moment**, or lying on a hard surface.	Rhus Tox 200

SCIATICA

An abnormal pressure on a part of the sciatic nerve can cause trouble in the back and in the limbs. A sudden pain runs down from the lower back to the legs.

Refer under '*The Extremities*'.

SLIPPED DISC

Degeneration and protrusion of the spinal disc from its position between the vertebrae. The protruded disc puts pressure on spinal nerves, generating pain in the area served by the specific nerve.

Symptoms: Can appear suddenly or develop over a period. Severe pain, tingling, numbness in a leg or in an arm. Stiffness. Restricted movement of the affected limb. Relieved by rest. Made worse by movement, climbing stairs, sneezing, coughing, and even sitting.

Consult an orthopaedic surgeon and a physiotherapist.

The medicines indicated below are of great help.

Distinguishing symptoms of the patient	Medicine and potency
• **Pain with numbness** and tingling in the feet and the legs.	Aconite 30
• **Acute** onset	
• Hip joint and thigh feel **lame** while lying down.	
• **Violent** pain in **sacro-lumbar** region	Antim Tart 200
• Sensation of a **weight at coccyx**. Feels being dragged down.	
• **Gradual onset**.	
• Stitching pain in the **neck and back.**	Berberis Vulgaris 30
• **Numbness** in legs and feet.	
• **Stiffness** with pain. **Worse on movement**.	Bryonia 200
• Slipped disc in the **neck**. Stiffness.	Cimicifuga 200

- Rheumatic pain in the back, **neck, shoulder blades,** lumbar region, through hips, down thighs.
- Severe pain in the **lower back spreading down** one or both legs.   Colocynthis 200
- **Stiffness and numbness** of joints.
- Pain in **lumbar, coccyx**, with stiffness
- **Temporarily better on movement** or lying on a hard surface.   Rhus Tox 200

STIFFNESS

Difficulty in bending or flexing resulting in pain on making such an effort. Uncomfortable rigidity of a part of the body.

Distinguishing symptoms of the patient	Medicine and potency
• Stiff neck with **swollen glands**.	Belladonna 200
• Back stiff with tearing pain.	Berberis Vulgaris 30
• **Post operative pain** in lumbar region.	
• Stiffness **worse on movement.**	Bryonia 200
• In nape of the neck, in small of the back.	**The first medicine in**
• Stitching pain.	**stiffness**.
• Stiff neck and back. Muscles feel as if **bound with a rope.**	Causticum 200
• Can scarcely move the head.	
• **Chronic rheumatic pain. Deformed joints**.	
• Stiffness in the neck with **fixed pain under** the inner and lower angle of the right scapula.	Chelidonium 30
• Stiffness and spondylosis.	Cicuta 200
• **Spasms and cramps** in neck muscles.	
• Stiffness and contraction in **neck and back.**	Cimicifuga 200
• Upper spine sensitive. Severe pain.	
• **Unbearable giddiness**. Cervical spondylosis	

- **Numbness and tingling** in fingers.
- Stiff and painful neck from **catching cold**   Dulcamara 200
  in wet weather.
- **Ice-cold sensation** down spine. Back stiff.   Strychninum 30
- Cervical **muscles rigid**. Sharp pain in
  the neck.

SWELLING

Distinguishing symptoms of the patient	Medicine and potency
• Swollen glands in the **nape of the occiput.**	Baryta Carb 200
• **Cervical glands** enlarged and hardened.	Heckla Lava 30
• **Veins** in the neck swollen.	Opium 200
• **Chronic** swelling in glands of the cervix. **Hard and cold.**	Silicea 200
• Diseases of the **bones in the spine**.	

THE URINARY SYSTEM

The Urinary System performs the function of removal of chemical wastes, excess water etc. from the body in the form of urine. These wastes are produced when enzymes act upon various nutrients to release the energy from the food we take.

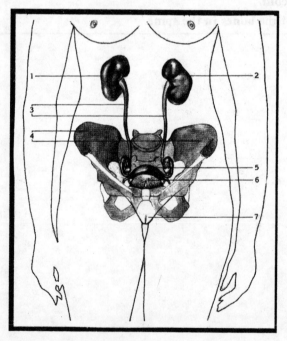

FEMALE URINARY SYSTEM
1. Right kidney. 2. Left kidney. 3. Ureters. 4. Hip bone. 5. Uterus.
6. Urinary bladder. 7. Urethra.

The urinary system is made up of the kidneys, the ureters, the bladder, and the urethra. The ureters, narrow pipes, connect each kidney to the bladder. Urine flows through them, collects in the bladder and from time to time leaves the body through the urethra.

The bloodstream brings the chemicals for filtration to the kidneys where the waste products and excess water are removed. If this process is interrupted, it can be life-threatening.

The kidneys are situated on either side of the spinal cord immediately above the waist. A million filtering units called glomeruli carry out the purification of blood.

While filtering the blood the kidneys produce urine. Further, they keep the blood levels of water, salts, and acid at a proper and constant level.

The purification of blood is a round the clock process. A little less than 1.5 litres of urine are passed from the human body in a period of 24 hours.

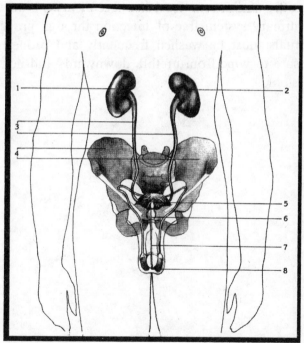

MALE URINARY SYSTEM
1. Right kidney. 2. Left kidney. 3. Ureters. 4. Hip bone. 5. Urinary bladder.
6. Prostate gland. 7. Urethra. 8. Urethral opening.

The kidneys can be inflamed or damaged by external injury. This reduces the efficiency of the filtering mechanism. Bladder infections too can travel to the kidneys.

The kidneys can fail leading to serious consequences.

Cancerous or benign tumours can form in the urinary tract. Stones form in the bladder and the kidneys.

In women, the length of the urethra is short. It lies above the vagina and is subject to frequent infection.

In men, the urethra is larger. It passes through the prostate gland and the penis. It carries semen as well.

An enlarged prostate gland obstructs the flow of urine. Retained urine is a fertile base for bacteria to multiply. Bladder control is exercised by nerves and the brain. An injury to the spine or the brain can lead to loss of bladder control.

Listen to your body. A severe pain in the lower back beneath the rib cage can indicate an infection of the urinary system. Passing blood in urine is a matter of concern. Total stoppage of urine is an emergency.

Keep the urinary system free of infection through proper hygienic care. The genitals must be washed frequently and properly. Women should make sure to wipe from urethra downwards and not vice versa after passing stool.

BED-WETTING

Sometimes the nervous system that controls the bladder movement matures slowly in a child. Hence, even after the age of three the child continues to pass urine at night.

Distinguishing symptoms of the patient	Medicine and potency
• **Repulsive odour** in the urine. • Colour often **brown** but changeable. • Involuntary.	Benzoic Acid 30, 200 4 times a day for a fortnight or more. If a cure occurs, discontinue after 3 days.
• Involuntary. In the **first part of the night.** • Offensive odour.	Kreosote 200

BLOOD IN URINE/INFLAMMATION OF THE KIDNEYS

The kidneys can be inflamed due to bacterial infection.

Symptoms: Fever over 38° C [100° F]. Painful and frequent passing of urine. Urine stained with blood, cloudy, fetid. Nausea, vomiting. Intense pain in the kidney region: begins in the back just above the waist and then moves to the side and the groin.

Consult a specialist. Kidney problems cannot be taken lightly.

Distinguishing symptoms of the patient	Medicine and potency
• Inflammation of the kidney. Severe pain. • **Burning** urine. Intolerable urge. • Tenesmus. **Never get done feeling**.	Cantharis 200
• Bleeding because of **urinary stones.** • **Brick red** sediment • Severe pain from **kidney to bladder.**	Coccus Cactii 30
• **Acute** Bright's disease. **Albuminuria**. • High **blood pressure.**	Phosphorus 200

- **Turbid brown** colour. Red sediment.
- **Odour of violets.**   Terebinthina 30
- Burning pain in the kidney region.
- **Slow and painful discharge.**

Refer '*Bright's disease/Nephritis*' below as well.

BRIGHT'S DISEASE/NEPHRITIS

An acute or chronic infection of the delicate glomeruli [the blood-filtering parts of the kidney].

Symptoms: Urine contains albumin or protein leaked into it from the damaged kidneys. In acute cases, urine red or smoky, frothy, face puffy, swelling around the eyes in the morning, swollen feet and legs in the later part of the day, severe headache and backache.

In chronic cases, the face and limbs are swollen. Urine is passed in large quantity. Patient is always thirsty.

In **acute kidney failure**, where both the kidneys cease to function, the quantity of urine is greatly reduced. There is nausea and vomiting, reduced quantity of urine, back pain, and headache.

In **chronic kidney failure**, where the loss of function of both the kidneys is progressive, cramps and numbness in the legs, muscular twitching, short breath, skin pale and itchy, easily bruised and very frequent urination.

All the above conditions require immediate medical attention. Acute kidney failure is a life-threatening situation.

Distinguishing symptoms of the patient	Medicine and potency
• **Acute. Extremities swollen.** **Face puffy.**	Apis 200
• Pain in kidneys. Headache. Backache.	
• High concentration of albumin.	
• **Scanty but frequent** urination.	
• Very effective in later stages when **watery diarrhoea** sets in.	Arsenic Alb 200

- Thirst for sips of water at **short intervals.**
- Face puffy.
- Fear of death. Restlessness.
- Urine **loaded with albumin** and casts.
- **Skin pale** and waxen.
- **Paroxysmal, burning,** and cutting pain   Cantharis 200
  in the region of kidneys.
- Tenderness.
- **Pure blood** in urine. Gravel.
- **Painful urge** but urine passes **drop by drop.**
- Pain in **tip of penis, in testes**, in loins.
- Inflammation of kidney **following any**   Terebinthina 30
  acute disease.

BURNING

Distinguishing symptoms of the patient	Medicine and potency
• Scalding, **extending to bladder.**.	Cannabis Sativa 30
• Acute stage of gonorrhoea. **Mucous and pus** in the urethra	
• **Violent paroxysms** of burning and cutting pain in the renal region.	Cantharis 200
• Painful urge but urine passes **drop by drop.**	
• **Bloody urine**.	
• In the urethra. With sharp pain in the **loins.**	Hydrangea
• **Heavy mucous**. White amorphous salts.	Mother tincture, 10 drops,
• **Stones. Bloody** urine.	4 times a day.
• Smarting continues a **long time after** passing urine. Urethra scalded. **Every drop burns** to touch.	Sulphur 200
• Great quantity of **colourless urine.** **Must hurry.**	

• Burning and inflammation especially in the right kidney, after any acute disease.	Terebinthina 30

COLOUR/SEDIMENT

Distinguishing symptoms of the patient	Medicine and potency
• **Red, hot,** painful, and **scanty.** • **Retention with screaming** and restlessness. • Tenesmus.	Aconite Nap 30
• **Albuminous**. Globules of **pus and blood.** • Scanty, burning, involuntary. Bladder as if **paralysed.** • **Extreme restlessness**.	Arsenic Alb 200
• **Dark**, loaded with **phosphates.** • Acute urinary infection.	Belladonna 200
• Almost **black**. With **diabetes**.	Carbolic Acid 30
• **Yellow, like beer**. Foaming. **Jaundice** present. • **Dark, turbid**.	Cheledonium 30
• Liver enlarged. **Bile and sugar** in urine. Very dark urine. • Jaundice with diabetes mellitus.	Chionanthus 30
• Black, red sediment in cases of **urinary stones.** • Severe pain from kidney to bladder.	Coccus Cacti 30
• **Acetones** and acetoacetic acid in urine.	Cup Arsenic 30
• Dark red sediment with **throbbing pain** in the **neck of the bladder.**	Digitalis 30
• Urine loaded with sugar. Diabetes mellitus. • **Rheumatic pain in joints**. • **Voracious hunger**.	Lactic Acid 30 Over a long time.
• Specific for albuminuria in **pregnancy**.	Merc Cor 30
• Profuse milky urine with diabetes.	Phosphoric Acid 30

CONVULSIONS-URAEMIC

Distinguishing symptoms of the patient	Medicine and potency
• **Brain oedema. Vertigo.** • Deficient functioning of the kidneys. • **Unconsciousness.** • Increased **acetones** in urine.	Cup Arsenicum 30

DIABETES MELLITUS

A chronic inability of the pancreas to produce sufficient insulin leads to the body accumulating sugar in the blood because it cannot use sugar and starch properly. This causes severe malfunctioning in different parts of the body.

Symptoms: Abnormal thirst which is not reduced by liquids intake. Abnormal passing of urine, day and night. Blurred vision. Fatigue. Increased appetite, yet weight loss. Itching on the penis or on the vulva. Ulcers on the feet, numbness in hands and feet.

If you have a family history, go for regular blood sugar tests at an early age.

The disease develops suddenly. Hence, **it is important to look for symptoms and seek medical advice immediately.**

If you are obese, reduce your weight. Diet control is necessary. Seek guidance.

A regular, daily, brisk walk for sixty minutes helps a lot. It reduces the chances of your developing a heart problem, besides controlling blood sugar.

For strenuous exercise, work under the guidance of an instructor.

Diabetes is not curable. However, it is controllable. If you smoke, stop. If you drink, either stop or be moderate. Get your eyes examined and blood pressure monitored regularly.

Follow your doctor's advice. However, the following remedies help.

Distinguishing symptoms of the patient	Medicine and potency
• Abundant sugar. Copious urine.	Acetic Acid 30
• Extreme prostration. **Pale, waxen skin**.	
• **Great thirst but a cold drink feels heavy.**	
• **Bruised feeling** in muscles. Debility.	Acid Phos 200
• Milky urine, copious.	
• **Boils** on the body.	
• **Swelling** of feet and scrotum.	Argentum Met 30
• Profuse, turbid, sweetish urine.	
• Emaciation. Face pale and sallow.	
• Diabetic patient **dwindling fast**.	Arsenic Alb 200
Emaciated. Dry brittle skin	To be used alternately
• Appetite lost. Unquenchable thirst	with Syzygium
• Mouth, tongue, trachea dry.	Jambolanum, Mother Tincture
• Diabetes with **rheumatic pain in joints.**	Lactic Acid 200
• **Voracious** hunger. Thirsty.	
• **Constant dribbling.**	Rhus Aromatic
• Urine pale, **albuminous.**	Mother Tincture 15 drops,
• Copious urine of **low specific gravity.**	4 times a day.
• **Sugar in urine and blood.**	Syzygium Jambolanum
• Diabetic **ulceration.**	Mother Tincture, 15 drops, 4 times a day,
• **High specific gravity**. Copious urine.	indefinitely
• Great thirst. Emaciation.	

DIFFICULT/CONSTRICTION/RETENTION/STRICTURE IN URETHRA

Medical consultation is necessary. However, the remedies as indicated below are of immense help.

For a stricture, cystoscopy is advisable.

Distinguishing symptoms of the patient	Medicine and potency
• Retention with screaming. **Restlessness.**	Aconite Nap 30
• Urine **red, hot, and painful.**	
• **Muscles** of the bladder **paretic**. Must urge to stool in order to pass urine.	Alumina 30
• With **acute** urinary **infection.**	Belladonna 200
• Urine dark, loaded with phosphates.	
• **Iron band** constriction of the neck of the bladder.	Cactus 30
• **Clots** of blood in urine.	
• Painful, **spasmodic** urination.	
• **Acute prostatitis.**	Chimaphila Umb 30
• Urinary problems of **chronic alcoholics.**	
• Urine has **ropy, bloody mucous**. Sugar. Copious sediment. Muddy. Offensive.	
• **Stoppage** of urine. Slow and difficult.	Morphinum 30
• **Enlarged** prostate.	
• Acute or chronic **uraemia**.	
• Urine stopped **after fright.**	Opium 200

ENURESIS

Involuntary discharge of urine at night.
For remedies, refer '*Inability to control/Incontinence*' below.

INABILITY TO CONTROL/INCONTINENCE

Distinguishing symptoms of the patient	Medicine and potency
• Stinging pain. **Last drops burn and smart.**	Apis 200
• Inflammation of the kidneys.	

- **Scanty**, highly coloured urine.
- Unable to control.
- Urine passes **unconsciously** day and night.   Arg Nitricum 200
- Urine scanty and dark.
- Inflammation of the urethra. **Burning. Itching. Splinter pain.**
- Involuntary urine at night   Benzoic Acid 30
- **Repulsive odour**. Brown colour
- **Bed-wetting** in children.
- **Constant urge** to pass urine.   Digitalis 30
- Enlarged prostate.
- **Scalding** urine with a never-get-done feeling.   Cantharis 200
- **Severe cutting** pain before, during, and after urination.
- Nocturnal, involuntary discharge in children **with worms.**   Silicea 200
- **Red, yellow** sediment

INFLAMMATION OF THE KIDNEYS

Refer '*Blood in urine etc.*' above.

KIDNEY STONES

Hard, soft, sharp, or smooth stones [crystal deposits] present in one or both the kidneys.

Symptoms: Excruciating, sudden pain low down in the back, reaching the abdomen and the groin, sometimes felt in the genitals, with nausea, vomiting, chills, and sweating. Blood in urine. Increased frequency of urine. Painful urination.

A severe pain because of kidney stones requires immediate medical attention.

Distinguishing symptoms of the patient	Medicine and potency
• Pain extends from **kidney to urethra.** • **Burning, cutting, piercing** pain in bladder, in urethra. • Constant urge to pass urine. • Urethra burns **even when not making** water. • Bright red sediment. Urine hot, dark, bright yellow.	Berberis Vulgaris 30 **Primary remedy for renal colic.**
• Renal colic extending from **right side to the bladder.** • **Severe backache**. Relieved by urine. • Abdomen **bloated, rumbling.** • Frequent urge. • Urine scanty. Highly coloured. Red sand sediment.	Lycopodium 200
• With black, bloody urine full of **mucous.** • **Violent pain in the back**, in the bladder. • Urine comes in **drops** in spite of straining although **urge constant**. Bladder feels **full**.	Pereira Brava 30
• Kidney **stones and gravel**. Thick urine.	Urtica Urens 30 Expels gravel and stone from kidney.

NEPHROSIS

The kidneys leak a large amount of proteins into the urine. The sufferer becomes anaemic. His face gets puffed. Dropsy occurs in all the body tissues.

A high protein and low salt diet is recommended.

For remedies, refer '*Colour/sediment*' and '*Bright's disease*' above. **Consult a specialist.**

NEWBORN—STOPPAGE OF URINE

Distinguishing symptoms of the patient	Medicine and potency
• No urine because of **shock suffered during birth.**	Aconite Nap 30

ODOUR

Distinguishing symptoms of the patient	Medicine and potency
• **Repulsive odour.** Brown or dark colour.	Benzoic Acid 30
• **Bed wetting children.**	
• Smelling like horse urine. Dark.	Nitric Acid 200
• Stitching pain.	

OLD PERSONS

Distinguishing symptoms of the patient	Medicine and potency
• **Dribbling. Prostate enlarged.**	Conium 200
• Urine **drops vertically. Slow, without force.** Tenesmus.	Hepar Sulph 200
• **Paralysis** of bladder.	Secale 30
• **Involuntary** discharge of urine **during sleep** in old age.	

PAIN

Consult a surgeon if pain does not subside soon. It maybe a stricture which medicines do not dissolve.

Distinguishing symptoms of the patient	Medicine and potency
• Stinging pain. **Stoppage** of urine.	Apis 200
• **Last drops** burn and smart.	

- **Inflammation** of urethra. Burning, cutting pain. — Arg Nit 200
- Scanty and dark.
- **Unconscious** discharge day and night.
- Fine stitches in the **orifice** of the urethra. — Asparagus 30
- Frequent urine.
- Pain in **thighs and loins** while urinating. — Berberis Vulgaris 30
- **Thick mucous**. Bright red sediment.
- Kidney painful.
- **Carbuncle** in urethra. Obstinate **constriction**. — Cannabis Sativa 30
- **Violent spasms** of cutting, burning pain. — Cantharis 200
- Renal region is on fire.
- As if, a **straw is being thrust back and forth** through urethra. Throbbing pain. — Digitalis 30
- Renal colic. Bloody urine. **Stones. Heavy mucous**. — Hydrangea 30
- **Inflammation of the urethra** with prostate problems. **Itching**. — Pereira Brava 30
- **Renal colic**.
- **Black, bloody** urine. Thick with **mucous**.
- Pain **down the thigh**.
- Pain from **right kidney downwards**. — Sarsaparilla 30
- **Screams** before and after passing urine.
- **Thin, feeble stream**. Slimy, bloody, scanty urine.

PROSTATITIS

Refer under '*The Male Genital System*'.

PUS

Distinguishing symptoms of the patient	Medicine and potency
• Pus with cystitis. **Tenesmus.** • Burning, piercing pain in the **urethral opening**.	Asparagus 30

- **Thick** mucous with **bright red** sediment.   Berberis Vulgaris 30
- Kidney, urethra sore.
- **Continuous burning** in urethra.
- Frequent urination.
- Pus in urethra with **obstinate constriction**.   Cannabis Sativa 30
- **Scanty** urine full of **ropy mucous and blood.**   Chimaphila Umb 30
- Acute prostatitis.
- **Ropy, green mucous** in urine.   Kali Bichrome 200
- Pain in **coccyx before** making water.
  Relieved thereafter.
- At the end a drop remains that **cannot
  be expelled**.

STONES IN KIDNEY, BLADDER

Excess of salt in the blood stream or infection of the urinary tract can cause formation of stones in the kidney or the bladder. A stone on its journey from the kidney to the bladder and onwards causes excruciating pain spreading to the vulva, or scrotum, as the case may be. The pain is spasmodic.

Refer '*Kidney stones*' above.

TENESMUS

Distinguishing symptoms of the patient	Medicine and potency
• Severe, **persistent tenesmus** of the bladder	Merc Cor 30
• Bloody, greenish discharge.	
• Bloody, hot, slimy dysentery.	
• Tenesmus in the rectum.	

URETHRITIS

An inflammation of the urethra in men or in women.

In women, the problem is usually acute because the length of the urethra is small. There is burning while passing urine. White or yellow discharge from the vagina. Intercourse is painful.

In men, discharge of pus from the penis.

For medicines, refer '*Burning*', '*Pain*', and '*Pus*' above and '*Gonorrhoea*' under the '*Female Genital System*.' Also, see the listing under '*The Male Genital System*.'

THE FEMALE GENITAL SYSTEM

The female genital system includes the external genitalia, that is, the vulva and the clitoris, the internal genitalia which encompass the vagina, the cervix, the uterus, the Fallopian tubes, and the ovaries.

The system also includes the breasts and nipples which play an important role in sexual arousal as well as in producing milk on the birth of a child.

Puberty is a milestone in the life of a woman because at this time the release of a hormone called oestrogen, leads to the enlargement of the breasts, the womb, the vagina etc. Hair grows under the armpits and in the pubic area. The female body develops curves.

The female sexual system conceives and gives birth. For this, ovaries produce sex cells, called ova or eggs, one every month. From here, the egg is carried to the womb by the Fallopian tube. At times, before the egg has reached the uterus, it is fertilized in the Fallopian tube by a male sperm which has travelled from the male genital system via the vagina and the uterus.

A fertilized egg is implanted in the wall of the womb. An unfertilized egg is washed away in the menstrual blood.

The clitoris is a gland covered by prepuce. It lies at the top of the vulva and at the centre of the labia. It plays a significant role in female arousal. It induces female orgasm. It becomes erect during sexual intercourse.

The vagina provides a passage for intercourse as well as birth. It is a muscular canal extending from the lower part of the uterus to the

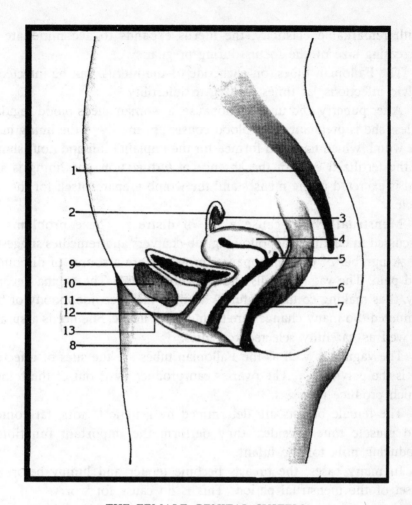

THE FEMALE GENITAL SYSTEM
1. Sacrum. 2. Fallopian tube. 3. Ovary. 4. Uterus. 5. Cervix. 6. Rectum.
7. Vaginal canal. 8. Anus. 9. Urinary bladder. 10. Bone. 11. Urethra.
12. Urethral opening. 13. Clitoris.

vulva. It lies between the bladder and the urethra in front, and the rectum
and the anal canal behind.

Semi fluid acids secreted by the vagina during the reproductive
period of a woman, mixed with a secretion from the cervix, often
prevent an infection of the vaginal canal.

The uterus is a pear-shaped organ and lies in the pelvic cavity with
the bladder in front and the rectum behind. Its neck, called the cervix,
opens on one side into the uterine cavity and on the other into the vagina.

With remarkable elasticity, the uterus expands to accommodate the increasing size of the foetus during pregnancy.

The Fallopian tubes, on each side of the uterus, can be infected by pelvic infections, at times leading to infertility.

After puberty and until menopause, a woman sheds blood regularly unless she is pregnant. This blood consists primarily of the lining inside the womb which has been formed for the implantation and nourishment of the fertilized egg. In the absence of fertilization, the lining is shed and is excreted in the menses and the womb prepares itself for the next cycle.

Menstrual cycles cause a lot of distress. These problems are discussed in detail in the following sub-chapters and remedies suggested.

A number of post-menopausal problems are a source of discomfort and pain. The vaginal walls and the vulva shrink. The vagina becomes dry, thus making coitus painful. A woman may become moody or bad-tempered. So many changes are taking place inside. She needs assurance as well as carefully selected remedies.

The vagina as well as the Fallopian tubes are the sites of infection. So is the pelvic area. The ovaries can produce cysts out of the follicles which produce the eggs.

The female breasts are determined by genetic factors, fat content, and muscle tone. Besides, they perform the important function of producing milk for the infant.

In many cases, the breasts become tender and lumpy before the onset of the menstrual period. This is no cause for worry.

However, the female breast is a site of cancer. Any lump which does not disappear within a few days ought to be investigated by a doctor. Self-examination can be easily learnt from your gynaecologist. It may save your life.

Women may develop cancer in the uterus after or around the age of fifty. Cervix cancer affects women who are unusually active sexually.

Prolapse of the uterus requires attention because it is most bothersome. The uterus at times hangs out of the vagina. Do not feel shy of seeking advice and help.

Proper personal hygiene is essential. Women should wipe from front to back after passing stool. They should avoid wearing tight underwear particularly that made with synthetic material.

It is advisable to have a cervical smear test taken every two or three years in order to detect an approaching sickness, not apparent otherwise.

Menstruation, pregnancy, and menopause ought to be part of a healthy living.

Every woman should exercise, of course under proper guidance. The earlier you start the better it is. Otherwise, the old age can be distressing.

ABORTION

Spontaneous or habitual termination of pregnancy before the twentieth week.

Symptoms: Obvious. Vaginal bleeding. Blood bright red if fresh. Brown, if it has been retained in the vagina for some time. At times, pain at regular intervals like short labour pains.

Consult your gynaecologist if you feel that an abortion is threatened. A pregnant woman must take adequate rest.

Distinguishing symptoms of the patient	Medicine and potency
• **Habitual** tendency to abortion.	Aletris Farinosa 30
• Suffers from **nervous indigestion.** Tired. Anaemic. Dislikes food.	
• **Prolapse** of the uterus.	
• Threatened abortion because of an **injury**.	Arnica 200
• Threatened abortion especially when haemorrhages are **dark and stringy**.	Crocus 30
• **Frequent** and **very early** miscarriages.	Viburnum Opulus 30
• **Excoriating leucorrhoea**.	
• Colic pain in pelvic region.	
• **False labour pains**. Pain from back to loin and womb.	

ABSCESS

A collection of pus formed by tissue disintegration and surrounded by an inflamed area.

Distinguishing symptoms of the patient	Medicine and potency
• **Of breasts**. Hard, hot and painful.	Bryonia 200
• **Of labia**. Acute pain..	Hepar Sulph 200

- Extremely **offensive leucorrhoea**, smelling of old cheese
- Of labia. **Chronic** cases. Itching of vulva and vagina.   Silicea 200
- **Milky**, **acrid** leucorrhoea.
- Vaginal **cysts**.

AMENORRHEA

When a woman's menstrual period does not start on time and within at least three months of the due date unless she is pregnant, it can be a symptom of some other problem. It can occur because of deficiency of hormones or because of tumours or disorders of the pituitary gland. There can be several other reasons.

Distinguishing symptoms of the patient	Medicine and potency
• **Anaemic. Emaciated.**	Ferrum Met 30
• Palpitation.	
• **Indigestion**. Abdominal **cramps.**	Kali Carb 200
• Palpitation.	
• Delayed menstruation at **puberty**.	Lycopodium 200
• **Breasts underdeveloped.**	
• Headache, **sour** vomiting, **swollen feet**.	
• Delayed menstruation at **puberty.**	Pulsatilla 30
• Emotional. **Weeps easily.**	
• Late menstruation.	
• Accompanied by **severe hysteric headache**, leucorrhoea, even toothache.	Sepia 200
• Of **delicate constitution**. Yellow spots on the face.	
• Suffers shivering and heat alternately.	

AVERSION/FRIGIDITY

Diminished desire for sex. Or, no desire at all.

Distinguishing symptoms of the patient	Medicine and potency
• Desire diminished. **Cutting pain** during intercourse.	Berberis Vulgaris 30
• Vagina sore, burning, **constricted**, has neuralgic pain.	
• **Scanty** menses.	
• Aversion with **constipation** and late **menses.**	Graphites 200
• Timid.	
• In **hysterical** and moody women.	Ignatia 200
• Desire destroyed.	Onosmodium 200
• Severe **uterine pain.**	
• **Early and prolonged menses.**	
• Weak muscles. Tired.	

BACKACHE

Distinguishing symptoms of the patient	Medicine and potency
• Violent pain with late menses. **Dark blood.**	Calcarea Phos 30
• Leucorrhoea like the **white of an egg**.	
• In **young** girls whose menses are **retarded or absent**.	Senecio Aureus 30

BLADDER—IRRITABLE

Distinguishing symptoms of the patient	Medicine and potency
In young, **newly married** women.	Staphysagria 200

BLEEDING/PROFUSE MENSTRUATION/MENORRHAGIA

Abnormal vaginal bleeding not due to menstruation.
Menorrhagia is heavier than normal menstrual periods.

Distinguishing symptoms of the patient	Medicine and potency
• Profuse menstruation. Premature. • **Labour like pains**.	Aletris Farinosa 30
• Blood between periods **with every little accident.**	Amber Grisea 30
• Menses early, copious. Blood bluish.	
• Too frequent. Excessive flow. **Clotted** blood.	Ammonium Carb 30
• Pain in the **thighs.**	
• **Aversion to sex**.	
• **Excoriating**, foul leucorrhoea.	Arg Met 30
• Haemorrhage at the time of **climacteric**.	
• Profuse menstruation.	Arsenic Alb 200
• **Burning pain** as from **hot wires** inserted in the pelvis.	
• Blood **bright red. Foul** smell. **Too early**. Too profuse.	Belladonna 200
• Profuse with **membrane shreds**.	Bromum 30
• Menses profuse. Long duration. Early.	Calcarea Carb 30
• **Vertigo**. Toothache.	
• Heavy **sweating on vulva**.	
• One period **runs into another. Non-stop** bleeding.	Carbo Veg 200
• Debility.	
• Profuse. Early. Dark clots.	China 200
• **Abdominal distension.**	
• **Bloody leucorrhoea**.	
• Uterine bleeding caused by **lifting a weight.**	Cinnamon 30
• Bright red blood literally running out.	
• Large **clots** of blood from vagina **while passing urine.**	Coccus Cacti 30

- Menses early, profuse, black, thick, **intermittent**.
- Blood clots **with long strings.**   Crocus 30
- Menstrual blood dark, frequent, slimy, abundant.
- Haemorrhage from uterus occurring **midway** the periods. Dark. Copious.   Hamamelis 30
- **Abdomen sore**.
- Bleeding from **fibroids** in uterus.   Hydrastinum Mur 30
- Profuse bright blood with **nausea**.   Ipecac 200
- During climacteric with **palpitation.**   Lachesis 200
- Vertex headache. **Fainting spells.**
- Between periods with **sexual excitement.**   Sabina 30
- Profuse, bright flow.
- **Pain** from sacrum to pubes, **shooting up** the vagina.
- Ice-cold all over the body.   Silicea 200
- During first few weeks **after childbirth.**   Trillium Pendulum 30
- From uterine **fibroids.**
- During climacteric
- Sensation as if **hips and back falling to pieces**.

BLEEDING/SCANTY MENSTRUATION

Distinguishing symptoms of the patient	Medicine and potency
- Menses too early, short, scanty. Exhaustion thereafter.	Alumina 200
- After menses, **burning,** profuse and **transparent** leucorrhoea.	
- Suppressed menstruation with **splitting headache**.	Bryonia 200
- **Breasts** hard, **painful**.	
- **Complete absence** of menstruation with **ophthalmia.**	Euphrasia 200
- Painful, scanty flow.	

- **Uterine prolapse** with dark, clotted, scanty menses.   Lilium Tig 200
- Brown, excoriating leucorrhoea.
- **Pain in ovaries. Itching** in vulva.
- Suppressed menses. **Delayed** menses in **young women**. Painful.   Pulsatilla 200
- Blood thick, dark, clotted, late, scanty, intermittent.
- **Gentle disposition**. Sheds tears easily.
- With **pain in the back**. Flow scanty, late, irregular.   Sepia 200
- Vagina **painful during coitus.**
- Uterine, vaginal **prolapse**. Constant weighing down sensation.
- **Yellow**, greenish, **itching** leucorrhoea.
- Vagina **burns**. Vulva **sore.**   Sulphur 200
- Menses late, scanty, thick, black, and acrid
- Unhygienic habits.
- Patient has **early miscarriages.**   Viburnum Opulus 30
- Menstruation early, scanty, lasting a few hours, not days.
- **Early morning pain** from back to **womb**, to loins.

BREAST ABSCESS

An uncommon problem.

Symptoms: Red and painful abscess. Severe, stabbing pain. Fever. For medicines, refer '*Abscess*' above and '*Breasts: Nipples/Cancer/ Fissures/Inflammation/Pain/Tumour*' below.

BREAST CANCER

A tumour that can be benign or malignant. Responsible for almost twenty percent deaths from cancer in women. **It is a serious problem**

and should be attended to immediately. Do not ignore any change in the appearance or texture of your breasts.

Women after forty-five are in greater danger than others are. In malignant cases, surgery is required to remove the affected breast. If taken care of in time, the survival rate is good.

Symptoms: To begin with a hard, painless lump in one breast. The skin looks like an orange peel and dimples. Inverted nipple. Blood stained discharge from the nipple.

Sometimes just a patch of dry, flaky skin on the nipple.
Consult a cancer specialist at the earliest.

Distinguishing symptoms of the patient	Medicine and potency
• Painful **swelling.**	Asterias Reubens 30
• Ulceration with piercing pain.	Excellent in early stages.
• Worse left side.	
• Tumour in women with **large breasts.**	Chimaphila 30
• Sharp pain runs through the tumour.	

BREASTS: NIPPLES/CANCER/FISSURES/ INFLAMMATION/ PAIN/TUMOUR

Consult a doctor.

Distinguishing symptoms of the patient	Medicine and potency
• Glands in armpit **swollen, hard, knotted.**	Asterias Rubens 30
• Neuralgia of the left breast which is swollen, painful and feels pulled inwards.	
• Cancer of the left breast with acute, piercing pain.	
• Cancer at an **ulcerated** stage.	
• Cancer of the **uterus or of breasts** with severe **burning** and restlessness.	Arsenic Alb 200

• Breasts hard, painful **during menstruation**.	Bryonia 200
• Abscess.	
• **Hard knots** in the breast. Non-malignant.	Calcarea Fluorica 200, 1000
• Piercing pain, burning sensation in the **right breast**.	Carbo Animalis 30
• Painful tumour of breast in women with **large breasts**.	Chimaphila 200
• Stitching pain in nipples. Wants to **press hard to get relief.**	Conium 200
• Breasts become large and painful **before menstruation**.	
• **Cracks** in nipples. **Burning fissure**. Stitching pain.	Graphites 200
• Numbness. **Oozing** honey-like.	
• **Dwindling** breasts with **nodosities** in their skin.	Iodum 30
• Breasts swollen, painful.	Lac Caninum 30
• Better on **appearance of menses**.	
• Breasts inflamed and bluish.	Lachesis 200
• Small **ulcers around nipples.**	Phytolacca 30
• Breasts sore, hard, and sensitive.	To be used externally as well. Apply Mother Tincture to reduce inflammation.
• Breasts shrivelled. Underdeveloped.	Sabal Serrulata 30
• **Young female neurotics.**	
• Suppressed sexual inclination.	
• **Chronic fissures** or ulcers of the breasts.	Silicea 200
• Nipples sore, drawn in.	

BURNING

Distinguishing symptoms of the patient	Medicine and potency
• In **leucorrhoea**, that is acrid, profuse, and ropy.	Alumina 200
• **Menses early, scanty,** exhausting.	
• Hot wires **in pelvis**. Sensation extending to thighs.	Arsenic Alb 200
• Menstruation profuse, red.	
• **Burning, swollen labia**. Stinging pain. Burning eruptions.	
• **Herpes** of the labia.	
• Painful burning in **ovaries.**	Cantharis 200
• **Scalding urine**. Bladder inflamed.	
• Urethritis.	
• Intolerable urge.	
• Burning in **right ovary.**	Eupion 30
• **Gushing** leucorrhoea.	
• **Labia swollen**, itching.	
• Early, copious menstruation.	
• Burning in **vagina**. Severe itching.	Hydrocotyle 30
• Granular **ulcers** on the womb.	
• Labia swollen; violent, **corrosive itching.**	Kreosotum 200
• Haemorrhage after coition.	
• Vagina burns **during and after** intercourse.	Lycopodium 200
Dry. Painful coitus.	Sulphur 200
• **Vagina and vulva burn and itch.**	
• **Copious leucorrhoea that excoriates genitals.**	

CANCER OF THE UTERUS

Consult a doctor.

Distinguishing symptoms of the patient	Medicine and potency
• With burning pain piercing down thighs. • Cancer of uterus. Palliative.	Carbo Animalis 30 Caltha Palustris Mother Tincture, 10 drops, 4 times in a day.
• Of the left ovary that is swollen, hard, and painful.	Lachesis 200

CERVICITIS

Inflammation of the uterus.

Symptoms: Vaginal discharge, white, or yellow, green, occasionally brown. Pain, low down in the back.

Distinguishing symptoms of the patient	Medicine and potency
• **Granular ulceration** of the neck of the uterus. Redness. Swelling. • **Vagina hot**, intensely **itching**.	Hydrocotyle 30
• Inveterate ulcers on the cervix which **bleed easily. Fetid, acrid** discharge. • Cervix sore, burning.	Kreosotum 30

CLIMACTERIC/MENOPAUSE

The cessation of the menstruation cycle in the life of a woman when she is in her forties. It is a normal happening and need not be a cause for worry. Symptoms that appear can be looked after with the following remedies.

Distinguishing symptoms of the patient	Medicine and potency
• Flushes of heat and headache.	Amyl Nitrosum 30
• **Anxiety. Palpitation**.	
• Flushes with convulsions	Glonoine 200
• **Surging** of blood to the head.	
• Worse in heat, in the sun, stooping.	
• Constriction. Palpitation. Flushes.	Lachesis 200
• Vertex headache. Burning. **Fainting spells.**	
• Uterine **haemorrhage**.	
• Terrible **bearing down** sensation.	Sepia 200
• **Ulcers** in the cervix.	
• Vagina painful during coitus.	
• Flushes, perspiration, faintness.	

COLDNESS

Distinguishing symptoms of the patient	Medicine and potency
• **Vagina** cold as if packed with ice.	Boric Acid 30
• Climacteric flushing.	

CONSTRICTION/VAGINISMUS/COITUS PAINFUL

Distinguishing symptoms of the patient	Medicine and potency
• Constriction of the vagina. **An iron band feeling.**	Cactus Mother Tincture, 10 drops,
• Coitus painful.	4 times in a day.
• Vaginismus with weakness. Wants to be **left alone**.	Gelsemium 200
• Vagina **dry**. Emaciation.	Lycopodium 200
• **Constipation.**	
• Breasts hard.	

CONVULSIONS

Distinguishing symptoms of the patient	Medicine and potency
• During **menstruation or labour pains.** • Violent onset. All muscles tremble. • Cramps in **sleep, in toes and calves**.	Hyoscymus 200

CYSTITIS

Inflammation of the bladder. In newly married women or in pregnant women.

Symptoms: Severe pain in urethra while passing urine. A never-get-over feeling. Loss of control. At times, blood in urine.

Distinguishing symptoms of the patient	Medicine and potency
• With **pus**, mucous and **tenesmus.** • Burning. Fine stitches in the **urethral** orifice. • Frequent desire.	Asparagus 200
• Intolerable **tenesmus. Scalding** urine. • **Cutting** pain before and after urine. • Blood in urine.	Cantharis 200 In acute as well as chronic cases.

CYSTS, VAGINAL

Distinguishing symptoms of the patient	Medicine and potency
• Projecting out of vagina or upwards. Size of a pea.	Silicea 200

DEFICIENT MILK

Distinguishing symptoms of the patient	Medicine and potency
• Deficient milk in **oversensitive** mothers.	Asafoetida 30

DESIRE—INCREASED/NYMPHOMANIA

Distinguishing symptoms of the patient	Medicine and potency
• Insatiable desire for sex accompanied by **intolerable urge to pass urine** and tenesmus.	Cantharis 200
• With **intolerable itching** in vulva and vagina.	Moschus 30
• **Hysterical** women. **Early, copious** menstruation.	
• In **nervous, lively, affectionate** women.	Murex 30
• **Least touch** excites a violent desire.	
• In women of a **mild, tearful disposition**.	Pulsatilla 30
• With vulva **dry, hot. Severe itching**.	Tarantula Hispanica 200
• Erotic **spasms during** copious menstruation.	

DYSMENORRHOEA

Cramping pain in the lower abdomen and pelvis just before and during the periods.

Symptoms: Cramping lower abdominal pain which comes in waves. Radiating to the lower back and down the legs. Pain in the pelvis as if being dragged.

Refer *'Pain/Inflammation/Painful menstruation'* below.

EPILEPSY

Distinguishing symptoms of the patient	Medicine and potency
• Epilepsy during menstruation.	Bufo 30

Refer '*Epilepsy*' under '*The Brain, The Mind, The Emotions and The Head*' and under '*Extremities*'.

FIBRO-ADENOMA OF THE BREAST

A soft lump which slips away from the examining fingers. Usually benign.

Distinguishing symptoms of the patient	Medicine and potency
• **Hard, stony knots** in the breast.	Calcarea Fluorica 200, 1000
• Painful tumour in women with **large breasts.**	Chimaphila 30
• Stitching pain **in nipples.**	Conium 200
• **Pressing hard** gives relief.	
• **Swelling** before menstruation.	
• **Abscess** in a tumour in the breast.	Phytolacca 30

Also refer '*Breasts*: N*ipples* above.

FIBROID TUMOUR IN UTERUS

Benign tumours in the uterine walls. Common in women above the age of thirty-five.

Usually accompanied by excessive and painful menstruation. **Seek medical guidance.**

Distinguishing symptoms of the patient	Medicine and potency
• Womb packed with fibroid tumours. • **Hot, burning feet.** • Limbs feel tired, sleepy. At times, shivering all over.	Kali Iod 200
• Fibroid tumours in uterine wall **near the cervix.**	Pulsatilla 1000 every 15 days.

FRIGIDITY

A woman shuns sex. She does not want it. Cannot achieve orgasm. Most of the time a psychological and environmental problem. Consult a psychiatrist.
Refer '*Aversion/frigidity*' above.

GONORRHOEA

A bacterial inflammation that causes genital swelling, heat, redness and discharge. A serious, sexually transmitted disea Affects men as well as women, even unborn babies.

Symptoms: Often no symptoms for a few days after infection. Purulent inflammation of the urethra or vagina. [In men from penis.] Yellowish green discharge of pus from the vagina. Pain in lower abdomen. Pain while passing urine. Irregular bleeding from vagina.

Distinguishing symptoms of the patient	Medicine and potency
• **Burning** in urethra. Painful urine. Tenesmus. • **Urine scanty, red.** • Restlessness.	Aconite 30 In acute stage, alternate with Pulsatilla 30, five times each, every day. As the disease abates, eliminate Aconite.

• Terrible pain. **Yellow pus. Copious** discharge.	Ars Sulf Flavum 30
• **Burning day and night** along urethra.	
• **Acute**. Urethra **blocked by pus.**	Cannabis Sativa 30
• Burning, smarting, and swelling in urethra.	
• Urine **white and turbid.**	
• Walks with **legs apart**.	
• **Chronic.**	Silicea 1000
• Discharge from urethra **bloody, full of pus**. Fetid, thick.	One dose in a day.

HEMICRANIA

Pain in a part of the head.

Distinguishing symptoms of the patient	Medicine and potency
• **After menopause.** • Pain in **unbearable shocks.** • Cannot control **jerking** of the head.	Sepia 200

HYSTERIA

Refer '*Hysteria*' in the chapter on '*The Brain, The Mind, The Emotions ad The Head.*'

IRREGULAR MENSTRUATION

Wide variations in a menstrual cycle, its onset and duration, or the flow of blood.

Distinguishing symptoms of the patient	Medicine and potency
• Irregularity of time and quantity. • Menses long, dark, thick. • Frequent **fainting attacks. Drowsy** all the time.	Nux Moschata 30

- **Bloody leucorrhoea.**
- Start early and stay long. Blood black.   Nux Vomica 200
- Menstrual cycles **overlap**.
- Suppressed from **fright**.   Opium 200
- Scanty, irregular, painful   Pulsatilla 30
- **Delayed. Suppressed. Intermittent.**
- Blood thick, dark, clotted.

ITCHING

Distinguishing symptoms of the patient	Medicine and potency
• Itching, soreness and swelling of vulva.	Ambra Grisea 30
• **Copious bleeding** for any reason.	
• During **pregnancy**, pruritis of vulva and vagina.	Caladium Seg 30
• **Voluptuous** sensation.	
• Intolerable itching of vulva with **urinary problems**. Burning and inflammation.	Cantharis 200
• **Yellow** leucorrhoea. Itching on the vulva.	Fagopyrum 30
• **Between** the vulva and the thigh.	Kreosotum 200
• **Corrosive** itching.	
• With yellow or greenish leucorrhoea. **Chronic**.	Sepia 200
• Pain in the **small of the back**.	
• Itching vulva, burning vagina.	Sulphur 200
• Burning leucorrhoea.	

LABOUR PAINS

Distinguishing symptoms of the patient	Medicine and potency
• Weak or false labour pains.	Caulophyllum 30
• Revives and furthers the progress of labour.	
• Improves the tone of the womb and after labour **strengthens muscles**.	

• Unbearable labour pains with **numbness.**	Chamomilla 200
• Night sweats.	
• Helps the patient to **gain strength after delivery**.	Kali Carb 200. Once a day, for a few weeks.

LEUCORRHOEA

A thick, whitish discharge from the vagina or cervical canal. Odourless, transparent discharge in moderate quantity is normal. Otherwise, the problem requires medication.

Distinguishing symptoms of the patient	Medicine and potency
• **Yellow** or transparent. Scanty menstruation.	Agnus 30
• **Acrid, fetid,** burning.	Arg met 30
• **Milky**.	Calc Carb 200
• Offensive smell like **rotten cheese**.	Hepar Sulph 200
• Yellow, **tenacious, ropy**.	Kali Bi 200
• Acrid, **brown**.	Lilium Tig 200
• **Thick, profuse** like menstruation blood.	Magnesia Sulph 30
• **Pain in the small of the back**, in thighs.	
• Early menstruation.	
• Yellow, green **following gonorrhoea**.	Nat Sulph 30
• Thick, yellow, **green, easy flow**.	Pulsatilla 30
• Vagina raw.	
• Mild, gentle, tearful disposition.	
• Thin, protracted, **offensive** vaginal discharge during **first few weeks after childbirth**.	Rhus Tox 200
• Pain shooting upwards in vagina.	
• Excoriating, milky, **thick like curds**, like cheese. Yellow, greenish, with **intense itching**.	Sepia 200
• **Pain** in the small of the back, in vagina, during intercourse.	
• Copious, excoriating with **intense burning** in genitals. Itching in vulva.	Sulphur 200

MASTITIS

The breast feels full because a lump has formed. A harmless condition that comes and goes.

Malignancy should be ruled out if the condition lasts. **Consult a doctor**.

Refer '*Breasts: nipples/cancer* etc.' above.

MENORRHAGIA

Excessive bleeding during menstruation cycle.

Refer '*Bleeding*' above.

METATARSALGIA

Pain across the ball of the feet in middle-aged women who are overweight. Caused by excess weight, lack of exercise and tight fitting shoes.

Distinguishing symptoms of the patient	Medicine and potency
• Pain in soles while walking.	Aloe 200
• Specific for pain in heels.	Antim Crud 200
• Pain in the ball of the **foot and in the toes**.	Cannabis 30

MILK DEFICIENT

Distinguishing symptoms of the patient	Medicine and potency
• Absence or failure of secretion of milk.	Agnus 30

NAUSEA

Distinguishing symptoms of the patient	Medicine and potency
• In **pregnancy**. Run down condition. No appetite.	Carbo Veg 200
• Nausea and vomiting during pregnancy.	Ipecac 200
• **Nausea for any reason**.	
• **Persistent** nausea during pregnancy.	Symphori-Carpus 200
• Nausea during menstruation.	
• Aversion to all food.	
• **Constipation**. Worse motion.	

OVARIAN CYST

No apparent symptoms are noticed for a cyst in the ovary. It is a swelling full of liquid, sometimes cancerous. **Seek advice from your gynaecologist**.

Symptoms: During menstruation, pain in the lower abdomen. Pain during coitus.

Distinguishing symptoms of the patient	Medicine and potency
• Round, small cysts in the ovaries. **Boring pain. Must draw up double.**	Colocynthis 200
• Restlessness.	
• Ovarian cysts. Vagina **dry**. Coitus painful.	Lycopodium 200
• Worse **right side**.	

PAIN/INFLAMMATION/PAINFUL MENSTRUATION

Distinguishing symptoms of the patient	Medicine and potency
• Pain during menstruation. Like labour pain.	Belladonna 200
• Comes and goes **suddenly**. Of short **duration**.	

- During **coitus, cutting** pain.   Berberis Vulgaris 30
- Vagina **constricted**, tender, burning, sore.
- **Neuralgic** pain in vagina.
- **Inter-menstrual** pain with **abdominal and**   Bryonia 200
  pelvic soreness.
- Early, copious menses. **Worse on movement**.
- **Ovarian** neuralgia.   Cimicifuga 200
- Pain across pelvis from **hip to hip**.
- **Cervical** inflammation. Redness.   Hydrocotyle 30
- **Granular ulceration.**
- Vagina hot, itching.
- Pain in **ovaries**. Like a **wedge piercing**   Iodum 30
  into uterus.
- **Dwindling breasts**. Emaciation
- Irregular menses.
- Neuralgic menstrual colic. **Stops with**   Mag Phos 200
  onset of flow.
- **Cramps** during menstruation.
- Pain from **pubes to sacrum**, from **below**   Sabina 30
  upwards, shooting through vagina.
- Pain in **uterus**, running into **thighs**.
- Copious, bright menstruation. Worst
  least motion.
- Persistent sharp pain **up vagina**, in the   Sepia 200
  small of the back, from pelvis into back.   Great uterine remedy.
- Vaginal pain during **coitus**. Violent stitches
  upwards.
- Menstruation profuse, bright, or too late
  and variable.
- **Coldness. Cold feet** during painful menses.   Veratrum Alb 200
- Faints from least exertion.

PLACENTA

Distinguishing symptoms of the patient	Medicine and potency
• Placenta retained. Intense pain **afterwards**.	Sabina 30

PREGNANCY

Distinguishing symptoms of the patient	Medicine and potency
• **Run down condition**.	Carbo Veg 200
• Offensive flatulence. Acidity.	Prepares for a smooth confinement.
• **Varicose veins** full, enlarged, sore as if bruised. Stinging pain.	Hamamelis 200
• Skin dusky, purple.	
• Woman becomes weak **from nursing**.	
• **Albuminuria** during pregnancy.	Merc Cor 30
• Specific for **nausea** during pregnancy.	
• Varicose veins.	

PROLAPSE OF THE UTERUS/BEARING DOWN SENSATION

The uterus shifts out of its position when ligaments holding it, the bladder, and the rectum become weak.

Symptoms: A physical protrusion of the uterus through the vagina or a sensation of bearing down. As if, everything will fall through the vagina.

Distinguishing symptoms of the patient	Medicine and potency
• **Constant, violent, bearing down sensation.**	Belladonna 200
• Relieved by standing. Worse on lying down.	
• **Enlargement and prolapse** with pelvic pain running **towards breast**.	Murex 30
• Uterus has to **be physically** stopped from falling out.	Sepia 200
• Sensation as if everything would slip out through vulva.	
• **Inflammation**. Ulceration. Leucorrhoea. At times a **malignant growth. This requires medical investigation and advice.**	

SWELLING

Distinguishing symptoms of the patient	Medicine and potency
• Swollen, itching, and sore vulva.	Ambra Grisea 30
• **Early, copious menses**.	
• **Oedema** of the labia. **Stinging, burning** pain.	Apis 200
• Comfortable washing with cold water.	
• **Breast** painfully swollen. Ulceration.	Asterias Rubens 30
• Worse left side.	
• Swelling of the **cervix**, of the **ovaries.**	Aurum Mur 30
• **Chronic** inflammation of the **womb**. Ulceration.	
• Uterine **tumours**.	
• **Chronic prolapse. Seek medical advice**.	
• Swelling and stabbing pain in cracked **nipples**.	Aurum Sulph 30
• Uterus enlarged. Prolapse. Pelvic pain extending to breasts.	Murex 30
• **Pulsation in the neck** of the womb.	
• Aching in **sacrum.**	
• Leucorrhoea **green or bloody.**	
• **Easily excited** for coitus.	

SYPHILIS

A chronic, infectious venereal disease. The origin is often venereal. However, it can be congenital. It affects every organ or tissue in the body. Refer under '*Male Genital System.*'

THICKENING OF THE SKIN

Distinguishing symptoms of the patient	Medicine and potency
• In **middle aged women**. Thickening of the skin and of the tissues beneath.	Thyroidinum 30

TUMOURS IN WOMB/IN OVARIES/POLYP

This requires a thorough gynaecological examination.

Distinguishing symptoms of the patient	Medicine and potency
Uterine tumours. Chronic inflammation of the uterus.	Aurum Mur 30
Ulcers in the neck of the womb, in vagina.	
Prolapse of uterus which fills up the whole pelvis.	
Polyps and tumours in the womb.	Bufo 30
Uterine polyps with **slight haemorrhage**.	Phosphorus 200
Pus in breasts.	

ULCERATION OF CERVIX

Distinguishing symptoms of the patient	Medicine and potency
Ulcers in the cervix	Sepia 200

URETHRITIS

Inflammation of the urethra. A common disorder in women. Because the length of the female urethra is small, infection travels from the bladder above or from the vagina below.

Can be acute or chronic.

Symptoms: More than normal frequency of urine. Burning and pain while passing urine. Sexual intercourse painful.

Distinguishing symptoms of the patient	Medicine and potency
• **Tenesmus and burning** in the neck of the bladder, in urethra.	Aconite 30 In acute cases.
• Urine **red, hot,** and painful.	
• Frequent and involuntary urine. Stinging.	Apis 200
• **Oedema of labia** relieved by cold water.	
• **Last drops burn and smart**.	
• Bladder inflamed. **Violent paroxysms** of cutting pain and burning in the entire area in and around urethra.	Cantharis 200 **Use this medicine to begin with. Plus Aconite 30**
• **Urine scalds.** Passes **drop by drop.**	
• **Intolerable** urging and **tenesmus**.	
• Urinary stream **split and small.**	Thuja 200
• Urethra swollen, inflamed.	
• Painful and **frequent** passing of urine in **small quantities**. Followed by severe, cutting pain.	
• **Desire sudden, urgent, cannot be controlled.**	
• Coitus painful.	

VAGINITIS

Inflammation of the vagina.

Symptoms: Burning, itching discharge. Can be yellow or green, frothy and offensive. Increased frequency of urine.

Refer under respective symptoms, particularly under '*Abscess*' and '*Burning.*'

VARICOSE VEINS

Swollen and distorted veins, quite visible, lying just beneath the skin, mainly in the legs.

Distinguishing symptoms of the patient	Medicine and potency
• During **pregnancy**. Purple. Sensitive to touch.	Lachesis 200
• **Pressure relieves**.	
• On **vulva**.	Lycopodium 200
• Varicose veins with ulcers **oozing black blood that coagulates easily**.	Pulsatilla 30

WARTS

Small, hard, abnormal growth on the skin.

Distinguishing symptoms of the patient	Medicine and potency
• On **vulva**, on the pelvic flour.	Thuja 200
• **Cauliflower excrescences** on vagina, on cervix.	
• Spongy tumours. Carbuncles.	
• Ulcers on **genitals**.	

THE MALE GENITAL SYSTEM

The male genital system consists of testes, the scrotum, the urethra, and the penis. Most of it lies on the outside of the body. Inside the body are the prostate gland, the vas deferens, and the seminal vessels.

When a man is sexually excited, the penis which normally lies limp, gets erect. The inside spongy tissues become gorged with blood.

Sperm is produced in the two testes contained in the scrotum and released through a tube called vas deferens.

Seminal vesicles, two small glands are connected with the vas deferens through a duct. This combination is known as the ejaculatory duct. These two ducts ultimately enter part of the urethra passing through the prostate gland immediately below the bladder.

During sexual intercourse, sperm travels from the testes through the vas deferens, the seminal vesicles, the ejaculatory duct, the urethra, through the penis into the vagina. Seminal vesicles and the prostate gland add fluids to make up the quantity of semen released on ejaculation.

Urethra is also a channel for passing urine from the bladder out of the body. It is about 200 mm long and passes through the penis.

At the outer end of the penis is glans penis which has a functional and peculiar shape of its own. The glans is covered by the foreskin called the prepuce.

One ejaculation of semen may contain about 250 million sperms. These are minute, tadpole-like cells, with a flattened head and a long tail. Only a few hundred of these actually reach the egg high up in the Fallopian tube. Ultimately, only a single sperm penetrates the egg to fertilize it.

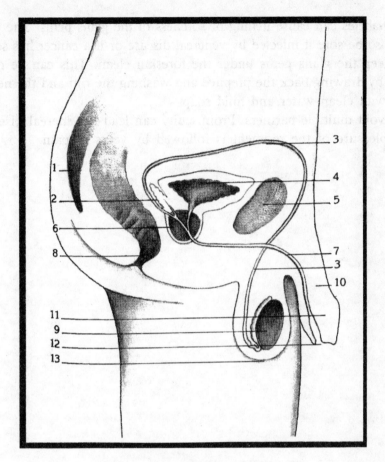

THE MALE GENITAL SYSTEM
1. Sacrum. 2. Seminal vesicle. 3. Vas deferens. 4. Urinary bladder. 5. Bone.
6. Prostate gland. 7. Urethra. 8. Rectum. 9. Testes. 10. Penis. 11. Glans penis.
12. Urethral opening. 13. Scrotum.

While a woman may be sometimes infertile, the childlessness is due to male sterility forty per cent of the time.

A man's failure to perform can be due to drugs taken for other sicknesses. At times, it is a result of emotional or psychological factors.

Disorders of the male sexual system require immediate medical attention. Sexually transmitted diseases are most unpleasant. AIDS is most often fatal in the end.

After sixty, in most of the men the prostate gland is enlarged. **Proper medical advice is required.**

Diabetes can cause itching or soreness of the glans penis. The penis can also be sore if infected by venereal disease or if a cancer has set in.

Keep the glans penis under the foreskin clean. This can be easily done by drawing back the prepuce and washing the rim and the nearby area with clean water and mild soap.

Avoid multiple partners. Promiscuity can lead to venereal diseases. The pleasure of the moment is followed by years of pain.

AVERSION

Distinguishing symptoms of the patient	Medicine and potency
• Disinterest in sex. • Too **early or no** ejaculation.	Graphites 200

BACKACHE

Distinguishing symptoms of the patient	Medicine and potency
Pain in the back after intercourse.	Cannabis Indica 30

BALANITIS

Inflammation on the tip of the penis and the foreskin.

Symptoms: Pain and burning on the tip of the penis. Foreskin swollen. Discharge of pus.

Distinguishing symptoms of the patient	Medicine and potency
• Discharge of pus from under the foreskin. • Inflamed prepuce with **severe itching.** • **Burning** in urethra while passing urine.	Merc Sol 200
• Swollen prepuce is **dark red**. Like erysipelas, swollen, red, hot spots.	Rhus Tox 200
• **Gonorrhoea**. Inflammation of glans penis and prepuce.	Thuja 200

BOILS

Distinguishing symptoms of the patient	Medicine and potency
• On the **scrotum**. which perspires.	Cup Arsenicum 30

BREATHING, LABOURED

Distinguishing symptoms of the patient	Medicine and potency
• Laboured breathing after coitus.	Staphysagria 200

BURNING

Distinguishing symptoms of the patient	Medicine and potency
• **Herpes** of the foreskin. Offensive discharge. • Penis swollen. **Burning, stinging** pain. • Burning in scrotum.	Arsenic Alb 200

CHANCRE

Symptoms: In the first stage of syphilis, ulcers form on the genitals, on the lips, the tongue, and the fingers or on the anus.
Seek medical advice.

Distinguishing symptoms of the patient	Medicine and potency
• **Soft, red ulcers** spreading inwards. • Yellowish, fetid discharge. At times, blood.	Merc Sol 200
• **Hard** chancre.	Merc I. R. 30

DESIRE

Distinguishing symptoms of the patient	Medicine and potency
• Strong desire. • **Painful erection**. Pain in glans penis.	Cantharis 200

- In gonorrhoea when the erection does not subside.
- Strong, long lasting **morning** erections.   Pulsatilla 30
- **Lasciviousness** bordering on insanity.   Tarentula Hispanica 30

ECZEMA

Distinguishing symptoms of the patient	Medicine and potency
• Eczema of the **scrotum.**	Acid Phos 30
• Herpes on the prepuce.	
• Glans penis and prepuce **swollen**.	
• Scrotum **thick and hard**. Eczema. Swelling	Rhus Tox 200
• Severe itching. Restlessness.	

EJACULATION, PREMATURE

Semen is ejaculated before or immediately after penetration because of excitement or otherwise.

A common sexual problem, particularly for young men. Nothing much to worry about. **Wait until you get used to the company of a woman**. Everything becomes normal. An extended foreplay helps.

If it does not happen, consult a doctor.

Distinguishing symptoms of the patient	Medicine and potency
• Penis **relaxed** during intercourse.	Acid Phos 30
• Early, **premature** ejaculation.	
• Deficient sexual power.	
• Premature ejaculation.	Calcarea Carb 30
• **Irritability and weakness after intercourse**.	
• Semen **thin, odourless.**	Selenium 30
• Emission rapid.	
• Discharge on **mere contact**.	Sulphur 200

GONORRHOEA

A venereal, purulent inflammation of the genitals, caused by gonococcus.

A sexually transmitted disease. **Consult a doctor**.

Symptoms: Copious yellow discharge from the penis. Pain and burning while passing urine. Symptoms develop many days after infection.

Distinguishing symptoms of the patient	Medicine and potency
• Urethra burning. **Painful** urine.	Aconite 30
• Urine scanty, at times red.	
• **Tenesmus. Restlessness.**	
• **Acute**, inflammatory stage.	
• Copious discharge of **yellow pus.**	Ars Sulf Flavum 30
• Terrible pain. **Burning day and night** along the entire urethra.	
• Restlessness.	
• Acute gonorrhoea.	Cannabis Sativa 30
• Urethra **blocked by pus**. Burning, smarting, and swelling in urethra.	
• Walks with legs apart.	
• Urine **white and turbid**.	
• **Chronic** cases. Yellowish, greenish discharge	Natrum Sulph 200
• **Inflammation of prepuce**.	
• **Stricture of the urethra. Urine passes in drops.**	Pulsatilla 30
• Burning. Pain. Worse lying on back.	
• **Chronic.**	Silicea 1000
• Pus thick, fetid.	One dose every day.
• **Bloody** discharge.	

HYDROCELE

A harmless accumulation of fluid in the scrotum. A painless swelling which, however, is quite uncomfortable.

Distinguishing symptoms of the patient	Medicine and potency
• With **hardening** of testicles.	Calc Fluor 30
• Scrotum enlarged like a **bladder**.	Digitalis 30
• Testicles swollen, hard, **shining**.	Merc Sol 200
• Testicles **retracted**, enlarged, dark red, sensitive to touch.	Pulsatilla 30

IMPOTENCE

Inability of the male to have sexual intercourse because of failure to have or maintain an erection or failure to ejaculate.

It is mostly a psychological disorder. Certain drugs can cause temporary impotence.

Consult a doctor.

Distinguishing symptoms of the patient	Medicine and potency
• No erection. Parts **cold, relaxed.**	Agnus 30
• No desire. **Depression.**	
• **Testicles swollen, hard.**	
• Erection **fails when coitus is attempted.**	Arg Nit 200
• **Shrivelled** genitals.	
• Fearful, nervous, **melancholic**.	
• **Spasm** during coition.	Bufo 30
• **Diabetes** with impotence.	Coca 30
• Discharge **without erection**.	Gelsemium 200
• **No erectile power.**	Lycopodium 1000.
• Discharge **on mere contact.**	Sulphur 200
• Burning, itching in genitalia.	
• Unhygienic habits.	

INFLAMMATION

Distinguishing symptoms of the patient	Medicine and potency
• Inflammation and pain in testicles from catching **cold or from mumps**.	Pulsatilla 200
• Inflammation and constriction of the orifice of the foreskin.	Sulphur 200
• **Herpetic eruptions** under the foreskin.	
• Of **foreskin, of glans penis** in gonorrhoea or otherwise.	Thuja 200

ITCHING

Distinguishing symptoms of the patient	Medicine and potency
• **Voluptuous itching** of the scrotum.	Ambra Grisea 30
• Glans penis red, **itching, puffed, relaxed,** sweating.	Caladium Seg 30
• Skin of scrotum **thickens**.	

ORCHITIS

An inflammation of the testicles causing fever and pain. Refer under *'Inflammation', 'Pus', and 'Swelling'* in this chapter.

PAIN

Distinguishing symptoms of the patient	Medicine and potency
• Neuralgia of the **spermatic cord and testicles**. Stitching pain in prepuce.	Berberis Vulgaris 30
• **Painful**, prolonged **erection** of penis. [Priapism.]	Camphor 30

- Pin in testicles with supra-orbital pain in eyes.   Lycopus Virg 30
- Testicles feel seized and **pulled** forcefully **upwards**. Neuralgia in spermatic cord.   Oleum Animale 30
- Violent pain in **glans penis.**   Pareira Brava 30
- Renal colic.
- Acute inflammation of the **prostate.**   Pulsatilla 200
- Pain and tenesmus **on passing urine.**
- Worse lying on back.

PHIMOSIS

Tight foreskin. Swollen.

Distinguishing symptoms of the patient	Medicine and potency
• **Acute, inflammatory** Phimosis.	Aconite 30
• **Swelling** most prominent. Acute.	Apis 200
• With **soreness and burning** in glans and beneath prepuce.	Nitric Acid 200

PROSTATITIS

An acute inflammation of the prostate gland accompanied by high fever and chills.

Symptoms: High fever. Pain and burning on passing urine. Urine fetid, bloody, and brown.

Refer *'Pain'* and *'Prostate gland, enlarged'*, in this chapter.

PROSTATE GLAND, ENLARGED

Enlargement of the prostate gland, mostly non-cancerous. An enlarged prostate constricts the urethra, making urination difficult. A normal occurrence during old age.

Symptoms: Frequency of urine increased day and night. A times the patient just cannot pass urine. Starting delay, particularly at night or when the bladder is full. Flow weak, intermittent. Dribbling at the end. Bladder does not feel empty even after passing urine.

Worse in cold weather, after taking lot of liquids or on taking drugs that increase the flow of urine.

Malignant prostate requires immediate medical attention.

For enlarged prostate, consult a surgeon about Photoselective Vaporization of the Prostate which uses the Green Light laser system. It is better than other surgical interventions used so far. It is a bloodless procedure.

Medicines alone do not help.

Distinguishing symptoms of the patient	Medicine and potency
• Prostrate enlarged.	Baryta Carb 200
• **Straining and dribbling** of urine after passing.	
• **Numbness** in genitals after urine.	
• Frequent urine in old age but in small quantities.	
• Acute. Excessive **itching**, painful irritation of the urethra from end of penis to neck of bladder.	Chimaphila 30
• Urine **retained.**	
• **Thick, bloody, ropy mucous** in urine.	
• Inability to pass urine without standing feet wide apart, body inclined forward.	
• Urine **starts and stops** in old persons with enlarged prostate.	Conium 200
• Pressure in the neck of the bladder. Stitching pain.	
• **Fruitless effort** to pass urine.	Digitalis 30
• Dribbling discharge. Feels full all the time.	
• **Throbbing pain** in the neck of the bladder while passing urine.	
• **Cardiac cases.**	

- **Urethritis with** prostate enlargement.   Pareira Brava 30
- Pain **down thighs** during effort to pass urine.
- Constant urging, great straining.
- **Violent pain in glans penis.**
- Black, bloody, thick mucous urine.

PUS

Distinguishing symptoms of the patient	Medicine and potency
• Purulent **white discharge** from urethra. • Gonorrhoea with thick, **yellow** discharge.	Cup Arsenicum 30 Pulsatilla 200

RHEUMATISM

Distinguishing symptoms of the patient	Medicine and potency
• **Gonorrhoeal** rheumatism.	Thuja 200

SWELLING

Distinguishing symptoms of the patient	Medicine and potency
• **Testicles swollen**, cold, hard, painful.	Agnus 30
• **No erection.**	
• Swollen glans penis and prepuce.	Acid Phos 30
• **Herpes** on prepuce.	
• **Chronic** hardening of testicles. Swelling. Hydrocele.	Aurum Met 30
• **Right half** of scrotum swollen.	Clematis Erecta 30
• Pain in spermatic cord.	
• **Violent erections**.	
• Penis, testicles enormously swollen.	Merc Cor 30

- **Gonorrhoea, advanced stage**. Greenish, thick discharge.
- Persistent tenesmus to pass urine.
- Testicles swollen, painful to touch.   Rhododendron 30
  Chronic inflammation.
- Soreness extending to abdomen and thighs.
- Gland feels as **if being crushed**. Worse left.
- Chronic swelling and hardening of testes   Thuja 200
  with enlarged prostate.
- Burning and pain in neck of bladder.

SYPHILIS

A venereal disease common to men and women. It is a bacterial infection affecting the genitals. If left untreated, syphilis can damage other parts of the body later.

The symptoms develop in three stages.

Symptoms: **Primary stage:** Chancres, highly infectious, painless, and hard sores, appear on penis or vulva. Can occur in mouth or rectum because of oral or anal sex. Lymph nodes in the groin or neck are enlarged but there is no pain.

Secondary stage: After 6-24 weeks following the appearance of chancres, fever, skin eruptions, iritis, baldness, mucous patches and severe pain in the head, joints and muscles. Contagious rash over the whole body, on the palms, on the soles. Wart like patches on the folds of genitalia and anus.

Third stage: After 4-12 weeks, the above symptoms disappear and the disease enters its final symptomless and long phase. Ten to 20 years after the initial infection unless a patient has been treated well, he may develop diseases of the nervous and cardio-vascular systems and of other organs and tissues including the bones.

Consult a doctor at the earliest.

Distinguishing symptoms of the patient	Medicine and potency
• **Second stage** of syphilis: when a few months after the healing of primary ulcers, the **whole body** gets affected. Skin **rash inside the mouth** and all over the body. No itching. Fever. Sufferer highly infectious.	Aurum Met 200
• **Iritis** with pain around the eyes. Putrid smell from mouth. **Caries of palate.**	
• Syphilitic cerebral or **meningeal tumours.**	
• Melancholic. Sleepless because of pain.	
• Syphilitic **ulcers in the mouth.**	Calc Fluorica 200
• Caries and **decay** of the bones.	
• Bruised aching in **sacral bones.**	
• Spasmodic burning and digging pain.	
• Bones of **arms and legs** affected.	
• Congenital, hereditary syphilis.	
• Syphilis of infants.	
• Syphilis and gonorrhoea **together.**	Cinnabaris 30
• Tiny ulcers on the palate, on the tip of the tongue.	
• **Penis and testicles swollen**. Prepuce red, painful, itching.	
• Fan shaped **fig warts.**	
• Stringy mucous down the throat.	
• Swollen **ulcers with hard edges**.	
• The **third stage** of syphilis: Slow-growing **abscess involving nervous tissues.**	Kali Iod 30
• Papular **eruptions on scalp** and **down the back**	
• **Deep-eating ulcers. Chancres with hard edges and cheesy.**	
• Severe, continuous, burning, throbbing pain in nasal and frontal bones.	
• Greenish yellow, excoriating discharge from nose.	

- Swollen glands.
- Violent headache.
- Symptoms given under Merc Sol but **more severe.**   Merc Cor 30
- Mouth, gums, throat, tonsils, nose, glans all affected.
- Syphilis **in women.**   Merc Dulc 30
- Warts and other growths in and around vulva and anus.
- **Copper coloured** eruptions over body with dry papules in the centre. Skin peels off.
- **Red chancre** on prepuce. Open, highly infectious, **deep penetrating ulcers** on glans and prepuce.
- Painless pimples. Nodules break and form **ulcers on penis, on vagina,** or at other points of sexual contact like arms, fingers, lips.

    Merc Sol 30, 200
The **best remedy for all stages** of non-congenital and acquired syphilis. Low potency in acute stages and high in chronic cases.

- Painful, bloody, yellow, fetid discharge.
- **Swelling in lymph glands** in the groin.
- **Infantile labial** ulcers.   Nitric Acid 200
- Fig warts around arms.
- Copper-coloured ulcers around **chest.**
- Stinging pain in ulcers spreading irregularly.
- Dorsal **nerves of spinal cord destroyed** by syphilis.
- Shooting, red-hot needles pain in legs.

    Syphilinum 1000
Start treatment with one dose. Repeat every week.

- **Locomotor ataxia.** Walks with stamping gait, lifts legs high, and keeps these wide apart.

TESTICLES, NOT DESCENDED

In case one or more testicles are not descended from the scrotum, consult a doctor immediately. Delay can cause total infertility, even malignancy in the testicles.

Distinguishing symptoms of the patient	Medicine and potency
• Testicles not descended in **boys who have girlish tendencies and appearance**.	Aurum Mur 1 Five drops daily in water.
• **Pain** along spermatic cord. Testicles **retracted**. Worse right side.	Clematis 30
• Worse left side. **Painful swelling**.	Rhododendron 30

ULCERS

Distinguishing symptoms of the patient	Medicine and potency
• Ulcers **externally** on the foreskin.	Hepar Sulph 200
• **Small ulcers** on glans penis, on prepuce. Pimples, crusts on prepuce.	Nitric Acid 200
• Splinter-piercing pain	
• Gonorrhoea.	

URETHRITIS

Inflammation of urethra, acute or chronic.

Symptoms: Pain as if broken glass is being passed through the penis. Burning on passing urine. Discharge of pus at times.

Distinguishing symptoms of the patient	Medicine and potency
• **Acute. Scanty, red, hot,** painful urine.	Aconite 30
• Burning in urethra.	
• **Screaming pain** and restlessness when urine retained.	
• **Slimy mucous** in urine. Stitches with burning.	Cannabis Indica 30
• Must strain. **Urine dribbles**.	

• **Violent inflammation** of the urethra.	Cantharis 200
• Intolerable urging. Never-get-done feeling.	**Think of Cantharis first**
• Violent, spasmodic, cutting, burning pain.	**in urinary problems.**
• Blood and pus in urine.	
• **Tenesmus of bladder** with bloody urine full of pus.	Merc Cor 30
• Intense burning.	
• **Urethra swollen**, painful.	Thuja 200
• Feeling of **broken glass** being passed through urethra.	
• Desire sudden, urgent, uncontrollable.	

WARTS

Distinguishing symptoms of the patient	Medicine and potency
• Warts on **prepuce**. Swollen, **bleeding easily**.	Chimaphila 30
• Obstinate gonorrhoea.	Hepar Sulph 200
• Fig warts with **offensive odour**.	

THE RECTUM AND THE ANUS

The rectum and the anal canal form a part of the digestive system running from the mouth to the anus. The rectum is almost the last portion of the large intestine. The anus is the opening of the rectum on the body surface.

When food is digested, all the nourishing components are absorbed into the bloodstream via various parts of the digestive system.

However, a good deal remains which is an absolute waste. Fibrous matter and dead bacteria are passed through the rectum and the anal canal out of the body.

The roughage though discarded at this stage, plays an important role in the digestive process. It helps in the movement of the bowels. It prevents certain diseases, even cancer of the rectum.

Faeces, the waste matter, enter the rectum shortly before evacuation. The brain sends messages to the muscles of the anal canal to open the passage for evacuation.

The entire process is natural. Yet it will help if we take certain precautions to keep this system running well.

Train a child to pass stool at a fixed time each day.

Diet management ought to be a priority. Include fibre, a variety of vegetables, fresh fruit, and other roughage in your diet. Substitute wholemeal bread for white bread.

Do not live with constipation. **Seek medical advice if constipation persists** even after taking the medicines corresponding to the symptoms as outlined below.

Maintain proper hygiene and cleanliness of the anal region. Wash with water and mild soap. Wiping with paper tissue is not very hygienic unless water is used thereafter.

Last but not the least, exercise regularly. Walk. Cycle. Swim. Run, jog. Exercise the abdomen under guidance.

ANAL FISSURES

A fissure or a crack in the lining of the anal canal. Caused often by constipation.

Symptoms: Severe pain during and after stool. Bleeding anus. Constipation.

Distinguishing symptoms of the patient	Medicine and potency
• Internal, blind fissures.	Berberis Vulgaris 30
• Thick, **yellow pus** with burning sensation.	
• Anal fissures with **oozing eczema** around anus.	Graphites 200
• Rectum torn, bleeding.	Nat Mur 200
• Constipation. **Dry, crumbling stool**.	
• **Splinters piercing** into the anus.	Nitric Acid 200
• Constriction. Tenesmus.	
• **Persistent foul oozing**.	
• Burning, soreness. Violent, cutting **pain lasts hours** after stool.	
• Rectum as if full of **broken glass.**	Ratanhia 200.
• At times protruding haemorrhoids.	Mother Tincture, on local
• Constriction.	application, renders
• **Burning** continues **hours after** stool.	relief.

ANAL ITCHING

Also known as pruritis ani. Usually caused by poor hygiene.

Symptoms: Inflamed skin around anus. Itching.

Distinguishing symptoms of the patient	Medicine and potency
• Stitching pain with **nightly itching**.	Aconite Nap 30
• Persistent **uneasiness** in the rectum.	Nux Vomica 200

• Itching in **blind haemorrhoids.** **Unsuccessful urge** to stool.	
• Dry itching. **Scratches till the anus bleeds.**	Sulphur 200
• Skin around the anus red.	One dose a day early
• Unclean, dirty habits.	morning.
• Worse in the warmth of the bed and while washing.	

BALL, SENSATION OF

Distinguishing symptoms of the patient	Medicine and potency
• Pain shoots up the rectum and the vagina with a sensation of a **ball in the rectum**.	Sepia 200
• Persistent **oozing** from anus.	

BLEEDING

Distinguishing symptoms of the patient	Medicine and potency
• From bowls in **debilitated constitutions**.	Carbo Veg 200
• Dysentery with mucous, **blood** and **tenesmus**.	Merc Cor 30
• **Bright red blood**. From **haemorrhoids** or otherwise.	Millefolium 30
• Haemorrhage from **bowls**. **Bright red** blood in large quantity.	Nitric Acid 200
• **Chronic** diarrhoea with blood and mucous.	Trillium 30
• Flow of almost **pure blood in dysentery.**	
• Bleeding causes **dizziness**.	

BURNING

Distinguishing symptoms of the patient	Medicine and potency
• Sensation of a coal **fire in the rectum.**	Arsenic Alb 200
• Hot needles in haemorrhoids.	
• Pain with pressure in rectum and anus.	
• Dysentery with **tenesmus** and burning. Stool hot, slimy.	Merc Cor 30
• Tenesmus not relieved by stool.	
• Anal **fissures** on fire. Oozing anus.	Ratanhia 30
• Rectum full of **broken glass.**	
• Burns for **hours afterwards**.	
• Itching, burning, **redness** around anus.	Sulphur 200

CANCER

Distinguishing symptoms of the patient	Medicine and potency
• Cancerous growth in the rectum.	Alumina 30
• Palliative in **painful cancer** in the rectum.	Nitric Acid 200

CONSTIPATION

Difficult and delayed passage of stool. A common problem. Over a period, constipation results in tears in the rectum. It leads to headache and overall uneasiness.

Change dietary and stool habits. In your diet, include fibre, a variety of vegetables, fresh fruit, and other roughage. Substitute wholemeal bread for white bread.

Do not suppress the urge. Time it to a regular schedule.

Exercise, preferably long, brisk walks regularly.

Drink a lot of water.

Avoid the use of laxatives except *isbagol* [psyllium or *Plantago ovata*] husk.

Distinguishing symptoms of the patient	Medicine and potency
• No desire for days though the rectum is full of **marble like masses**.	Alumen 200
• Violent, ineffectual urging.	
• Complete inertia of the rectum. **Even soft stool is expelled with great difficulty**. No peristatic action. Intestinal tract dry	Alumina 30
• Mouth dry. No appetite. Tongue irritated.	
• Stool hard, knotty, and dry. Accumulates inside.	
• Of women during **pregnancy**, with sedentary habits. Of infants. Of **old** persons.	
• Stools **dry as if burnt**. No secretions in the intestines. Absolutely no desire.	Bryonia 200
• Can pass stool **only when standing**. Face turns **red straining.**	Causticum 200
• Swollen **piles, moist, raw**, and burning.	
• Tenesmus	
• Worse on walking.	
• With **haemorrhoids and fissures** which burn and itch severely.	Graphites 200
• No stool for days. No urging.	
• **Blotches** on the face.	
• **Obese persons**. Sensitive. Sad. Unable to concentrate.	
• With **flatulence**, obstinate constipation.	Lycopodium 200
• Inside full, yet no desire.	
• First stool **hard**; then **gushing**.	
• Of infants during **dentition**.	Magnesia Mur 200
• Stool hard. **Crumbles** at the anus.	
• Frequent desire, yet each time expels only a small quantity.	Nux Vomica 200
• In persons **leading a fast life**, indulging in alcoholic drinks, fond of late nights.	
• Stools **hard, dark balls**. No urge for days.	Opium 200

- **Chronic** constipation with **haemorrhoids**.   Paraffin 30
- Obstinate constipation of children.
- **Dysentery and diarrhoea alternate.**   Pulsatilla 200
- No two stools alike.
- Blind haemorrhoids with stitching pain.
- Stool has to be **physically removed** in   Sepia 200
  children.
- Stool **protrudes, and then slips back.**   Silicea 200
- **Teething children.**
- Chronic cases.
- Acts as a **catalyst** for other remedies.   Sulphur 200
  Renders instant help.   One dose early morning.

CONSTRICTION

Distinguishing symptoms of the patient	Medicine and potency
- In anus with severe **constipation, with piles.**	Cactus Mother tincture 10 drops four times a day.
- Feeling of **an iron band**. Severe pain.	
- Painful constriction of anus **after** stool. Stitches deep into rectum.	Ignatia 200
- Pressure as if a sharp instrument is **digging from within outwards**.	

DIFFICULT FAECES

Distinguishing symptoms of the patient	Medicine and potency
- Has to **strain to evacuate**.	Ruta 200

FISTULA, ANAL

A painful channel created between the rectal canal and the skin around the surface of the anus.

Symptoms: Pain. Pus. Slight bleeding.

Distinguishing symptoms of the patient	Medicine and potency
• For **comfort and healing**.	Calendula Mother tincture for local application.
• **Aborts** formation of pus.	Myristica 200
• **Heals** when pus has formed.	
• Anal fissures, rectum torn. **Splinters** in the rectum.	Nitric Acid 200
• Constipation. Constriction.	
• Violent, cutting **pain after stool, lasting for hours**.	
• **Chronic** cases.	
• **Chronic**. Severe pain. **Spasm** of sphincter.	Silicea 200
• Heals **deep pus filled** pockets.	

HAEMORRHOIDS/PILES

Swollen veins inside or outside the anus.

Symptoms: Sometimes protruding like tiny balloons or like small grapes. Silent piles stay inside but obstruct the stool.
Frequent bleeding while passing stool or otherwise. Sometimes mucous. Itching, burning, and pulsation in the anal region. Tenesmus.

Distinguishing symptoms of the patient	Medicine and potency
• Protruding like **grapes.**	Aloe
• **Pulsation** in rectum, or near naval.	
• Intense itching, burning. Insecurity of rectum.	

• With continuous **oozing of mucous**.	Antim Crud 200
• Protruding while **passing urine**.	Baryta Carb 200
• **Violently painful and red**, greatly swollen, burning and sensitive to touch or otherwise.	Belladonna 200
• With **constipation**.	Causticum 200
• Swollen, moist, raw, itching, burning.	
• Look like **bunches** of grapes or red cherries.	Dioscorea 30
• Darting pain in the **region of the liver** and in anus.	
• Copious flow of dark blood.	Hamamelis 200 Mother tincture for external application.
• In patients of **chronic liver** problems and **flatulence**.	Lycopodium 200
• During **pregnancy. Bluish, hot**, painful to touch	Muriaticum Acid 30
• Violent stitching pain.	
• **With anal fissures**. Bleeding internally as well as externally.	Nitric Acid 200
• Copious blood and pus.	
• Severe **splinter** pain.	
• **Blind piles** with itching.	Nux Vomica 200
• Ineffectual urge to pass stool.	
• Protruding and burning like **fire.**	Ratanhia 30
• **Fissures**. Rectum feels as if full of **broken glass**.	

INFANTS

Distinguishing symptoms of the patient	Medicine and potency
• Total loss control Yellow/white mucous diarrhoea	Aloe 30
• Constipation. **Straining before and during motion**	Alumina 30

- Hard, dry, **knotty** stool.
- Cannot expel **even soft stool**.
- Spinach green loose stool   Arg. Nit 300
- Constipation **alternating** with diarrhoea.   Collinsonia 30
- Stool hard. **Crumbles** at the verge   Magnesia Mur 30
  of anus.
- **Cholera**. Early morning diarrhoea.   Podophyllum 200
- Teething diarrhoea.
- Stool **of yellow, green colour. Copious.**
  Gushing.
- Severe **gastroenteritis**. Retching.   Veratrum Alb 200, 1000
- Uncontrollable gushing of **white,**
  thin stool.
- **Cold sweat**. Cold limbs
- Pain. Fever. **Collapse**.

INSECURITY

Distinguishing symptoms of the patient	Medicine and potency
• **No control over motion**. Not sure whether will pass urine or stool.	Aloe 200
• Feeling **as if rectum would fall out.**	
• **Mucous**. Constant bearing down of wind or stool. **Spluttering** motion.	

INVOLUNTARY

Distinguishing symptoms of the patient	Medicine and potency
• Diarrhoea involuntary as if the **anus were wide open**.	Apis 200

PAIN

Distinguishing symptoms of the patient	Medicine and potency
• Rectum feels full of **small sticks**. Prolapsed.	Aesculus Hip 30
• **Swollen** haemorrhoidal veins. Painful. **Not bleeding**. Burning.	
• Backache. **Chill** in the spine.	
• **Rheumatic pain** in the rectum area.	Asclepias Tuberosa 30
• Catarrhal dysentery.	
• **Stitches deep into** rectum. Sharp instrument pushing **outwards.**	Ignatia 200
• Constriction of anus.	
• Stitching pain in **haemorrhoids**. Blue piles.	Muriaticum Acid 30
• Even toilet tissue hurts.	
• Worse during **pregnancy**; in damp weather.	
• Sharp, splinter like pain in **anal fistula, in fissures**, in piles or in **cancer** of the rectum.	Nitric Acid 200
• Foul odour.	
• **When wounds** do not heal. Chronic cases.	
• **Neuralgic** pain in the rectum. Anus drawn up with constriction.	Plumbum Met 30
• Rectum full of **broken glass**. Feels as if being knifed.	Ratanhia 200
• **Anal fissure**. Constriction.	
• **Protruding** piles on fire.	
• After stool ache and burning for hours.	

POLYPS OF COLON, OF RECTUM

Non-malignant growths in the colon or rectum.

Symptoms: Bleeding while passing stool. Pus in the rectum, anus, and mild diarrhoea.

Distinguishing symptoms of the patient	Medicine and potency
• **Blood and shreds of mucous** in the stool.	Merc Cor 30
• **Tenesmus**. Cutting pain.	
• Stool **and urine** bloody. Haemorrhoids.	Millefolium 200
• Polyps of rectum with **pus and inflammation**.	Phosphorus 200
• Itching with **restlessness at night**.	Teucrium 30
	Start treatment here.Apply Teucrium 3 or 6 powder locally.

PRESSURE

Distinguishing symptoms of the patient	Medicine and potency
• Constant **uneasiness, pressure** in the rectum.	Nux Vomica 200

PROLAPSE OF THE RECTUM

Protrusion of the anus or part of the rectal lining.

Distinguishing symptoms of the patient	Medicine and potency
• Prolapse with sharp pain shooting upwards.	Ignatia 200
• Rectum **protrudes on straining**.	
• Prolapse **before or with** stool in diarrhoea.	Podophyllum 200, 1000
• **Green, yellow**, watering, **gushing**, fetid stool.	
• **Dentition** diarrhoea.	
• **Every time** stool is passed.	Ruta 200
• In women **after** childbirth.	
• Of rectum with uterine and pelvic congestion.	Sepia 200
• Sensation of a **ball in the rectum**.	
• Constant, excoriating **oozing**.	

SPASM

Distinguishing symptoms of the patient	Medicine and potency
• Painful fissures with **spasm of the sphincter.** • Stool **comes out and recedes** again.	Silicea 200

TENESMUS

Distinguishing symptoms of the patient	Medicine and potency
• **Incessant**, of stool. A never get over feeling • **Blood dysentery** with mucous. Hot stool.	Merc Cor 30

UNEASINESS

Distinguishing symptoms of the patient	Medicine and potency
• Constant uneasiness in the rectum. **Pressure downwards.**	Nux Vomica 200

THE STOOL

AMOEBIC DYSENTERY/AMEBIASIS

An intestinal infection that causes diarrhoea. It can spread to the liver.

Symptoms: Initially diarrhoea with mild abdominal pain. Later, profuse bloody diarrhoea with intestinal ulceration. Severe abdominal cramps. Fever.

If the infection spreads through the blood stream to the liver, it can cause high fever, painful liver abscess, loss of appetite and total fatigue. **Consult a doctor**.

A patient needs guidance in his diet.

Distinguishing symptoms of the patient	Medicine and potency
• Effective for amoebic dysentery.	Emetine 200
• Amoebic dysentery with **tenesmus.**	Ipecac 200
• Cutting and **nauseating** pain on straining.	
• Pain worse **down the navel**.	

BIG SIZE

Distinguishing symptoms of the patient	Medicine and potency
• Size of faecal mass **big.**	Natrum Sulf 30
• Alternatively, stool **watery and yellow**.	

BLOODY/BLACK

Distinguishing symptoms of the patient	Medicine and potency
• **Dark, small, offensive** stool with prostration and restlessness. • **Food poisoning.** • Worst at night from over indulgence and **alcoholic abuse**.	Arsenic Alb 200
• Dark, **bloody, offensive**, thin. • Ulcers in bowels, in stomach. • Dysentery in **old age**.	Baptisia 30
• **Hard** stool followed by **blood.** • Dentition diarrhoea in children.	Calc Phos 30
• **Bleeding piles**. Anus sore. • Bloody **mucous with burning** and tenesmus.	Capsicum 30
• Severe **gastroenteritis with dark**, liquid stool. • **Violent pain** in abdomen.	Cuprum Ars 200
• Dysentery with **profuse blood.** • Sore **haemorrhoids** bleeding copiously.	Hamamelis 200 Mother Tincture for external application.
• **Bloody, hot** dysentery. • **Persistent tenesmus.** • **Shreds** of mucous membrane in stool. **Burning** in rectum.	Merc Cor 30
• Pure blood in dysentery and diarrhoea. **Chronic cases**.	Trillium 30

BURNING

Distinguishing symptoms of the patient	Medicine and potency
• Excoriating, burning stool. • **Involuntary**. Comes out spluttering, thundering. Total **loss of control**. • Full of mucous.	Aloe 200

- **Shivering** while burning stool is expelled.   Cantharis 200
- Tenesmus and shivering **even after** stool.
- **Mucous shreds in blood** dysentery.

CHOLERA

Bacteria in water, in uncooked food, in contaminated fruit and vegetables can cause an epidemic, acute and infectious disease known as cholera. If not taken care of in time the patient can collapse. **It as an emergency**.

Symptoms: After a few days of infection, cholera starts suddenly with rice-white, thin, loose motions. Uncontrollable vomiting. The loss of fluids from the body leads to dehydration, cramps in the muscles and if not taken care of well within time, collapse.

Dehydration must be avoided by continuously replacing lost fluids with a solution made by adding a tablespoon of sugar and a pinch of salt to a litre of water that has been boiled for five minutes and then cooled.

The patient should be administered a dose of Veratrum Alb 1000 on the tongue as soon as vomiting and/or stools start. Ordinarily one dose will stop vomiting. If not, administer another dose after one hour.

If you cannot handle the situation, get to the nearest hospital. Delay can lead to serious consequences.

Distinguishing symptoms of the patient	Medicine and potency
- Severe **food poisoning** cases.	Arsenic Alb 200
- Intense **burning thirst, prostration**, agony.	
- **Violent vomit** of watery, bilious, slimy, green, **black** masses.	
- Lips, tongue, **dry, black** and cracked.	
- Skin ice-cold. Sudden death like collapse with drowsiness verging on stupefaction.	
- **Early stage** of cholera with coldness, blue skin, **scanty vomiting**, and burning.	Camphor 200 On collapse, make the

- Scanty stool.
- **Collapse.**

patient smell Mother Tincture on a kerchief to revive. Further, administer 15 drops of the same on sugar every 15 minutes until he revives.

- Stool red. Flatulence. **Haemorrhage inside.**

Carbo Veg 200

- Frequent, involuntary, **cadaverous-smelling** stool, followed by burning. Vomiting.
- Collapse. **Lips blue**. Nose, cheeks, fingertips **cold like ice**. Breath **cold**. Tongue cold.
- Oppression of chest. **Weak respiration**. Asks to be fanned.
- With **cramps** in abdomen and calves.

Cuprum Met 200

- Painful, black, bloody stool.
- Offensive stool. **Jelly-like** mucous.

Podophyllum 200

- Painlessly **gushing** stool. Excessive. **Yellow or greenish**.
- **No cold sweat.**
- Colic. Rumbling in the abdomen.
- **Ineffective** retching.
- Stool olive **green, putrid**, bloody, thin.

Secale Cor 200

- **No sensation when passing stool**.
- Body **ice-cold**. Exhaustion. Does not want to be covered.
- Coldness and cramps.
- **Rice water, copious** stool with cutting pain.

Veratrum Alb 1000

- **Chronic vomiting.**

First remedy. Immediate effect.

- Cold sweat. Cold discharge. Skin cold and blue. **Whole body ice-cold.**
- Asks for a cold drink but cannot retain it.
- **Collapse**. Face pale, sunken.

COLLAPSE IN CHOLERA

Refer *Cholera* above, particularly *'Veratrum Alb'*, *'Camphor'*, and *'Carbo Veg'*.

COLOUR/MUCOUS

Distinguishing symptoms of the patient	Medicine and potency
• Yellow, bloody, transparent. Jelly-like mucous. Spluttering.	Aloe 200
• **Complete loss of anal control**.	
• **Green like chopped spinach**. Has shredded mucous. Offensive. Loss of control.	Arg Nit 200
• Stomach distended.	
• **Brown**, bloody, putrid. Looks like **brown yeast.**	Arnica 200
• Straining. Tenesmus.	
• **Undigested food** in stool.	Asarum Europum 30
• Strings of odourless, yellow, **tough** mucous.	
• Acrid, corrosive, **glutinous moisture from rectum**.	Carbo Veg 200
• Green, hot, slimy, watery, fetid. Sometimes white and yellow mucous like **chopped eggs** and spinach.	Chamomilla 200
• **Dentition diarrhoea** in children.	
• **Bright, yellow**, pasty, clay-coloured stool.	Chelidonium 30
• Jaundice. **Liver upset**.	
• Light-coloured, watery, undigested, painless.	China 200
• Abdomen **bloated like a tent**.	
• White mucous, like small pieces of **popcorn**.	Cina 200
• Greenish. Undigested food.	Iodoformum 30
• Suspected cases of **tuberculosis**.	
• **Nausea prominent.**	Ipecac 200
• Pitch-like, green as grass. Like frothy molasses.	
• Amoebic dysentery.	
• Indigestion caused by **fatty food**.	
• **Mucous most prominent** with **cutting pain.**	Merc Sol 200
• Greenish, bloody, slimy.	**First medicine in mucous dysentery.**
• **Blood, and mucous** in dysentery.	Merc Cor 30

• **Tenesmus** all the time.	**First medicine in blood dysentery with tenesmus**.
• **Yellow, green, gushing, copious,** rumbling, fetid with colic. In dentition.	Podophyllum 200
• Olive green, bloody, fetid, watery with ice-coldness and cramps.	Secale Cor 30
• **No sensation in rectum**. Effortless.	
• Thin, white, **rice-coloured, copious** stool.	Veratrum Alb 1000
• **Retching or vomiting** most prominent.	
• **Body cold**	
• Collapse.	

DENTITION DIARRHOEA

Distinguishing symptoms of the patient	Medicine and potency
• Hard stool followed by **blood**.	Calc Phos 30
• Child cross and **peevish.**	Chamomilla 30
• Stool hot, green, and slimy. Mucous **chopped, white, or yellow**.	
• In infants with **painful dentition**.	Kreosote 30
• Green stool.	
• Child is **exhausted**. Has nausea.	
• Stool yellow, greenish. Gushing out **painlessly.**	Podophyllum 200
• Offensive, **jelly-like** mucous.	

DIARRHOEA

Passing of copious stool with different symptoms. Must be attended to immediately.

For remedies, refer according to symptoms in this chapter. In particular, look at *Veratrum Alb, Podophyllum, Aloe, Arsenic Alb, and Argentum Nitricum.*

DESIRE

Distinguishing symptoms of the patient	Medicine and potency
• Constant desire to defecate. **Pressure in the rectum.** • Dysentery with mucous and blood.	Lilium Tig 200
• **Unending tenesmus**. A feeling of never being over with it. • Tenesmus of the bladder. • Blood dysentery.	Merc Cor 30

DESIRE, INEFFECTUAL

Distinguishing symptoms of the patient	Medicine and potency
• Constipation with **frequent but ineffectual urging**. A feeling that some matter is **still to be expelled**.	Nux Vomica 200

DYSENTERY

A common disorder of the intestine. Inflammation of the colon. Can be amoebic or bacillary.

Do not neglect. It can become chronic and weaken your body immensely.

Homoeopathy provides the best cure.

Symptoms: Diarrhoea, abdominal pain, tenesmus. The stool contains mucous, blood or both. *Frequent motion but in small quantity. Debilitating.*

Distinguishing symptoms of the patient	Medicine and potency
• Large quantity of jelly-like mucous. • **Prolapse** of the rectum. **Pain** in rectum after stool.	Aloe 200

- **Violent** tenesmus
- **Loss of control**.
- **Amoebic**, with slimy, green, frothy stool.   Ipecac 200
- **Nausea** prominent.
- **Griping pain at the navel.**
- Severe pain while trying to pass stool.
- With **cramps**, with colic.   Mag Phos 200
- Blood and mucous. **Pure blood.**   Merc Cor 30
- **Persistent tenesmus**. Constant urge to   **First remedy in blood**
  pass stool and urine.   **dysentery.**
- Shreds of mucous membrane in stool.
- **Burning in the rectum**.
- Stool **full of mucous**.   Merc Sol 200
- Cutting pain. **Acute. Chronic.**   **First remedy in mucous**
- Frequent but small defecation.   **dysentery, however old.**
- Pain and tenesmus continues **after** stool.
- Mucous dysentery.   Nux Vomica 200
- Constant **uneasiness in the rectum.**
- The more he strains, the harder it is to
  defecate. Urine **ceases on straining**.
- Mucous dysentery with **pain in the thighs**.   Rhus Tox 200
- Blood and mucous. Constant straining.   Sulphur 200

Further, refer *'Amoebic dysentery'* above.

FETID

Distinguishing symptoms of the patient	Medicine and potency
• **Fetid eructation. Fetid flatus. Fetid stool**. • Result of overeating or of a slow digestion.	Antim Crud 200
• .Excessively fetid stool and flatus. • Stool **narrow, hard,** constipated.	Phosphorus 200

GASTROENTERITIS

The medical term for food poisoning. An acute infection, inflammation of the stomach and the intestinal tract.

Symptoms: Severe vomiting. Diarrhoea. Abdominal cramps. Colic. At times fever.

Distinguishing symptoms of the patient	Medicine and potency
• Stool green like **chopped spinach. Shredded mucous**. Watery, noisy, flatulent stool.	Arg Nit 200
• Persistent vomiting.	
• Sharp pain below ribs, **radiating in all directions** from the centre.	
• Pain of **ulcers.**	
• Enormous **distension.**	
• Diarrhoea immediately after taking food or drink.	
• **Food poisoning** diarrhoea.	Arsenic Alb 200
• Nausea after eating or drinking. Throws up **acrid and bitter vomit. Blood, bile and mucous** in vomit.	
• Total **debility, restlessness**, exhaustion. Anguish.	
• Effects of taking rotten fruit or stale meat.	
• Oesophagus seems shut.	
• Burning pain. Unquenchable thirst.	
• **Collapse**.	Veratrum Alb 1000
• Non-stop diarrhoea of **watery, white, copious stool.**	
• **Violent vomiting**. Cholera.	
• Shooting pain radiates from stomach upwards. Abdomen swollen.	
• **Cramps** in abdomen and legs. **Extremities cold. Cold sweat**.	

GURGLING SOUNDS

Distinguishing symptoms of the patient	Medicine and potency
• Copious watery stool **forcibly shot out**. Sudden. **Gurgling** in intestines.	Croton Tiglium 30

HARD

Distinguishing symptoms of the patient	Medicine and potency
• **Marble like** masses.	Alumen 200
• Obstinate constipation. Violent, ineffectual urging.	
• Rectum sore after stool. Severe itching.	
• **Hard, knotty** stool. No desire. Painful urging before.	Alumina 30
• Constipation **of infants, of women** with sedentary habits.	
• Hard lumps **mixed with watery** discharge.	Antim Crud 200
• **Dry, hard as if burnt.**	Bryonia 200
• Mucous surfaces dry. Great thirst.	
• Hard stool, difficult to take out.	Lycopodium 200
• **Haemorrhoids** painful to touch.	
• Stool knotty like **sheep dung. Crumbling** at the edge of the anus.	Magnesia Mur 200
• Constipation of infants during dentition.	
• **Round, hard, black balls.**	Opium 200
• No desire even though inside is full.	

INVOLUNTARY

Distinguishing symptoms of the patient	Medicine and potency
• Solid stool, in large balls, passing involuntarily and unnoticed.	Aloe 200
• **Loss of control**. Insecurity of rectum.	
• Defecation **with every motion** of the body as if the anus were wide open.	Apis 200
• Copious, watery stool, **always forcibly shot out**. Gurgling intestines.	Croton Tig 30
• **No sensation** of passing faeces.	Secale 30

MENTAL SHOCK, CONSTIPATION AFTER

Distinguishing symptoms of the patient	Medicine and potency
• Constipation after **mental shock or severe nervous strain**.	Mag Carb 30

MILK DIARRHOEA

Distinguishing symptoms of the patient	Medicine and potency
• **Infantile** diarrhoea, worse from boiled milk.	Sepia 200

PAIN

Distinguishing symptoms of the patient	Medicine and potency
• Dysentery with **muscular pain**.	Arnica 200
• **Griping** pain in amoebic dysentery.	Ipecac 200

• Cramping colic in dysentery.	Mag Phos 200
• Cutting pain in blood dysentery.	Merc Cor 30
• Cutting colic in mucous dysentery.	Merc Sol 200
• Dysentery with pain in thighs and legs.	Rhus Tox 200

Further, refer '*Colic*' in the chapter '*Digestive System.*'

SHIVERING/SHUDDERING

Distinguishing symptoms of the patient	Medicine and potency
• Tenesmus and shuddering **after stool**. • Shivering with **burning** in stool, in urine.	Cantharis 200

THE LOCOMOTOR SYSTEM

Consisting of 206 bones, the human skeleton is a marvel of engineering skill. The bones consist of protein soaked with mineral substances, such as phosphorus and calcium, of which they act as a reservoir as well. They give the body shape and support its structure.

A bone is a living tissue that is being constantly renewed. The bones have elasticity and tension. They can resist compression. Their cavities are filled with a soft and fatty substance called marrow which in turn produces most of the body's blood cells.

Wherever the bones meet in the human body, there is a joint performing a special function. Some joints such as the one in the hip or in the shoulder are multi-functional. Their power and capacity to move has to be experienced to be believed. On the other hand, certain joints like those in the skull bones are immobile.

The central nervous system makes the body move through an interaction of muscles, bones, and joints. A muscle connects two bones and crosses the joint between them. When it contracts, it pulls on the bone to which it is attached. This contraction produces movement. A muscle can pull, not push. Hence, a paired muscle provides for the opposite movement.

Some bones play a protective role such as the vertebral column protecting the spinal cord. The human skeleton protects the internal organs. The brain, the spinal cord, the heart, and lungs are taken care of by the axial skeleton consisting of the skull, spine, and the rib cage. It is formed of eighty bones. The rest of 126 bones form the limbs, the collarbones, the shoulder blades, and the bones of the pelvis.

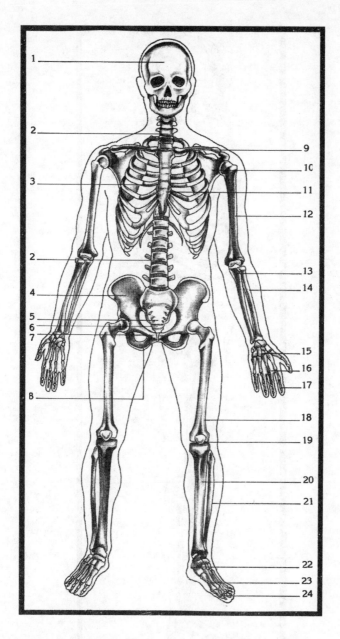

THE HUMAN SKELETON—FRONTAL VIEW

1. Cranium. [Skull] 2. Vertebrae. 3. Ribs. 4. Ileum. 5. Sacrum. 6. Coccyx. 7. Pubis.
8. Ischium. 9. Clavicle [Collarbone]. 10. Scapula [Shoulder blade]. 11. Sternum.
[Breastbone]. 12. Humerus. 13. Ulna. 14. Radius. 15. Carpus. 16. Metacarpus.
17. Phalanx. 18. Femur. 19. Patella [Kneecap]. 20. Tibia. 21. Fibula. 22. Tarsus.
23. Metatarsus. 24. Phalanx.

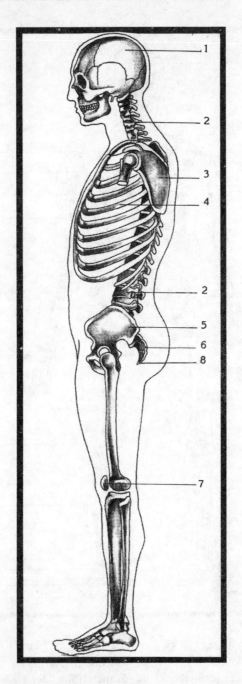

THE HUMAN SKELETON—SIDE VIEW

1. Cranium [Skull]. 2. Vertebrae. 3. Scapula. [Shoulder blade.] 4. Ribs. 5. Ileum.
6. Sacrum. 7. Patella [Knee cap]. 8. Coccyx.

The bones in a male skeleton are larger and heavier than the bones in a female skeleton. On the other hand, the male pelvic cavity is smaller· than the female pelvic cavity. The latter needs a larger size for a normal delivery.

The human legs and feet carry weight during a lifetime. The fingers of a hand can catch hold of an object, manipulate it in a delicate fashion and with these, an artist can create immortal paintings and sculpture or play a melody on a sitar, violin, or a piano. Their versatility is beyond description.

An inflammation of the joints causes arthritis. Repeated attacks deform the joints. Wear and tear of the joints and loss of cartilage lining leads to osteoarthritis. The joints in the neck, hands, hips, and knees are more susceptible to osteoarthritis than the other joints.

A derangement of the immune system affects the fibrous tissue around the joints. This results in stiffness, distortion, and dislocation. This disease is known as rheumatoid arthritis.

The locomotor system in the human body is working most of the time. Naturally, it is subjected to fatigue, pain, stiffness and swelling.

It is, therefore, necessary to keep the locomotor system fit and toned up. Regular, well directed exercise makes the muscles supple, strengthens and gives power to the arms, the trunk, and the legs. Many problems of the system can be avoided or at least put off by years by regular workouts. The latter need not be strenuous. Seek guidance for good results. Start early in your life. However, it is never too late to begin.

Obesity puts a strain on the legs and other parts of the body. It is a risk factor for a heart attack, or a stroke. Therefore, reduce weight through proper exercise and diet control. Seek help from a dietician and a gym instructor. Exercise your will-power besides exercising your body.

ACHES/PAIN/SORENESS/BRUISED FEELING/ RHEUMATIC, ARTHRITIC PAIN/GOUT PAIN

Distinguishing symptoms of the patient	Medicine and potency
• With **numbness, tingling**, shooting pain in limbs.	Aconite Nap 30
• Limbs **ice-cold**. Insensibility of hands, of feet.	
• Rheumatic inflammation of joints which are **red, shining and swollen.**	
• Acute. Comes suddenly but violently.	
• On exposure to dry cold air.	
• **Irrational fear**.	
• Pain because of injury **anywhere**.	Arnica 200
• Limbs ache as if beaten, **bruised. Sore**, lame feeling. Even bed feels hard.	
• **Bleeding** in injury, even internal.	
• Darting pain with **caries in bones**.	Asafoetida 30
• Inflammatory rheumatism. **Joints swollen, red, hot, sensitive**. Localised inflammation.	Belladonna 200
• **Violent cramps.**	
• **Sudden** inflammation on **exposure.**	
• Worse motion, even slight jolt.	
• Inflammatory rheumatism. However, **pain comes slowly**. Severity increases gradually. **Spreading** from one joint to another.	Bryonia 200, 1000 **First medicine for stiffness.**
• Joints inflamed, red, hot.	
• **Stiffness for any reason**, anywhere.	
• **Better from pressure**, firm and strong.	
• **Worse on movement**.	
• Feels as if parts of the body are **twisted with a wrench. Tearing, sticking** pain.	Calcarea Carb 30
• Lower extremities **cold. Cramps** in calves. Knees cold, swollen.	
• Excessive **deformity** of the joints. Enlarged, soft.	Causticum 200

- **Progressive loss of muscular strength.**
- Benumbing, tearing pain in joints and muscles. Lingering pain.
- Restlessness at night.
- Better by heat of bed or warm applications.
- Severe, violent, rheumatic **pain at night** with **burning soles**.

Chamomilla 200

- Pain like **electric shocks** in any part of the body. Cramps in muscles. Large muscles affected.
- Pain of **neurotic origin.**
- **Cervical pain and stiffness**.

Cimicifuga 200
First remedy in cervical spondylosis

- Intense, deep, aching in **bones of extremities**, with soreness of flesh.
- Moans with pain.
- Calves of legs as if beaten, bruised.
- In influenza, bronchitis, malaria etc., where **bone pain is prominent**.

Eupatorium Perf 200
In pain of bones, think of this remedy first.

- **Neuritis** of fingers, fingertips, and toes. Burning. **Tingling**, crawling.

Hypericum 200

- Ascending acute or chronic rheumatism. **Pain shoots up from feet.**
- **Gout.**
- **Swelling and heat in face**, shoulders, hands, knees, ankles, feet, soles or great toe. Looks pale or purple, **besotted.**
- **Hard nodes** first in foot-joints, then in hands.
- **Ankles sweat.**
- Patient unnaturally cold. **Lacks body heat**. Yet feels relieved putting feet into cold water. Worse at night. Takes off cover.

Ledum 200

- **Rheumatic pain and stiffness** in fibres, tissues, joints, tendons and sheaths. In nape of neck, loins, thighs, and knee joint.
- **Limbs stiff and paralysed.**

Rhus Tox 200, 1000
In sprains, when Arnica has reduced swelling, administer Rhus Tox to complete the cure.

- **Muscles: Chronic cutting or dull pain**. Sore. Bruised. Limbs numb.
- Caused by exposure to damp cold or on suppression of sweat, by advancing age.
- **By straining to lift weight. By wrong exercise.**
- Cannot tolerate cold, fresh air.
- Feels **better for sometime on movement**, from change of position.
- Worse at night.
- **Oedema of the legs. Obese** persons.   Thyroidinum 30
- Extremities cold. Cramps.
- Acute. Fever.   Veratrum Viride 30
- Violent, **electric-like shocks** in limbs.
- Severe pain in cervical bones, in shoulders, in joints and limbs.

Further, refer '*Pain*' under respective limbs under this chapter.

ACROCYANOSIS

Cold and blue hands and fingers.

Because of poor circulation of blood, in some young women hands and fingers are cold and blue. The condition may last for years.

Distinguishing symptoms of the patient	Medicine and potency
• Skin **blue. Body ice-cold.**	Arsenic Alb 200
• All pervading debility, exhaustion, and restlessness.	
• Exhausting discharge.	
• **Imperfect oxygenation** of blood. Poor digestion	Carbo Veg 200
• **Hot sweat**.	
• Cold, blue nails with **sweating palms**.	Nitric Acid 200

• Cyanosis with **cold sweat** on the forehead.	Veratrum Alb 200
• Skin cold as in death. Clammy.	
• **Wrinkles** on hand and feet.	

ACROPARAESTHESIA

An abnormal sensation of itching, tingling caused by pressure on a nerve in the fingers or toes or other extremities. Numbness. Throbbing.

Distinguishing symptoms of the patient	Medicine and potency
• **Acute** numbness and tingling.	Aconite 30
• On **exposure to dry, cold air.**	
• Because of shock, grief, fear or for any other reason.	
• Of hands and fingers.	Lachesis 200
• **Worse by heat**, after sleep, or in the morning.	
• Arms and hands numb, crawling.	Phosphorus 200
• **Ascending sensory and motor paralysis.** from ends of toes or fingers.	
• In case of **heavy smokers**. Violent cramps in fingers.	Secale Cor 30
• Tingling, crawling in fingers. Insensitive to touch and cold.	

ANKLES

Distinguishing symptoms of the patient	Medicine and potency
Inflammation/Pain/Swelling	
• Tearing pain in ankles, in bones of the feet.	Ammonia Carb 30
• **Worse cold, wet weather**.	
• Ankles swollen, legs **weak, trembling.**	Arg Met 30

- Rheumatic pain in joints.
- **Worse touch, at noon**.
- **Gout**. Ankles **sweat**. Soles painful.   Ledum 200
- **Ball** of the great toe **swollen**.
  Joints swollen.
- **Hard nodes** on joints.

Sprain

- Due to **injury**.   Arnica 200
- **Dislocated**, swollen ankle, easily sprained.   Ledum 200
- **Severe pain** in soles on **taking a step**.
- Sprained and swollen ankle. **Foot**   Nat Carb 30
  bends under.
- In sprain when Arnica has reduced   Rhus Tox 200
  swelling, **to complete cure**.

Weak

- Ankles weak. Turn in easily.   Natrum Mur 200
- Lower extremities **numb**.

ARTHRITIS

Inflammation of a joint, usually accompanied by pain, swelling, and stiffness. It results from infection, trauma, degenerative changes, metabolic disturbances, or other causes. It occurs in various forms as indicated in this chapter.

Refer '*Aches/Pain*' etc. above and other sub-chapters that follow.

ARTHRITIS-GOUT

An acute inflammation of the joints because of deposits of uric acid crystals. Commonly big toe joints are affected. However, it can affect the wrists, the elbows, the knees, and the ankles as well.

Symptoms: Excruciating pain that comes suddenly. Swelling, redness, and tenderness. Mild fever.

Distinguishing symptoms of the patient	Medicine and potency
• **Acute**, shooting, gout pain. Redness and swelling of joints.	Aconite Ferox 30
• **Chronic** inflammation of the **knee joint**.	Calcarea Fluorica 200
• Specific for swelling of the left **big toe**.	Eupatorium Perf 200
• Headache when joints are sore.	
• **Excruciating bone pain**.	
• Specific when gout pain travels **from down upwards**.	Ledum 200
• Deposits of chalk stone in finger joints, wrist, and toes.	
• The patient is chilly but feels **relieved by cold application**.	
• Toes and fingers contracted in chronic gout. Chalky deposits.	Lycopodium 200
• Pain in heel on treading as from **a sharp pebble**.	
• Painful **callosities on soles**.	
• Pain **shifts from limb to limb**.	Pulsatilla 30
• Pain at night.	
• Better in open air, by warm application.	
• Knees, ankles, and small joints of hands and feet affected.	

ARTHRITIS-RHEUMATOID

A chronic inflammatory disease in which there is a progressive and destructive swelling of joints. The disease starts in the small joints of the hands and the feet and moves on to cover the larger joints.

Rheumatoid arthritis lasts a lifetime. Not much can be done by way of prevention. However, the medicines indicated below will alleviate discomfort and pain.

Symptoms: Swelling, pain and stiffness in the affected joints, all worse in the morning. The skin at the affected areas is red and shiny. Painless, small nodules.

Progressively the joints are deformed and destroyed.
Loss of weight, fever in some cases.

Distinguishing symptoms of the patient	Medicine and potency
• Rheumatism of **small joints**.	Actea Spicata 30
• Wrist, fingers, ankles, toes affected.	
• Swelling on slight exertion.	
• Tearing, tingling pain.	
• **Knees stiff** and hurting.	Bryonia 200
• Feet swollen and hot.	
• Every spot painful on pressure.	
• Better rest. **Worse motion**.	
• Excessive **deformity** of joints which are enlarged and have gone **soft**.	Causticum 200
• Benumbing pain that lingers.	
• Progressive **loss of muscular strength**. Worse right side; in dry weather.	
• Better in the heat of the bed or warm application.	
• Effective in rheumatism of **large muscles**.	Cimicifuga 200
• Pins and needles in **hands and wrists**. Fingertips numb.	Colchicum 200
• Joints stiff and feverish.	
• Gout in **heel. Big** toe inflamed. Cannot bear touch.	
• Shifting pain, worse at night.	
• Softens and **absorbs** nodes and other **abnormal growths** of the bones.	Fluoric Acid 1000
• Severe pain in **extended heel bone**.	
• Acute **gonorrhoeal** arthritis.	Formic Acid 30
• Pain spreads over a **large surface**, nape of neck, loins, and extremities.	Rhus Tox 200
• **Pain temporarily reduced on motion.**	
• Limbs stiff as if paralysed.	
• **Loss of power in forearm, fingers. Tingling** in fingers, in the feet.	
• Cannot tolerate cold, fresh air.	
• Better by warmth, in dry weather, on walking, changing position.	

ATAXIA-LOCOMOTOR

Loss of co-ordination of muscles, particularly of the extremities. Caused by a disease of the brain or of the spinal cord.

Symptoms: Clumsy movements. Inability to keep balance.

Distinguishing symptoms of the patient	Medicine and potency
• **Jerking, twitching**, trembling, and itching. • **Neuralgic pain**.	Agaricus 200
• Mind confused and **bewildered**. Depressed. Desires to be left alone. • **Cramps** of muscles in front of the leg while walking. • Loss of co-ordination and paralysis. • Worse in the morning.	Aragallus 200
• Rigidity and **debility of calves**. Unsteady gait and posture. • **Numbness** in the **arms**. • **Gastric** symptoms in locomotor ataxia.	Argentin Nitricum 200
• **Weakness in the small of the back as if paralysed.** • **Knees give** way when walking. Cracking. • Limbs straightened with difficulty, can be flexed only with great pain. • **Hands and arms** numb, **go to sleep**. Alternately hot and cold. • **Soles go to sleep** while sitting. • Worse after sleep.	Cocculus 200
• Flashes of pain. • **Neuralgia** of head and face. • **Vertigo**. Nervousness. **Brain fag**.	Zincum Phos 200

ATHLETE'S FOOT

An infection common to adults who use public changing rooms. A fungus infection caught generally on the toes and on the soles of the feet.

Symptoms: Irritation. Itching. Skin excoriated between the fourth and the little toe. Pulp-like cracks. Soles and heels inflamed bright red and covered with white scales.

Distinguishing symptoms of the patient	Medicine and potency
• A rapid action remedy.	Bacillinum 200 Daily one dose
• Pimp-like eruptions, **pustules**, and cracks.	Sulphur 200
• Folds of the skin excoriated	
• Itching, **burning**. Worse, while scratching.	

BROKEN BONES

Distinguishing symptoms of the patient	Medicine and potency
• Repairs broken bones. Speeds up joining.	Calcarea Phos 200

BRUISED FEELING

Refer '*Aches/Pain* etc' above and '*Injuries*' under '*Miscellaneous*'.

BUNION

Enlargement and deformity at the base of the big toe. The skin is tender, red, and hard.

Distinguishing symptoms of the patient	Medicine and potency
• **Specific**. Tearing pain in the big toe.	Benzoic Acid 30
• **Gouty inflammation** of the big toe-joint.	Rhododendron 30
• Tearing pain worse at rest.	

BURSITIS

An affliction of the elbow or of the knee cap.

Symptoms: Swelling with heat of bursa, a protective sac, between the skin, the muscles, and the bone, containing lubricating fluid.

Distinguishing symptoms of the patient	Medicine and potency
• If caused by an **injury**, nothing else may be required.	Arnica 200
• **Knees crack** on motion.	Benzoic Acid 30
• Tearing pain and swelling.	
• When **pus** has formed in the swelling. Chronic cases.	Silicea 200
• Housemaid's knee. Caused by **excessive kneeling.**	Sticta 200
• Bursitis in **elbow**.	

CALCANEAL SPUR

A sharp projection of heel bone. Use of specially made, flat-soled shoes with heel raised inside is recommended until the spur has been dissolved. Walk with weight shifted to the toes.

Symptoms: Acute pain on standing or walking. As if the bone will pierce the flesh and come out.

Distinguishing symptoms of the patient	Medicine and potency
• Piercing pain. Feels like a **nail jutting** out under the skin.	Calcarea Fluorica 1000 A **most effective remedy.** One dose daily for a few days.

CALLOSITIES/CORNS

Commonly formed on the sole of the foot because of pressure or because of friction on a part of the skin next to a bone.

Symptoms: The skin turns hard and thick. It loses sensitivity.

Distinguishing symptoms of the patient	Medicine and potency
• **Inflamed** corns. **Large, horny** formations.	Antim Crud 200
• Pain in heels. Feet tender.	
• Painful callosities **on the soles**.	Lycopodium 200
• Toes and fingers **contracted**.	
• Formed by **pressure of shoes**.	Sulphur 200
• Hard, thick, **insensitive**.	Thuja, Mother Tincture for local application.

CALVES/LEGS

Distinguishing symptoms of the patient	Medicine and potency
Cramps	
• In **old persons**. So severe that he feels paralysed. For anyone.	Anacardium 200
• **Knees cold**. Cramps in calves.	Calc. Carb 200
• In calves, soles and in palms. In **epilepsy**.	Cup Met 200
• Pain comes like an **electric flash**.	Veratrum Alb 200

Decay
- **Decay** of tibia.   Phosphorus 200

Inflammation/Pain/Swelling
- **Chronic gouty** paroxysms.   Colchicum 30
- Swelling with **coldness.**
- Pain worse at midnight.
- Calves painfully **stiff**. Difficult gait.   Conium 200
- **Sudden loss of strength**. Muscular weakness.
- **Ascending paralysis**.
- Violent gait as if **bound by a cord**.   Lolium 30
  Unsteady gait.
- Feet and legs swollen.   Merc Sol 200
- Cold, **clammy sweat** at night.
- Feet puffed.   Phytolacca 30
- Rheumatic pain flying **like shocks in
  legs**, ankles, feet, heels, toes and under-side
  of thighs.
- Worse in the morning.

Numbness
- Tingling. Numbness of **lower extremities**.   Natrum Mur 200

Stiffness/Paralysis
- Legs **emaciated**. Calves **rigid**. Joints   Arg Nit 200
  stiff and lame.
- Paralysis and stiffness of both legs.
  Feel heavy.
- **Failure of muscular co-ordination** in legs.   Sulfonal 30
- **No sensation in legs**.

CARTILAGE, DAMAGED

An injury to the knee, suffered generally by sportsmen.

Symptoms: The knee is swollen and painful because of a tear in one of the cartilages of the knee joint.

Distinguishing symptoms of the patient	Medicine and potency
• Severe pain caused by a **sudden twist** of the knee-joint.	Aconite Nap 30
• **Inflammation. Unsteady knees**. Foot turns in.	
• Weak, lax ligaments.	
• **Swelling** with stinging pain.	Apis 200
• Result of an **injury**. First medicine.	Arnica 200
• Pain **worse on movement. Stiffness**.	Bryonia 200
• The **knee is locked**. Does not straighten.	Causticum 200
• Stiffness and tearing pain in the knee-joint.	
• Better by warmth.	

CEREBRAL PALSY

A group of movement and posture disorders resulting from an injury to the immature brain.

Symptoms: Increasing tightness of muscles. Weak muscles. Lack of co-ordination. Movement with unusual postures and stiffness. Swallowing and speech difficulties. Chronic constipation.

Complications can follow. **Seek medical advice at the earliest.**

Distinguishing symptoms of the patient	Medicine and potency
• Palsy of upper and lower limbs from incipient **softening of spinal cord**.	Agaricus 200
• **Weakness all down the spine.**	
• **Paralysis** of lower limbs. **Slight spasm** in the arms.	
• Violent pain in the affected limbs, in the **lumbar region.**	
• Numbness in the upper and lower limbs.	
• Paralysis with agitating movements.	Bufo 30
• Idiotic, weak memory.	

- Twitching of the **whole body**, increasing
  rapidly in severity. Weakness in extremities.
- **Fainting fits.**
- Palsy of lips, of pharynx, of vocal cords,   Causticum 200
  of tongue. **Speech more or less destroyed**.
- One-sided paralysis. Muscles and **forearms
  unsteady.**
- Walks unsteady. **Falls easily**. Weakness in
  knees and ankles.
- Palsy and **concussion of the spine.**   Conium 200
  No spasm.   Once a day.
- Ascending paralysis. Hands unsteady.
- **Painless lameness**. Difficult gait. Legs
  stiff. Lower extremities weak.
- **Epileptic attacks** ending in **deep sleep**.   Hyoscymus 200
- Spasms and convulsions.
- Descending paralysis. **Upper extremities   Merc Sol 200
  affected first.**
- Twitching of hands, arms, and legs with
  tearing pain.
- Limbs rigid and immobile.
- Multiple cerebro-spinal meningitis.   Plumbum 200
- **Tremors followed by paralysis.**
- Palsy of tongue, of **organs of speech.**
- **Wrist drop.**
- Obstinate constipation.
- Right side affected more than the left.

COCCYX

Distinguishing symptoms of the patient	Medicine and potency

Inflammation / Pain / Swelling
- Tearing pain. Usually with **urinary problems**. Cantharis 200
- Tearing pain and **jerking** in coccyx, especially Cicuta 200
  during **menstruation**.

- Spinal **concussion**.   Hypericum 200
- **Neuralgic pain**. Must sit still.   Lachesis 200
- Worse rising.
Itching
- Intolerable itching at the tip of the coccyx.   Bovista 30

Also, refer *'Coccydynia'* and *'Pain'* in the chapter *'Back and Neck.'*

CONVULSIONS

An intense, paroxysmal, involuntary muscular contraction.

Distinguishing symptoms of the patient	Medicine and potency
• In **children** because of **cerebral congestion**.	Belladonna 200
• Sudden onset. Intense fever. Skin hot, face red.	
• The child **jumps in sleep**.	
• **Frightful and violent contortions**.	Cicuta 200
• Curved limbs cannot be straightened nor straight ones bent.	
• In children **cutting teeth or with worms**.	
• Because of a **concussion** of head or spine.	
• Convulsion with cramps in **epilepsy, in cholera, whooping cough. In dysmenorrhoea**.	Cup Met 200
• In **meningitis**, in **scarlatina**.	
• Cramps in calves, legs, in palms.	
• Epileptic fit. Aura begins at knee. Cyanosis sets in.	
• Of **all the muscles** of the body. With great violence.	Hyoscymus 200
• In **menstruation, in labour pains, during sleep**.	
• **Cramps in toes and calves**.	

See *'Convulsions'* and *'Epilepsy'* in the chapter *'The Brain, The Mind, The Emotions and The Head.'*

CRAMPS IN LEGS

Sudden, involuntary contraction of a muscle or a group of muscles.

Symptoms: Severe pain immobilises the sufferer. The cramped muscle feels tied in knots.

Immediate relief can be obtained by holding the toes and the upper part of the foot or the leg undergoing cramp and pulling it towards the body. Rub the affected part and apply a heating pad. Take a large liquid sip and eat a salty snack.

For medicines, see *'Calves/Legs'* above.

DECAY

Distinguishing symptoms of the patient	Medicine and potency
• Bone decay. **Bones sore.**	Aurum Met 200
• Bone decay in **secondary syphilis.**	
• **Fetid discharge** from nose which is ulcerated, obstructed, painful, and swollen.	
• **Caries of nasal, palatine, and mastoid** bones.	
• Better in open air. Worse at night.	

DEFORMED BONES, JOINTS

Distinguishing symptoms of the patient	Medicine and potency
• Crooked spine. **Deformed** extremities.	Calcarea Carb 200
• Irregular bone development.	
• **Softening** bones.	
• **Excessive deformity** of bones in rheumatism. **Chronic** cases.	Causticum 200
• Joints painful, enlarged, soft.	
• Better heat of the bed.	

- Reduces to normal size joints enlarged
  in acute rheumatism.   Kali Mur 200
- For **infants** whose bones are underdeveloped.   Sulphur 200
                                                          To follow Cal Carb.

ECZEMA

Distinguishing symptoms of the patient	Medicine and potency
• Itching eruptions on **joints**.	Aethusa 30
• Oozing skin	Arsenic Alb 200
• Of **hands**. Circumscribed **pigmentation** after inflammation.	Berberis Vulgaris 30
• Thin and **sticky fluid** coming out of ulcers in joints of hands, of legs.	Graphites 200
• **Crusty** eruptions in **raw, red, and inflamed** joints.	Nat Mur 200
• Of **hands**. Of **legs**. **Thick, greenish crusts.**	Petroleum 200
• Burning. Itching.	
• Cracks **bleed easily**.	
• Burning eczematous eruptions. **Skin red, swollen. Intense itch.**	Rhus Tox 200
• Tendency to scale formation.	

Refer '*Eczema*' under the chapter '*The Skin*', as well.

ELBOWS

Distinguishing symptoms of the patient	Medicine and potency
Inflammation / Pain / Swelling	
• Partial **paralysis** of forearm.	Arg Met 30
• **Rheumatism** of elbows and knees	
• Writer's **cramp**.	

• Tennis elbow. Sprain. Injury.	Arnica 200
• **Stitches** in the elbow-joint.	Phosphorus 200
• Arms and knees numb. **Can scarcely hold anything**.	

Numbness

• **Numbness around elbows**.	Pulsatilla 30

EPILEPSY

See under '*Convulsions*' above as well as the chapter '*The Brain, The Mind, The Emotions* etc.'

FEET

Distinguishing symptoms of the patient	Medicine and potency
Burning/Itching	
• **Feet and soles** burning, itching.	Calc Sulph 30
• Burning in soles and hands **at night**.	Sulphur 200
Inflammation/Pain/Swelling	
• **Swelling** with stiffness.	Apis 200
• **Stiffness. Worse on movement.**	Bryonia 200
• Joints red, swollen, hot.	
• Pain of **gout** in feet. **Ball** of great toe swollen, hot. **Ankles** swollen	Ledum 200
• **Hard nodes on joints** of feet.	
• **Progressive paralysis of the lower parts** of the body, of legs.	Manganum Aceticum 30
• **Rheumatism of the feet.**	
• Staggering gait. Tends to fall forward.	
• Pain and stiffness in feet and **fingers**.	Ruta 200
• **Pus** formation in **instep and soles**.	Silicea 200
Numbness/Crawling	
• Soles go to sleep **when sitting**.	Cocculus 200
• Numbness and tingling in lower extremities, **in knees, legs, in feet, and in toes**.	Nat Mur 200

Sweat
- **Profuse and offensive**.   Butyric Acid 30
- **Sour**. Feet cold and damp.   Calc Carb 30

FINGERS

Distinguishing symptoms of the patient	Medicine and potency

Fissures / Eruptions
- **Tips** of fingers cracked, **fissured** every **winter**. Petroleum 30
- **Eruptions** around fingers.   Psorinum 200

Inflammation / Pain / Swelling
- **Arthritic** pain.   Antim Crud 200
- Swelling of joints and fingers in **gout**.   Calc Fluorica 200
- Swollen, insensitive, in **chronic** rheumatism.   Carbo Sulph 30
- **Traumatic neuralgia** of fingers and nails.   Hypericum 200
- Fingertips accidentally crushed.

Numbness
- Fingers **blue and numb**. Ice-cold.   Aconite 30
- **Swelling** with numbness.   Apis 200
- Fingertips ice-cold while the **liver is sluggish**. Chelidonium 30
- Tingling, **burning and numbness** in fingers.   Hypericum 200

Also, refer '*Acroparaesthesia*' above.   Great nerve remedy.

Paralysis
- Sensory and motor paralysis of the fingers.   Phosphorus 200
  Cannot hold anything in hand.
- Paralysis **ascending** from toes upwards.
- Paralysis of arms and fingers in **chronic**   Rhus Tox 200
  rheumatism.
- **Tingling** sensation on grasping anything.
- Paralytic weakness. **Drops things.**   Stannum 30
- Fingers **jerk when holding a pen.**
- Typist's paralysis.

FIT

Refer '*Convulsions*' above.

FRACTURE

Cracking of a bone because of an injury or bone fatigue.
Consult an orthopaedic surgeon immediately.
The following medicines relieve pain and help in healing.

Distinguishing symptoms of the patient	Medicine and potency
• First medicine in an **injury** resulting in bone fracture.	Arnica 200 Repeat until pain and swelling subside.
• Promotes **repair, reunion** of broken bones.	Calc Phos 30 Continue until recovery is complete.
• Follows Arnica when fracture is a **result of sprain**.	Ruta 200

GANGRENE

Distinguishing symptoms of the patient	Medicine and potency
• Diabetic gangrene.	Arsenic Alb 200

HANDS

Distinguishing symptoms of the patient	Medicine and potency
Burning	
• Hot and sweating at **night**.	Sulphur 200
Cramps	
• In **hands and fingers**.	Ambra Grisea 30
• Cramps of fingers of sitarists, **violin players, writers**.	Mag Phos 200

Inflammation / Pain / Swelling

- In **rheumatism. In gout. Hard nodes** on joints.   Ledum 200
- Starting in feet and going upwards.
- Hands and feet stiff.
- Hands and **wrists stiff**.   Ruta 200

Numbness

- **Ice-cold. Shooting** pain. Insensitive to touch.   Aconite Nap 30
- Numbness with **swelling**.   Apis 200
- Fingertips, hands, and **wrists** numb.   Colchicum 200
- In chronic **rheumatism**. Paralysis of arm leading to numbness on grasping.   Rhus Tox 200

Paralysis Agitans

- **Involuntary shaking** of hands.   Mag Phos 200
- **Neuralgic pain** in hands and fingers.
- Fingers stiff and numb. Relieved by hot application.

Red

- **Bright red eminence** on both hands.   Aconite 30

Weakness

- **Unsteady** muscles of hands, of forearm.   Causticum 200

HEELS

Distinguishing symptoms of the patient	Medicine and potency
Pain	
• Piercing, **nail like protrusion** of the heel bone downwards.	Calcarea Fluorica 1000 **Excellent results.**
• Intolerable pain, as if pinched by too **narrow a shoe**.	Chelidonium 30
• Heels sore and weak. Worse on exposure.	Kali Bi 200

HIPS

Distinguishing symptoms of the patient	Medicine and potency
Cramps	
• **Cramps. Sciatica** pain, left side. Tearing pain.	Colocynthis 200
• Better from pressure and heat.	
Inflammation / Pain / Swelling	
• Hip and thigh feel lame, especially after lying down.	Aconite 30
• Pain as if the **hip is broken**, as if the pelvis was falling apart.	Aesculus 30
• Pain **worse on movement**, on pressure.	Bryonia 200
• **Rheumatic** pain in hips and thighs. Worse right side.	Chelidonium 30
• **Hip joint** painful as if sprained.	Pulsatilla 30
• Violent pain in left hip.	Stramonium 30

INGROWN TOENAIL

Nail of the big toe grows inwards in the front. It can be caused by tight fitting shoes or by close clipping of the nail.

Surgery may be necessary.

Distinguishing symptoms of the patient	Medicine and potency
• **Abscess formed. Shooting pain** even on slight pressure.	Hepar Sulph 200
• **Chronic** cases. Site of pain full of pus.	Silicea 200

KNEES

Distinguishing symptoms of the patient	Medicine and potency
Inflammation/Pain/Swelling	
• **Walking painful** in the knee. Stiffness.	Angustura Vera 30
• Weakness. Rheumatic or paralytic complaints.	
• **Swelling** with **stinging** pain. Shiny.	Apis 200
• Pain and swelling with **urinary problems**.	Benzoic Acid 30
• Stiff. Painful. Swollen feet. Joints red hot, swollen.	Bryonia 200 **Think of Bryonia first.**
• Worse on movement.	
• Chronic inflammation of the knee joint.	Calc Fluorica 200
• Sharp pain in **knees, calves, ankles, and soles**.	Cannabis Indica 30
• **Gout**. Hard nodes on knee joint.	Ledum 200
• **Chronic rheumatic** inflammation of the knee joint.	
• Inflammation with pus. **Chronic**.	Silicea 200
• **Housemaid's knee**. Shooting pain.	Sticta 200
• Muscles around red, swollen and hot.	
• Painful contraction of surrounding **tendons**.	Tellurium 30
Numbness	
• Knees cold. **Cramps** in calves.	Calc Carb 200
• Numbness and tingling in **knees, legs, and feet**.	Nat Mur 200
Stiffness	
• **Stiff** knee. Worse on movement.	Bryonia 200
• **Scalding** sensation with stiffness.	Petroleum 30

Further see '*Cartilage damaged*' above.

MYASTHENIA GRAVIS

A chronic condition in which muscles all over the body tire soon with activity. A rare condition.

Symptoms: The jaw and throat muscles tire so that the patient finds it difficult to eat. The vision deteriorates as the day advances. The lips retract and cause an involuntary smile.

In the worst of cases, the muscles controlling breathing are paralysed.

Hospitalization may be necessary. Seek medical counsel.

Distinguishing symptoms of the patient	Medicine and potency
• To **start** the treatment with • Abnormal exhaustion of muscles.	Causticum 1000 One dose every 4th day. Continue for a long time.
• Weakness of muscles with **anaemia**. • Weakness from **mere speaking**. • **Pallor** of skin, of mucous membranes, of face, **alternating with flushes**. • Face fiery red from least exertion, emotion, or pain • Pain in **hip joint, tibia, soles,** and heel. • **Extremities cold.**	Ferrum Met 30

NAILS

Distinguishing symptoms of the patient	Medicine and potency
Brittle/Splitting • Fingernails grown in **splits**, like warts. • Toenails **brittle**.	Antim Crud 200
• Crippled nails with **white spots**. • Brittle, **crumbling, distorted**.	Silicea 200 Thuja 200

Inflammation/Pain/Swelling
- **Neuralgia** of finger nails.
- Pus with **piercing pain**.
- Inflammation around the **roots**.
- **Chronic pus** formation.

Berberis Vulgaris 30
Hepar Sulph 200
Nat Sulph 30
Silicea

Thick, misshapen
- Fingers and toenails **thick and grown out of shape**.

Graphites 200

OSTEOMYELITIS

A bacterial infection of a bone. Normally affects children or teenagers.

Symptoms: High fever with shivering. Acute pain. Swelling.

Distinguishing symptoms of the patient	Medicine and potency
• High fever. Cold sweat. Face ice-cold.	Aconite Nap 30
• **Cold waves** pass through the body.	
• **Numbness.**	
• Restlessness. Fear without basis. Anguish.	
• Shooting pain in extremities.	
• **Acute, sudden and violent.**	
• Feels chilly if uncovered.	
• High fever. **Feet ice-cold. No thirst.**	Belladonna 200
• Joints and limbs swollen, shining with **red streaks radiating**.	
• Shooting pain.	
• Fever with **full, hard pulse.**	Bryonia 200
• Joints red, swollen. Stitching pain.	
• Chill with **external coldness.**	
• **Worse on motion**, warmth, or touch.	
• Fever with **pain in the back**.	Nat Mur 200
• Chill. Violent thirst. **Limbs weak**.	
• Broken **bone pieces in the pus.**	Silicea 200
• **Chronic**. Retarded healing.	

PALMS

Distinguishing symptoms of the patient	Medicine and potency
Cramps	
• Cramps.	Cup Met 200
Heat	
• Hot and **perspiring**.	Nat Mur 200
• Burning.	Sanguinaria 30
Nodules	
• Formed because of **holding tools** frequently. Skin **thickened**.	Ruta 200
Warts	
• Warts on the palms.	Anacardium 200

PARALYSIS

Loss or impairment of the ability to move a body part caused by damage to its nerve supply.

Symptoms: Inability to contract and move the muscles in a normal fashion.

Distinguishing symptoms of the patient	Medicine and potency
• Paralysis of the **lower limbs**.	Arsenic Alb 200
• All pervading debility. **Restlessness. Burning**.	
• Constant **nodding of the head**.	Aurum Sulph 30
• Appears **gradually**.	Causticum 200
• Of vocal cords. **Voice lost**.	
• Of muscles of **eyelids, of face, of tongue, of oesophagus, of bladder, of extremities.**	
• **Deformity** of joints.	
• Restlessness at night. Worse right side.	
• Of lower extremities, spreading upwards.	Conium 200
• Severe **pain in coccyx.**	

- Of **oesophagus**. Food does not go down.
- **Right side** paralysed.   Crotalus 200
- **Left side**. Later extending to the right.   Lachesis 200
  Start with this medicine.
- Persistent, involuntary **jerking** of limbs,   Mag Phos 200
  of hands, of knees.
- **Cramps** in fingers. Finger tips stiff and numb.
- Cramps of calves.
- **Ascending** sensory and motor paralysis   Phosphorus 200
  from ends of fingers, from toes.
- **Difficulty** in holding anything in the hands.
- **Numbness** of arms and hands.
- Stitching pain in shoulder-joint and elbow.
- **Infantile** paralysis. On exposure of a   Rhus Tox 200
  perspiring body to **damp cold**.
- With a weak spine. Chorea. **Anaemia of**   Strychnia Phos 30
  the spine.

PARKINSON'S DISEASE/PARALYSIS AGITANS

A chronic, progressive disease of the nerves occurring most often after the age of fifty. Caused by destruction of brain cells that produce dopamine.

Symptoms: The patient develops tremors in arms, hands, and legs. He experiences a weakening of facial muscles and lack of facial expressions. His stare is vacant, his mouth open. His hands tremble involuntarily. His head nods rhythmically.

For medicines, refer '*Hands*' and '*Paralysis*' above.

A medical consultation is advisable.

PARONYCHIA

An inflammation of the tissue surrounding the nail of a finger or toe.

Symptoms: Skin swollen, red, and full of pus. Throbbing pain. See under '*Nails*' above.

PERIOSTITIS

An inflammation of the thin layer of the tissue surrounding a bone.

Distinguishing symptoms of the patient	Medicine and potency
• Swelling. Inflammation. Pain. **For any reason**.	Apis 200
• Caused by **injury**.	Arnica 200
• Cracking of any joint. Pain, stiffness, swelling. **Shifting pains**.	Kali Bi 200
• Swelling of the **feet and legs.**	
• Cold, clammy, weak limbs. **Sweat at night**.	Merc Sol 200

RHEUMATISM

Any of the several pathological conditions of the muscles, tendons, joints, bones, or nerves, characterized by pain and stiffness, discomfort and disability.

For remedies, refer '*Arthritis-Rheumatoid*' above

SCIATICA

Excruciating pain along the sciatic nerve usually caused by a herniated disc of the lumbar region of the spine and radiating to the buttocks and the back of the thigh.

Symptoms: Sudden, severe pain running from the lower back down the legs. At times, it sets gradually.

Distinguishing symptoms of the patient	Medicine and potency
• Sensation of **ice water** poured along the course of the nerves. **Crawling**.	Aconite Nap 30
• **Baseless fear**, shock, anguish.	

• **Intermittent**, violent, **burning**, tearing pain in left hip, running into thighs.	Ars Alb 200
• **Restlessness. Prostration**.	
• Better warm application.	
• With **facial neuralgia**.	Carbo Sulf 30
• Left-sided with numbness.	Causticum 200
• Progressive **loss of muscular strength**.	
• **Unbearable** pain.	Chamomilla 200
• Painful **cramps** in hips, in knee joint with sciatic pain.	Colocynthis 200
• **Right side**. Shooting pain down the thigh.	Dioscorea 30
• **Cramps** in fingers and toes.	
• **Left side** with tearing **pain in tibia**.	Kali Bi 200
• **Right side**. Legs feel numb, paralysed.	Lac Caninum 30
• Rheumatic pain in the back, in extremities.	
• **Worse in bed at night** or resting.	Rhus Tox 200, 1000
• On **exposure to damp** cold while sweating.	
• Temporary relief on motion.	
• With **swelling of ankles.**	Strontium 30
• **Chronic spasms** of ankle-joint.	
• Better immersing in hot water.	
• Pain like **electric flashes.**	Veratrum Alb 200
• **Cramps** in extremities with **vomiting**.	
• Cramps in calves.	
• **Cold sweat**. Prostration.	
• Shooting pain in **both thighs.**	Viscum Alb 30
• Pain in upper extremities.	
• **Body on fire**. Heat rises from feet to head.	
• Worse in winter, in bed, on movement.	

SEIZURE

Please refer '*Convulsions*' above.

SHOULDERS

Distinguishing symptoms of the patient	Medicine and potency
Inflammation/Pain/Swelling	
• Rheumatic pain between shoulders.	Camphor 30
• Pain across **shoulder and spine.**	Cannabis Indica 30
• **Must stoop to walk**.	
• Constant pain **under right shoulder** bone.	Chelidonium 30
• **Liver disorder**.	
• Cervical pain spreading to shoulders	Cimicituga 200
• Throbbing pain in **right** shoulder.	Ledum 200
• **Ascending** rheumatism.	
• **Gout** pain in joints.	
• Shooting pain in the **right shoulder**.	Phytolacca 30
Numbness	
• Shoulders cold, **numb, tingling**.	Camphor 30
Stoop	
• **Stoop**–shouldered.	Sulphur 200

SOLES

Distinguishing symptoms of the patient	Medicine and potency
Burning	
• At night. Wants to uncover the feet.	Chamomilla 200
• In **soles and hands, at night**.	Sulphur 200
Corns	
• From **pressure**. Soles painful.	Antim Crud 200
Please see '*Callosities/Corns*' above.	
Inflammation/Pain/Swelling	
• Soles sore from **foot sweat**.	Baryta Carb 200
• **Severe pain** in soles and in heels.	Borax 200
• Pain in **gout.**	
• **Chronic. Hard nodes** formed in joints of the feet. Can hardly step on soles.	Ledum 200

SPRAIN

An injury to a ligament without fracture of bone or dislocation of joint. Literally, a painful wrenching or laceration of the ligament of a joint.

Symptoms: Acute inflammation. Pain worse on movement.

Distinguishing symptoms of the patient	Medicine and potency
• First remedy in an **injury** in acute as well as chronic cases. • **Injuries** to cartilages, tendons, periosteum, joints. • Painful wrist due to **overuse** of an arm in writing or in using the key board.	Arnica 200 Alternate with Ruta 200 Ruta 200 Follows Arnica to complete the cure.

STAGGER

Distinguishing symptoms of the patient	Medicine and potency
Gait without co-ordination. Please see '*Ataxia locomotor*' above.	Conium 200

STRAIN

Heavy lifting or severe muscular exercise may cause an injury to the muscles and the tendons. Literally, to injure or impair by overuse or overexertion: wrench, strain a muscle.

Symptoms: Pain and swelling.

Distinguishing symptoms of the patient	Medicine and potency
• Caused by an **injury**, acute or chronic. • Bruised and sore all over.	Arnica 200 Alternate with Rhus Tox 200.

• Strain of tendons and muscles from **heavy lifting** or severe muscular **exercise** or from **wrong posture** in lifting a weight.	Rhus Tox 200
• Pain all over. Temporary relief on movement.	

SWEATING

Distinguishing symptoms of the patient	Medicine and potency
• Sweating in armpits. • Smells like garlic.	Sulphur 200

TENDO ACHILLES

Snapping into two, of the tendon which attaches the calf muscle to the back of the ankle.

Symptoms: Sudden and excruciating pain at the back of the ankle. Cannot stand on tiptoe.

The lower leg has to be put in plaster for two months. Medically advised shoes ought to be worn.

Distinguishing symptoms of the patient	Medicine and potency
• Stiffness. Pain like electric shocks.	Cimicifuga 200
• Tendo-achilles swollen and painful.	Kali Bi 200
• Tender pain but **temporary relief from motion**.	Rhus Tox 200
• **Neuralgic** pain.	Ruta 200

THIGHS

Distinguishing symptoms of the patient	Medicine and potency
Inflammation/Pain/Swelling	
• **Spasmodic** pain in thigh muscles.	Plumbum Met 30
• **Shifting** pain in thighs and legs.	Pulsatilla 30
• Tearing down pain **with or without dysentery.**	Rhus Tox 200
• Temporary relief on motion.	

THUMB

Distinguishing symptoms of the patient	Medicine and potency
Inflammation/Pain/Swelling	
• **Throbbing** pain in the tip of the thumb.	Borax 200

TICK

Twitching of a muscle.

Distinguishing symptoms of the patient	Medicine and potency
• **Acute, sudden, violent**. A result either of exposure to dry cold or due to shock, nervous excitement, or fear.	Aconite 30
• **Jerking, twitching, and trembling.**	Agaricus 200
• Twitching during sleep.	**Try this first.**

TOES

Distinguishing symptoms of the patient	Medicine and potency
Cramps	
• Cramps in toes and calves.	Hyoscymus 200
Eczema	
• **Loss of nails**. Eczema of toes.	Borax 30
Inflammation/Pain/Swelling	
• **Swelling** in toes, fingers, ankles.	Actea Spicata 30
• Tearing pain. **Urinary** disturbance.	Benzoic Acid 30
• **Eczema and inflammation** of the ball of the toe.	Borax 200
• **Chronic gouty spasm** and inflammation..	Colchicum 30
• Gout in heel.	
• Arthritic **nodules** with pain in toe.	Elaterium 30
• **Numbness** alternating with pain. Gout.	Gnaphalium 30
• Pain in calves, in feet, in the sciatic nerve.	
• Toenail **grown into flesh** with pain.	Teucrium 30

ULCERS

Distinguishing symptoms of the patient	Medicine and potency
• Ulceration on extremities.	Arsenic Alb 200

VARICOSE VEINS

Swollen and twisted veins on the calves.

Symptoms: Visibly swollen veins. Dull aching pain after standing. Cramps in the legs at night.

Distinguishing symptoms of the patient	Medicine and potency
• Chronic. In old persons.	Calc Fluorica 200
• Varicosity with **offensive, excoriating discharge.**	Carbo Veg 200
• In genitals with blueness and burning. **Bluish tumours**.	
• Varicose veins during **pregnancy**. Veins enlarged with stinging pain.	Hamamelis 200 Mother Tincture for local
• Swollen, burning, and **bleeding piles**.	application.
• Of right leg. Of labia during pregnancy. Of **genitalia**.	Lycopodium 200
• Often the **liver is sluggish**.	
• Spongy and enlarged.	Millefolium 200
• **Congested veins break easily.**	
• Ulcerating veins on legs.	
• In **legs, on testicles**, blue, sore and stinging.	Pulsatilla 30
• Veins **ulcerate, rupture**, and bleed.	Sulphur 200 Give one dose a day in addition to other selected remedy.

Please refer under '*the Female Genital System*' as well.

WHITLOW

An infection of the soft pad of the fingertip of the thumb.

Distinguishing symptoms of the patient	Medicine and potency
• **Piercing pain.**	Hepar Sulph 200
• Nail suppurates and **comes off**.	
• Caused by a **needle puncture**.	Ledum 200
• Abscess. **Hastens suppuration and aborts** pus.	Myristica 200
• **Chronic cases**. Pus oozes intermittently.	Silicea 200
• When another medicine has stopped being effective.	

WRIST/ARM

Distinguishing symptoms of the patient	Medicine and potency
Cramps	
• In muscles of **forearm**. Loss of muscular control.	Gelsemium 200
• Excessive trembling.	
Inflammation/Pain/Swelling	
• **Pain** in wrists, arms, shoulders, and ankles.	Abrotanum 30
• **Coldness** in fingers and feet. **Crawling**.	
• **Violent pain** in wrist. Paralysis. Pain of sprain in the wrist.	Hippomanes 30
• **Pain deep in the bones** of the arms.Chronic.	Eupatorium Perf 200
• Neuritis of the right arm **in writers**. Very painful.	Merc I.F. 30
• Stiffness in the wrist and **inability to raise the arm**.	Phytolacca 30
• Shooting pain in the right shoulder.	
• Pain like **electric shocks**.	
Stiffness	
• Wrists and hands stiff. Sprained.	Ruta 200
• **Overuse in writing**.	
Tumour	
• Encysted tumours on the **back of the wrist**.	Calc Fluor 30
Weakness	
• Involuntary motion of **one arm and leg**.	Hellebores 30
• **Wrist drop**.	Plumbum Met 30

THE SKIN

While the skeleton gives the inner form to human body, the skin gives it the outer shape. It has an average surface area of two square meters. It provides with its strong and flexible covering, protection to various organs of the body from damage either by injury or by infection.

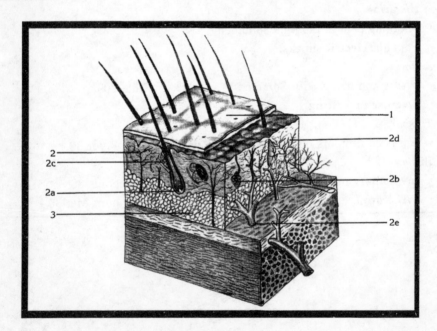

LAYERS OF THE SKIN
1. Epidermis. 2. Dermis: [a] Hair roots. [b] Sweat glands. [c] Sebaceous glands. [d]. nerve endings. [e]. Blood vessels. 3. Fat and subcutaneous tissue.

The skin has three layers: [1] the epidermis, the outer-celled layer, [2] the dermis which contains blood vessels, hair follicles, glands and [3] the innermost layer of subcutaneous tissue. It is not uniformly thick. It is thickest on the soles and the palms. It is thinnest on the eyelids.

Under the dermis lies a layer of fat which acts as an insulator and shock absorber. It is also a storehouse of energy.

The skin is a living organ although the uppermost layer of the epidermis is made of dead cells. It is a great receptor and communicator. It is sensitive to touch, pressure, heat, cold and pain. These sensations are conveyed to the brain by the skin through nerve endings. The lips and the fingertips have the highest concentration of nerve endings.

While a human being sheds more than thirty thousand dead cells every minute, the lower part of the epidermis constantly produces live cells to replace the dead ones.

Most parts of the skin have sweat glands. The maximum concentration lies in the palms and the soles. It is the function of the sweat glands to produce sweat to cool the body when it is too hot. Further, they produce a wax-like substance that helps prevent infection and keep the skin surface flexible and proof against water. That is why you can swim for hours and not soak a drop of water

When it gets too hot, our skin takes on a flushed appearance. The small blood vessels in the skin expand in order to lose heat. In cold weather, a constriction takes place so that heat is preserved. This results in the skin looking pale.

Exposed to sunlight, the skin produces vitamin D which helps in the absorption of Calcium and thus strengthens our bones.

The human skin is covered by hair all over, the maximum concentration being on the scalp, under the arms and in the pubic region.

Balding is a problem of the skin. It is generally hereditary. Not much can be done to grow hair on the scalp except by surgical grafting which is a reasonably successful procedure.

Fingernails and toenails are produced from under the skin.

A fibrous protein called keratin is the main component of the skin surface. As a part of hair, keratin provides warmth and protection. Nails which cover the delicate ends of fingers and toes, also contain keratin.

As we age, our skin develops wrinkles, loses elasticity, and may become rough if not taken care of. Our environment affects the colouring of the skin. People are fair in cold climates and darker under the African sun. The latter skin is, however, less susceptible to sunburn.

Mostly, the problems affecting skin are not life threatening. An unbroken skin is a highly effective barrier against bacteria and other harmful substances. However, a wound provides these micro-organisms direct access into the bloodstream. Infection sets in causing a rise in temperature, swelling, itching, and formation of boils or ulcers.

Besides, the skin can be infected by herpes, by warts. Burning and scalding of the skin can be painful. Eczema becomes chronic.

A cut or bruise triggers off a repair mechanism in the body. The capillaries on the site expand to allow more blood to flow into it. The skin turns red. The wounded tissue is swollen because of an excess of blood serum flowing into it. The white blood cells fight any invading bacteria.

While this process is on, formation of fresh skin starts simultaneously. Healing is normally quite a swift process.

To ensure a healthy skin, take a comfortable bath twice a day. You do not have to use soap unnecessarily except to wash away dirt, sweat, and grime. A walk under mild sunlight makes for a healthy skin. Avoid harsh sunlight. Pleasant outdoors are conducive to a healthy skin.

Avoid tension. Think well of everyone. Control anger. Be happy. Your skin will glow.

ABSCESS/SEPSIS

An abscess is a collection of pus under the skin caused by bacterial infection.

An abscess around a hair follicle is known as a boil. A collection of boils is called a carbuncle.

Symptoms: Swelling in the infected area with severe pain most of the time. Fever is caused by pus spreading into the bloodstream.

Distinguishing symptoms of the patient	Medicine and potency
• Prevents pus formation in **injuries**.	Arnica 200
• In **deep muscles** such as neck or thighs.	Calc Carb 200
• With callous, **hard edges**.	Calc Fluorica 200
• **Chronic** cases where a **discharge** from wounds, cuts, bruises **does not heal easily.**	Calc Sulph 200
• Pus is yellow and lumpy.	
• Pus formation **after surgery.**	Carbo Veg 200
• Any inflammation becomes purple.	
• With **piercing pain**, on any part of the body.	Hepar Sulph 200
• Suppuration with **easy bleeding.**	**First remedy**. Aborts pus
• **Tendency** to pus formation. Every little injury suppurates.	formation or bursts it.
• Hastens pus formation. Cuts its duration.	Myristica 200
• **Acute** as well as **chronic** cases.	Very powerful. Goes
• **Can avoid surgery**.	beyond Silicea.
• **Chronic** cases.	Silicea 200
• Old **fistulous** ulcers. **Moist** eruptions.	**Goes deeper than Hepar**
• **Deep-rooted** abscess in tendons, ligaments, in cavities.	**Sulph**.
• Severe pain and inflammation.	Tarentula Cubensis 200
• Tissues put on **blue colour**.	
• Carbuncles with **burning**, stinging pain.	

ACNE VULGARIS

An adolescence problem where a sebaceous gland meant to lubricate the skin is blocked by pus resulting from an infection. Pus forms below the blockage.

Acne cannot be prevented. However, it can be controlled. Keep the skin clean and sunbathe if you can.

Acne pimples should not be squeezed nor pinchèd.

Avoid dry fruit and chocolate. Eat fresh fruits and vegetables.

There is nothing to worry about acne. Everyone gets them. As you grow older, these disappear.

Symptoms: Small red pimples or blackheads on the face, neck, shoulders, chest, and back.

In severe cases, cysts form and there is painful inflammation.

Distinguishing symptoms of the patient	Medicine and potency
• **Red** pimples, on the side of the nose, chin, and mouth.	Asterias Rubens 30
• Pus with **piercing pain**. Unhealthy skin.	Hepar Sulph 200
• Pimples on face or anywhere on the skin. One dose early morning per week for a few weeks with other selected medicine.	Sulphur 200 To start the treatment with.

BALDNESS

Please refer '*Alopecia*' under the chapter '*The Brain, The Mind, The Emotions, and The Head*'.

BARBER'S ITCH

Rash on the site of the beard on a man's face.

Symptoms: Pus forms in hair follicles. Inflammation.

Distinguishing symptoms of the patient	Medicine and potency
• **Moist eczema** around mouth and chin.	Graphites 200
• Itching pimples.	
• Barber's itch and weeping eczema.	Sulphur 200
Pus in hair follicles.	
• **Intense itching**. Skin **red and swollen**.	Rhus Tox 200

BEDSORES

Skin ulcers caused by continuous pressure over the bones of the elbows and around buttocks in case of bed-ridden patients.

Symptoms: In the beginning a mild redness over the bony protrusions. Later, tenderness followed by cracks in the skin. Ulcers form. If not treated, they become infected.

Distinguishing symptoms of the patient	Medicine and potency
• A **prophylactic**. Prevents as well as heals.	Arnica 200
• For **local application**. Soothes and heals.	Calendula Mother tincture.
• Chronic ulcers below **coccyx, around sacrum.**	Paeonia 30
• Severe itching and burning.	
• Bedsores turning **gangrenous**.	Sulphur 200 One dose early morning for a week with other selected medicine.
• Skin livid, **red**, has **itching blotches.**	Sulphuric Acid 200
• **Carbuncles**, boils in bedsores.	

BLACKHEADS

Plugs of fatty material formed and hardened in a pore of the skin. Refer '*Acne*' above.

BLISTERS

When skin is injured by sunburn, heat, or friction, clear fluid, a part of blood, accumulates under the skin and a swelling is formed, This is called a 'blister.'

Do not burst a blister. Otherwise, an infection may develop.

Distinguishing symptoms of the patient	Medicine and potency
• Caused by **insect bite**.	Apis 200
• Crusty blisters which form in **typhoid**.	Acid Phos 200
• To ease **pain**, to subside **swelling.**	Cantharis 200
• Mother Tincture, diluted with water, one to four parts, for local application.	**A great remedy for blisters.**
• When **pus** has formed with stabbing pain.	Hepar Sulph 200
• Blisters formed during **intermittent fevers** like malaria, typhoid.	Natrum Mur 200

BLUE SKIN/CYANOSIS

Skin, fingers, and lips turn blue because of imperfect oxygenation. In children, this may indicate the presence of a heart problem.

Distinguishing symptoms of the patient	Medicine and potency
• With **palpitation, breathing difficulty** and dizziness.	Arsenic Alb 200
• **Heart dilated**.	
• Insufficient supply of oxygen for whatever reason. Skin turns **blue and cold**. The patient feels lifeless but his **head is hot.**	Carbo Veg 200
• **Puffy, blue face.**	
• Cyanosis of persons **continually** sick.	
• Wants fresh air, windows open.	

BOIL

A raised, tender area of the skin under which pus has formed. Abscess around a hair follicle.

To exclude the possibility of malignancy, consult a specialist.

Distinguishing symptoms of the patient	Medicine and potency
• Carbuncles. Succession of boils. **Burning.**	Anthracinum 30
• **Malignant** ulcers.	
• With stinging pain, burning, **swelling**.	Apis 200
• Ulcers with offensive discharge	Arsenic Alb 200
• **Malignant pustules**.	
• On **coccyx, shinbones, auditory canal**, recurring boils.	Calc Picrata 30
• **Chronic** cases.	
• Ulceration or carbuncles in **anus or the genital region**.	Thuja 200

BROWN SPOTS

Distinguishing symptoms of the patient	Medicine and potency
• On **abdomen**, in **chronic liver** condition.	Lycopodium 200
• Flatulence.	
• On **nose and arms**.	Thuja 200

BRUISE

Discoloration below the skin caused by an injury.

Symptoms: Blood leaks from damaged blood vessels. Skin turns purple or blue. Swelling on and around the injured surface.

Distinguishing symptoms of the patient	Medicine and potency
• Bruises. Traumatic injuries.	Arnica 200
• Skin turns **blue or purple.**	**The first medicine**.
• **Pain, swelling**, a bruised feeling.	
• For **local application** to heal, to soothe.	Calendula Mother Tincture or ointment.

Please refer the chapter *'Injuries/Bruises/Cuts'* etc. as well.

BURNING SENSATION

Distinguishing symptoms of the patient	Medicine and potency
• On **any surface**. In brain, in inner head, in throat, in lungs, in breasts, in stomach, in vagina, in bladder or on the skin. **Acute**.	Arsenic Alb 200
• **Prostration and restlessness.**	
• Better by hot bath, from hot food.	
• Worse at night; from cold application.	
• With **urinary irritation** and copious urine.	Cantharis 200
• **Biting heat** sensation on face, mouth, throat, oesophagus, stomach.	
• Burning in **soles at night.**	
• Erysipelas of **face. Large blisters**.	
• Intense. In lungs, **small intestines, up the spine, anus, and palms**.	Phosphorus 200
• **Chronic**, as against Arsenic that is acute.	Sulphur 200
• Burning with itching **anywhere**: inside head, margins of the eyes, nose, face, mouth, tongue, nipples, in stomach, while passing urine, vagina, rectum, in piles, hands, palms, feet, soles.	
• **Dry, scaly, unhealthy skin**. Persons of **unclean habits.**	
• Worse washing, scratching and at night.	

BURNS/SCALDS

Distinguishing symptoms of the patient	Medicine and potency
• By fire, by sunlight. **Sunburns.** • Painful burns. **Blisters anywhere.** • On soles due to walking • **Scalds by boiling liquids.** Immediate relief. No scars will be left if used in time. • Chronic old burns and scalds.	Cantharis 200 **Excellent first aid as well** **as a cure.** Take internally and apply Mother Tincture, diluted with water, 1 to 4, repeatedly. Causticum 200

CARBUNCLES

A cluster of boils. Commonly on the back of the neck.
Please refer '*Abscess/Sepsis*' and '*Boil*' above.

CELLULITIS

Rapidly spreading inflammation of the skin and subcutaneous tissue
due to infection.
Diabetics are more vulnerable than others are.

Symptoms: Blisters. Red swelling. May lead to formation of boils and
carbuncles.

Distinguishing symptoms of the patient	Medicine and potency
• Intensely painful swelling due to **insect** **bite. Even otherwise.** • Stinging pain. Skin red, shining and sensitive. • **Punctured wounds** leading to cellulitis.	Apis 200 Ledum 200

- Affected part swollen and cold. **First remedy for**
  Prevents tetanus. **punctured wounds.**
- Of the neck. Of the pelvis. About Rhus Tox 200
  the glands.
- **Pitting on pressure. Purple, inflamed,**
  skin hot and painful.

CHILBLAINS

An inflammation followed by itchy irritation, on the fingers, toes, back of the leg, sometimes buttocks, or ears. Results from exposure to moist cold.

Symptoms: Pain, sensation of heat, inflammatory swelling, itching. Swelling with ulceration in severe cases.

Distinguishing symptoms of the patient	Medicine and potency
• **Frostbites.**	Agaricus 200
• **Veins swollen with cold skin.**	
• Painful, intense itching, red swelling.	
• Skin hot, **dark red.**	Rhus Ven 30
• Severe itching. Relieved by hot water.	Mother Tincture for local use. Relief and cure.
• Erythema of fingers and toes caused by **frostbite.**	Terebinthina 30
• Muscles aching and sore.	
• Intense itching. **Pulsating pain.**	
• **Ulcers on skin with pus.**	

CHLOASMA

Temporary darkening of the skin because of hormones stimulating the skin pigment, melanin, during pregnancy or when using contraceptive pills or by use of a certain perfume.

The condition disappears usually after childbirth or when the particular perfume has been discontinued or with the stoppage of contraceptive pills.

Symptoms: Skin becomes temporarily dark on cheekbones, the bridge of the nose or the area around mouth.

Distinguishing symptoms of the patient	Medicine and potency
• Discoloration of the skin, particularly **purple**.	Sepia 200 Once a day

COLDNESS

Distinguishing symptoms of the patient	Medicine and potency
• **Internal burning** with external coldness. • Lack of vitality.	Carbo Veg 200
• **Ice-cold** in individual parts, **external as well as external**. • Coldness of legs, of feet.	Calcarea Carb 200

Please refer '*Numbness*', as well below.

COLD SORES/HERPES SIMPLEX

Primary cold sores

Small blisters occurring on the lips, on face, caused by herpes simplex.

Herpes simplex is a recurrent viral disease caused by the herpes simplex virus, type one, and marked by the eruption of fluid-containing vesicles on the mouth, lips, or the face.

The type two is marked by the eruptions on the genitals. Sexual intercourse can cause herpes on the genitals if one party is infected.

Symptoms: Tingling in the affected site. A feeling of feverishness. Blisters, bleeding ulcers on the lips and the inside of the cheeks, of the gums, the tongue, vulva, and vagina. The skin surrounding the blisters becomes inflamed. Later the blisters burst and the site becomes crusty. **Seek medical advice when genitalia are affected.**

Distinguishing symptoms of the patient	Medicine and potency
• Pricking sensation in the affected areas.	Hepar Sulph 200
• **Abscess** on the labia.	
• Herpes on the outside of prepuce.	
• Burning, stinging, bleeding ulcers. Painful to touch.	
• **Offensive exhalation** from the body.	
• Threatened pus formation.	
• **Bleeding ulcers. Black pores** on the face.	Nitric Acid 200
• **Genital herpes**. Glans penis and prepuce sore, burning. Pus. Stinging pain.	
• Vesicles of **bluish colour**. Burning. Stitching pain.	Ranunculus Bulbosus 30
• Terrible itching as vesicles dry.	
• Burning, itching with **fever.**	Rhus Tox 200
• Chronic suppurating eruptions on the face. Swelling.	Try first.

Recurrent cold sores

An acute disease. Comes suddenly. Blisters form on the lips and face. Painful eruptions develop on genitals.

For medicines, please refer '*Primary cold sores*' above.

COLOUR

Distinguishing symptoms of the patient	Medicine and potency
• Profound anaemia. Eyes sunken. **Dark rings around eyes.**	Acetic Acid 30

- **Face pale**, waxen, emaciated, or swollen.
- On account of injury, skin black or blue.   Arnica 200
- **Red, shining, throbbing**.   Belladonna 200
- Painful inflammation.
- **Erysipelas of the face**. Swollen, red.   Borax 200
- **Minute red spots** or eruptions on   Calc Carb 200
  the surface.
- **Face blue. Skin pale. Lack of oxygen**   Carbo Veg 200
  for any reason. Pulse intermittent.
- Skin **purple** with sepsis, **congestion**,
  inflammation.
- Yellow skin in **liver disorders**.   Chelidonium 30
- **Pink spots** on back, chest, and abdomen.   Colchicum 30
- Urticaria. **Sudden** rash.
- Yellow skin and nails. **Jaundice in heart**   Digitalis 30
  patients. Pulse slow.
- Liver swollen and hard.
- Haemorrhage below the skin. Skin **purple.**   Lachesis 200
- Purple face. Purple varicose veins.
  Purple breasts.
- Large blisters as from scalds.   Mancinella 30
- **Red vesicles**. Intense erythema.
- Urticaria **after rich food**. Red, raised rash. Pulsatilla 30
- **Red, swollen, itching eruptions**. Urticaria. Rhus Tox 200
- Blue. Cold as death. **Cold sweat.**   Veratrum Alb 1000
- **Pale, sunken face.**
- **Cholera. Collapse**.
- Blisters, red spots on the face, hands,   Viola Tricolour 30
  knees **of children**. Pus discharge.

CORNS/CALLOSITIES

A horny thickening of the skin on hands or feet. Caused by pressure or friction.

Distinguishing symptoms of the patient	Medicine and potency
• Corns from pressure.	Antim Crud 200
• Callosities from pressure of shoes.	
• Corns or bunions from tight shoes. On soles.	Sulphur 200
• **Itching, burning**.	

CRAB LICE

Crab lice infest the pubic hair and the hair around the anus. Quite often, these have to be physically picked out and killed.

Distinguishing symptoms of the patient	Medicine and potency
• Lice in pubic hair. Near the anus.	Staphysagria 200

CRACKS/FISSURES

Distinguishing symptoms of the patient	Medicine and potency
• Fissures **on palms**.	Calc Fluor 200
• In hands. Skin **hard, thick, and dry**.	Cistus Can 30
Deep cracks with itching.	
• Cannot sleep due to itching.	
• Around mouth, in nipples, at the ends of fingers, between toes, on labia, on anus.	Graphites 200
• **Burning, stitching pain** in fissures. Skin numb, sore.	
• Deep cracks, ulcers on hands and feet with **piercing pain and pus**.	Hepar Sulph 200
• **Ulceration, cracks**, swelling, splinter-like pain in canthi, nose, lips, or other **mucous junctions**.	Nitric Acid 200
• Cracks **worse every winter.**	Petroleum 200

- Skin dry, contracted. Wears a
  leathery look.
- **Ends of fingers** cracked.   Silicea 200
- Cracked and **burning** nipples.
- Burning and itching in vagina and   Sulphur 200
  around vulva.

CYST

A lump full of fluid or air on any part of the body. Different sizes. It can be near the skin or deep in an organ.

Symptoms: An infected cyst is red and sore. It is usually benign. However, sometimes it is cancerous.

For cancerous cyst, consult a doctor.

Distinguishing symptoms of the patient	Medicine and potency
• Stinging pain. Swelling. Red inflammation.	Apis 200

ECZEMA/DERMATITIS

A non-contagious inflammation of the skin.

Symptoms: Redness, itching, outbreak of lesions that may discharge serous matter and become encrusted and scaly.

Eczema is of five different types: atopic, contact dermatitis, seborrheic dermatitis, discoid eczema, and varicose eczema. **Seek advice of a skin specialist**.

Eczema is bothersome. There are no easy and quick cures. However, most of the problem disappears with time and treatment.

Distinguishing symptoms of the patient	Medicine and potency
• **Chronic, suppressed** eczema. Skin dry, scaly, burning.	Arsenic Alb 200 **Remarkable results in**

• **Oozing holes** with offensive discharge.	**oozing eczema**.
• **Malignant** pustules.	
• Of **eyelids**.	Bacillum 200
• Of **anus**. Of **hands**.	Berberis Vulgaris 30
• Of toes and fingers.	Borax 30
• Secondary eczema on **scrotum, genitals**, following excessive **perspiration.**	Cantharis 200 Apply Mother Tincture, diluted in water, 1 to 4,
• **Acute** cases.	locally as well.
• **Offensive oozing** eczema on head, face, nose, mouth and chin. Beyond ears. On legs. On genitals. Around anus.	Graphites 200
• Of eyelids with fissured margins	
• Sticky, **glutinous fluid** oozing.	
• On **cheeks**. Stinging pain when touched.	Ledum 200
• On bald patches **on the scalp**. Behind **ears.**	Lycopodium 200
• Copper coloured eruptions on face.	
• On **genitals with swelling**. Scrotum thick and hard.	Rhus Tox 200

ERYSIPELAS

A serious, acute bacterial infection of the skin spread by direct contact. It spreads rapidly to the surrounding tissues. It is also called Saint Anthony's fire.

Symptoms: Begins as a red spot on the face or the scalp. The spot grows larger with raised edges and a diameter of several inches. This area is hot, painful, and swollen. Temperature goes up. The patient has chills, nausea, and vomiting.

Seek medical advice. Erysipelas can lead to death.

Distinguishing symptoms of the patient	Medicine and potency
• **Severe swelling** of the throat. **Rosy** hue. **Pits on pressure.**	Apis 200

- Stinging pain. Scanty, painful urination.
- **Afternoon chill** with thirst.
- Better cold application.
- **Restlessness** with swelling. Dry, **rough,**   Arsenic Alb 200
  scaly skin.
- High temperature.
- Worse cold, scratching, after midnight.
- Of face, of head. Worse right side.   Belladonna 200
- **Glands of neck swollen.**
- Skin dry, swollen, hot. **Burns red. Hard**
  inflammation.
- High fever. **Pungent, steaming hot**. No thirst.
- **Visual hallucinations. Delirium**. Violent.
- Feet ice-cold.
- Of **face, beginning on nose.**   Cantharis 200
- Large blisters. Restlessness, burning,
  stinging pain.
- **Urinary complications**.
- **Pus** formation in affected areas. **Splinter**   Hepar Sulph 200
  pain in glands of the neck.
- In **old age**. On face.   Lachesis 200
- Skin swollen. Boils and ulcers with **bluish**
  or purple edges.
- Chill in the **back. Feet cold.**
- **Hot flushes and perspiration.**
- Cries violently sometimes. Uneasy, restless.
- **Large**, intensely burning blisters on   Rhus Tox 200
  face, **extending rapidly.**
- Skin purple, pits on pressure.
- Skin **dark and rough**, not red and smooth.
  Moist, not dry.
- Pain which tears apart. Pus under the
  swollen skin.

FOREIGN BODIES

Distinguishing symptoms of the patient	Medicine and potency
• **Expels foreign bodies under the skin**. • Creates inflammation and suppuration to remove tiny bodies that cannot be easily located.	Hepar Sulph 200
• **Chronic** cases.	**Silicea 200**

FROSTBITE

A prolonged exposure to severe cold, particularly at high altitudes, damages the extremities.

Symptoms: The parts affected are the ears, nose, the fingers, and the toes. They turn pale. Blisters form. The parts are numb, yet painful. Please refer '*Chilblains*' above.

GANGRENE

Death of skin tissue followed by bacterial infection and putrefaction. It sets in fingers, toes, limbs, and other parts of the body after their blood supply has been cut off.

Symptoms: The affected area becomes cold and pale. After a few days, it turns black. Severe pain at the edge of the affected part.

Distinguishing symptoms of the patient	Medicine and potency

• **Diabetic** gangrene.
• Gangrene in **internal organs**.
  Burning ulcers.
• Inflammation in gangrene.
  Blue-black base.
	Arsenic Alb 200

- In old age, beginning at the **toes.**   Carbo Veg 200
- On the margins. **Blue, cold skin**.
  Insufficient supply of oxygen.
- Easily bleeding **bedsores**.
- In old **age**, of the **lungs**.   Kreosote 30
- In **old persons. Shrivelled** skin.   Secale 30
- **Dry gangrene** developing slowly
- **Varicose ulcers.**
- Numbness. Burning sensation.

IMPETIGO

Highly contagious skin infection common in young children. It affects the face, hands, and the knees. It is caused by different bacteria.

Symptoms: Red spots appear on the skin and change into blisters. The blisters break down and the discharge forms a honey-coloured crust. More of red spots are formed by the oozing liquid.

Distinguishing symptoms of the patient	Medicine and potency
• **Malignant** pustules.	Arsenic Alb 200
• Eruptions dry, rough, scaly.	
• **Restlessness and prostration.**	
• Worse cold, scratching.	
• **Ulcerating** eruptions with thick scabs.	Mezerium 30
• **Oozing pus.**	
• Worse in cold air, at night, taking warm food, touch, and motion.	

INFLAMMATION/GLANDULAR INFLAMMATION/ NODULES

The body tissues react to an injury or infection by supplying extra blood so that more white blood cells are available to repair.

A nodule is a small node or rounded eminence which is solid and can be detected by touch.

Symptoms: The affected area becomes red, hot, swollen, and tender.

Distinguishing symptoms of the patient	Medicine and potency
• Glands of **armpits** swollen, hard and painful.	Asterias Rubens 30
• Glands of **neck** enlarged.	Bacillinum 200
• Skin is **hot, scarlet red,** gradually turning purple. It is smooth.	Belladonna 200
• **Throbbing** inflammation. Carbuncles.	
• **Acute** cases.	
• Feels better in a warm room.	
• Glands near **lower jaw and throat,** stone hard.	Bromum 30
• Glands in **neck, armpits, breasts, groin** swollen.	Carbo Ani 30
• Burning, **piercing pain**.	
• Rough nodules **all over**. Hard, enlarged.	Kali Hydro 30
• Worse on covering.	
• **Piercing pain** in swollen glands of neck, armpit, breast, or groin. In **bones, roots of nails, ends of fingers.**	Hepar Sulph 200
• **Hard red** swelling and **suppuration**.	
• The glands enlarge while the **body shrivels.**	Iodum 200
• **Goitre.**	
• Appetite great but flesh is lost.	
• Skin hot, dry, yellow, and withered.	
• **Breasts dwindle** while other glands grow.	
• Nodules on the skin of the breasts.	
• Enlargement of **thyroid, sub maxillary glands, uvula, liver, spleen.**	
• **Hard inflammation** beneath the tongue, in tonsils, glands of the neck, near the ears, in armpits, breasts, in the liver, in groin.	Merc Sol 200

- **Chronic**, prolonged suppuration in glands.   Nitric Acid 200
- **No tendency to repair**
- Piercing pain.
- **Chronic glandular or bony abscess**.   Silicea 200

In addition, refer under '*Inflammation*' under separate body parts.

INTERTRIGO

Inflammation because of excessive sweating and friction on skin surfaces which are in close contact like thighs, groin and armpits.

Symptoms: Foul smell. Itching inflammation.

Distinguishing symptoms of the patient	Medicine and potency
• Between thighs. Excoriation. Itching.	Aethusa 30
• Soreness between **folds of the skin**, anywhere.	
• Intertrigo during **dentition** of children	Causticum 200
• Better in damp hot weather and in bed.	
• Rawness on neck, **behind ears, in groin**.	Graphites 200

ITCHING/PRURITIS

It can be a symptom of a number of disorders. It is aggravated by heat and anxiety.

Avoid scratching if you can help it. Scratching can result in pus formation.

Application of Calamine lotion gives relief. So does dusting with herbal talcum powders.

At the anus, Calendula Mother Tincture soothes and cures.

Taking care of personal hygiene is of utmost importance.

Distinguishing symptoms of the patient	Medicine and potency
• Terrible, **allergic**, urticaria. Thirst, fever, and heat.	Aconite 30
• On exposure to dry, cold air.	
• Itching eruption around **joints**, between **folds** of thighs, on walking.	Aethusa 30
• Copious, excoriating sweat.	
• Intolerable when getting into a **warm bed**.	Alumina 30
• In **frostbite**.	Agaricus 30
• On tip of **coccyx.**	Bovista 30
• Urticaria on excitement.	
• On vulva during **pregnancy.**	Caladium Seg 30
• On glans **penis**.	
• Soreness in the **folds** of the skin, behind ears, between thighs.	Causticum 200
• Crusty eruptions **on head**. Ring worm of **scalp**.	Dulcamara 200
• Nettle rash. Pruritis worse in wet, cold weather.	
• **Chronic** or recurring urticaria.	Hepar Sulph 200
• Swelling, itching, piercing pain.	
• Intolerable itching **on soles**.	Hydrocotyle 30
• Small pustules **all over** the body, itching intolerably.	Magnesia Sulph 30 Apply mother tincture for relief.
• On **feet**.	Magnolia 30
• On **forehead, scalp**, edges of hair, corrosive itching.	Oleander 30
• Bleeding, **oozing eruptions**.	
• On **lower extremities**, violent itching on **exposure** to cold air, on undressing.	Rumex 30
• Voluptuous, itching eruptions.	Sulphur 200
• **Burning follows. Most prominent.**	
• **Excoriating moisture in folds**, in orifices like eyelids, ears, lips, urethra, and anus. Surface vermilion red.	

- **Chronic** cases
- Better dry, warm weather. Worse washing.
  At night.

LEPROSY

A chronic inflammation that affects nerves, skin, and the bones adjacent to the skin. It is not as contagious as it is believed to be.

Symptoms: Inflammation of nerves leads to acute loss of sensation, paralysis, and deformity. Fingers and toes drop. Glands are enlarged. Skin oozes and falls off in scales.
Consult a doctor.

Distinguishing symptoms of the patient	Medicine and potency
• **Dropping of fingers and toes.**	Arsenic Iod 30
• Enlarged glands. Pricking **numbness**.	
• **Scales** fall off profusely. The skin below is raw and exudes moisture.	
• To be used once a week with the other chosen medicine.	Bacillinum 200

LICE

Small parasites that live on the skin and suck blood. Transferred from person to person by contact or sharing clothes.

Symptoms: Severe itching. Scratching leads to infection.

Distinguishing symptoms of the patient	Medicine and potency
• Lice on the head.	Carbolic Acid 30
• Lice **anywhere**.	Lycopodium 200
• Lice in pubic hair.	Staphysagria 200

NUMBNESS/PINS AND NEEDLES

Deprivation of powers to feel or move normally.

Symptoms: A loss of sensation in a part of the body. It is caused by swelling or pressure on the nerve in that area. There is a tickling sensation called 'pins and needles'.

Distinguishing symptoms of the patient	Medicine and potency
• Numbness and tingling.	Aconite 30
• Sometimes shooting pain in the face and in extremities.	**First remedy.**
• Caused by fear, anguish, by sudden loss.	
• On exposure to dry cold air.	
• **Body ice-cold**.	Arsenic Alb 200
• **Skin cold, pale, blue**. Cannot bear to be covered.	Camphor 30
• Numbness **down the arm** with pain in glands in the armpit.	Conium 30
• In **lips, tongue, knees, legs, feet**. Tingling sensation.	Nat Mur 200
• Extreme **sensitivity to cold**. Desires warm clothing even in summer.	Psorinum 200
• **In collapse. In cholera**. Cold as death. Blue skin. Cold sweat.	Veratrum Alb 1000

ODOUR

Distinguishing symptoms of the patient	Medicine and potency
• Persistent offensive odour from the **body**.	Hepar Sulph 200
• Offensive odour in **pus, in perspiration, in saliva, urine, stool, in ulcers in the mouth, on gums, in ear discharge, in nasal discharge etc.**	Merc Sol 200

PAIN

Distinguishing symptoms of the patient	Medicine and potency
• Piercing pain. Because of **pus formation, indurations** in skin. In glands. In boils.	Hepar Sulph 200

PERSPIRATION/SWEATING

Distinguishing symptoms of the patient	Medicine and potency
• Copious perspiration when the patient is **debilitated** by sickness.	Calcarea Carb 200
• Internal or external parts of the body **ice-cold**.	
• **Persistent sweating** day and night. Sweat **offensive.**	Hepar Sulph 200
• Unhealthy, suppurating skin.	
• **Tendency to excessive** perspiration.	Merc Sol 200
• Skin **constantly moist**, oily, emanating unpleasant odour.	
• **Excessive salivation**.	
• Hot perspiration over **entire body surface** except lower limbs.	Opium 200
• Sweating excoriation **in folds,** in armpits etc.	Sulphur 200
• With **burning**.	

PRICKLY HEAT

Skin rash that develops in hot and humid weather. Blisters appear in folds.

Distinguishing symptoms of the patient	Medicine and potency
• In **folds** of the skin, between thighs.	Causticum 200
• In infants, around **neck, armpits, chest and groin**.	
• **Red, swollen** skin with intense itching.	Rhus Tox 200
• **Burning eruptions.**	
• Better in warm, dry weather.	
• Worse during wet weather, being drenched.	

PSORIASIS

A chronic skin eruption. Patches of red, thickened, scaly skin. Mostly, the scalp, eyebrows, fingernails, back, buttocks and the knees are affected.

Symptoms: Red patches which develop slowly, are covered with silver-white, hard, and dry scales. The lesions are rough, red, and permanent. There is no itching.

Talk to your skin specialist for help.

Distinguishing symptoms of the patient	Medicine and potency
• Symptoms as above. Four drops in water daily for a long time until a cure occurs.	Arsenic Bromatum Mother Tincture
• Symptoms as above. One dose every 15 days, early morning, for 6 months, besides the other medicine.	Sulphur 1000

RASH

A temporary eruption of the skin.

Distinguishing symptoms of the patient	Medicine and potency
• **Sudden, violent. On exposure** to dry cold air.	Aconite 30
• **Thick, rough**, rosy swelling anywhere.	Apis 200
• **Springtime rash** on exposure to open air. A **crust forms**.	Sarsaparilla 30

RINGWORM

A contagious skin infection caused by fungus.

Symptoms: Initially a small, round, scaly, itchy patch appears. It grows larger to form a scaly, red ring around a central area of normal skin. Later more patches form.

Largely, ringworm affects moist parts of the body such as the armpits, the surface beneath the breast, the groin, and the feet. However, it can occur anywhere.

Distinguishing symptoms of the patient	Medicine and potency
• Ringworm accompanied by swelling, itching, and intense burning.	Apis 200
• One dose once a week. Should clear the infection by itself.	Bacillinum 200
• Ringworm **worse every spring**.	Sepia 200
• With **dry, scaly and unhealthy skin**.	Sulphur 200
• Of the face	Tellurium 30
• Body **sweat** offensive **like garlic**.	

ROSACEA

A chronic dermatitis of the face caused by dilation of capillaries.

Symptoms: Permanent reddening of the skin on the face, on the nose and the cheeks. Blisters full of pus form on the affected area. Skin puffy. Visible tiny blood vessels. Stinging, burning or itching sensation. Avoid alcohol, strong spices, exposure to harsh sun or to cold winds.

Distinguishing symptoms of the patient	Medicine and potency
• Red acne with violet papules on nose.	Arsenic Bromatum Mother Tincture. One dose of 15 drops in water daily.
• Copper coloured eruptions. • **Worse in the spring.**	Carbo Animalis 30

SENSITIVE

Distinguishing symptoms of the patient	Medicine and potency
• Sensitive to touch, to cold, to pain. • **Suppurating boils** with piercing pain. It hurts to touch the boil.	Hepar Sulph 200
• Skin sensitive to heat or cold like a thermometer. • **Copious sweating** day and night. Foul odour in the sweat.	Merc Sol 200
• Face hot. Yet, **experiences a chill the moment he uncovers**.	Nux Vomica 200

SHRIVELLED

Distinguishing symptoms of the patient	Medicine and potency
• Looks prematurely old. Shrivelled, scaly skin. • Small, circumscribed, **hard, elevated, swollen lesions**.	Arsenic Alb 200
• Dry, emaciated, shrivelled skin **lies in folds**.	Sarsaparilla 30

SWELLING/DROPSY/OEDEMA

An abnormal accumulation of fluid in the body tissues.

Distinguishing symptoms of the patient	Medicine and potency
• **Pale, waxen**, swollen skin.	Acetic Acid 30
• Terrible, **allergic urticaria** with thirst, fear of death, anguish.	Aconite 30
• On exposure to dry cold air.	
• From **frostbite**.	Agaricus 30
• In **eczema. In urticaria**. Intense itching.	Anacardium 200
• Puffing **anywhere**. Stinging pain.	Apis 200
• Red, rosy hue.	**The first remedy.**
• Insect bites.	
• Urticaria. Erysipelas.	
• With eruptions which are small, and **circumscribed.**	Arsenic Alb 200
• **Solid, elevated lesions.**	
• Dry, rough, scaly skin.	
• **Stony** hardness.	Calc Fluor 30
• With **varicose ulcers**.	Carbo Veg 200
• Purple skin that pits on pressure. Inflammation extending rapidly.	Rhus Tox 200
• **Erysipelas** of the vesicular variety.	
• **Urticaria** of face.	
• **Large, burning blisters**.	
• Unbroken **chilblain** swelling.	Terebinthina 30
• Erythema of the ears, fingers, toes, caused by **mild frostbite**.	

TUMOUR

A non-inflammatory growth, circumscribed, serving no physiological function. It arises from existing tissue but grows independently of such tissue.

Tumours can be cancerous. **Seek medical advice at the earliest.**

Distinguishing symptoms of the patient	Medicine and potency
• Hard excrescences on the **skull**. Knots in **female breast**. On the back of the **wrist**.	Calcarea Fluorica 200
• Hard swelling on the **cheek**, with pain or toothache.	
• Painful and **enlarged tumours or glands**.	Conium 200
• Morning and night, offensive sweat and smarting skin.	
• **Spongy tumours.**	Thuja 200
• **Glandular enlargement** with piercing pain.	
• Bleeding **fungus growth.**	
• Tumours of **breast**. Nipple retracted.	

ULCER

A break in the skin or in the mucous lining of the alimentary tract caused by inflammation.

Symptoms: Severe biting pain. At times massive haemorrhage.

Distinguishing symptoms of the patient	Medicine and potency
• Burning like **hell-fire. Offensive oozing.**	Arsenic Alb 200
• **Diabetic gangrene** in extremities.	
• Blue-black base.	
• Ulcers on **heels**.	
• In the **mouth**. On **tongue**.	Borax 200
• With **hard elevated edges.**	Calc Fluor 200
• Skin purple and swollen.	
• With **varicose veins.**	Calc Iod 30
• Copper coloured eruptions.	
• **Easy bleeding**. Sensitive to touch. Burning, stinging.	Hepar Sulph 200

• With **regular edges** as if made with a punch.	Kali Bi 200
• In the **mouth**, on the tongue, on gums, inside of cheeks, on tonsils.	Merc Sol 200
• Fetid, painful, full of **pus**.	
• **Chronic**, in the mouth. Full of pus.	Nit Acid 200
• **Below coccyx**, caused by pressure. **Bedsores**.	Paeonia 30
• Near **genitals**, near anus.	Thuja 200

URTICARIA

Known as 'nettle rash' or 'hives'. A bothersome skin itching.

Symptoms: Tissues under the skin swell. Intense irritation. Formation of patches of pale skin surrounded by red.
Please refer '*Itching*' above.

VARICOSE VEINS

Abnormally swollen or knotted veins. Visibly so. Mainly in the legs.

Symptoms: Blue, swollen, distorted, easily visible veins, bulging beneath the skin. More prominent when standing. Discomfort, pain in the legs after prolonged standing.

Distinguishing symptoms of the patient	Medicine and potency
• **Chronic**. Burning intensely at night.	Arsenic Alb 200
• Of **legs, in women** who have had several pregnancies. Varicose ulcers as well.	Fluoric Acid 30
• With **inflammation during pregnancy**.	Lachesis 200
• **Easy bleeding** varicose veins. Enlarged and spongy.	Millefolium 30
• Stinging pain.	Pulsatilla 30
• Ulcers surrounded by varicose veins **bleed black blood which coagulates easily**.	
• In **extremities**. Ulcerate, rupture, and bleed.	Sulphur 200

VITILIGO/LEUCODERMA

A common problem affecting about one percent of human beings.

Symptoms: White patches form on the skin because of loss of pigment. There is neither pain nor loss of sensation.

The rate of cure is negligible, particularly in old cases.

Try

Arsenic Sulph Flavum 3, 30, 200

3: Four doses every day for the first two months.

30: Four doses every day for the next two months.

200: One dose per week. For a long time.

Hydrocotyle 30

If the Arsenic Sulph Flavum fails, give Hydrocotyle 30, four doses a day, for a long time.

Tuberculinum 200

One dose to start the treatment with. Later one dose every month.

In order to accelerate recovery, expose affected parts to mild sunlight for ten minutes, once a day, 30 minutes after the administration of the medicine.

WARTS

Small growth on the skin or on a mucous membrane.

Distinguishing symptoms of the patient	Medicine and potency
• On **hands**. Hard. Horny excrescences under nails and from the **ends of fingers**.	Antim Crud 200
• Chronic warts on face, eyelids, eyebrows, nose, tips of fingers.	Causticum 200
• Large, jagged, **easily bleeding**.	
• Large, smooth warts coming in **wet, cold weather**.	Dulcamara 200

- Warts on **back of hands**.
- **Bleeding easily** on washing. Moist oozing.   Nitric Acid 200
  Splinter pain. Large, jagged.
- Fig warts. Intolerable **itching and burning**.   Sabina 30
  Apply mother tincture
  locally.

- On margins of **prepuce**.   Sepia 200
- **Suppurating** warts and cavities.   Silicea 200
- Warty excrescences. Fig warts.   Thuja 1000
- On **genitals, cervix, anus**.

FEVERS

The body temperature, higher than the normal of 98.4°F or 37°C is known as fever. It is a nuisance but an unavoidable one. It indicates that the body is resisting an attack by organisms that cause disease.

An infection by carriers of disease is met with resistance by the white blood cells by surrounding the former. The blood cells signal the brain which, in turn, activates the thermostat of the body situated in the hypothalamus. The body is ordered to raise the temperature and the human being begins to shiver.

Shivering, being movement, generates heat. The blood vessels near the skin surface become narrow so that the heat loss is prevented. The fat stored under the skin breaks down and provides further heat.

A shivering patient is covered with heavy clothing. This helps in further raising the temperature.

When the body temperature rises, the defence mechanism operates more efficiently.

This is true of mild fevers which do not last long.

However, when the temperatures exceeds 40°C or 104°F, or if a child under one year runs a high temperature, get **immediate medical assistance. It as an emergency.**

Fevers lasting beyond three days in adults too require medical consultation.

A patient running a temperature must rest and take proper medication. He should stay snug and warm. He should take a light diet and plenty of cool fluids.

Medicines like aspirin should not be used casually or frequently. In adults, it irritates the stomach and the intestines. The fever should be diagnosed correctly and medicine taken according to symptoms.

BURNING

Distinguishing symptoms of the patient	Medicine and potency
• Burning in brain, in stomach, in **bladder**, **in lungs**. Acute sensation. • In malaria, typhoid. Last stages of pneumonia. • Nightly aggravation.	Ars Alb 200
• **High fever**. The body burns, **pungent, steaming hot.** • No thirst.	Belladonna 200
• **Frequent, violent flushes** of heat through the entire body.	Sulphur 200

CHICKEN POX

An acute, contagious disease, primarily in children, caused by the varicella-zoster virus.

Symptoms: Skin eruptions rapidly turning into fluid-filled blisters. Slight fever. Discomfort. The irritating rash spreads to the arms, legs, face, and the head. The Chicken Pox appears in severely itching clusters.

Apply calamine lotion to the rash several times a day to soothe the itching. Have plenty of liquids. Keep the rash dry and clean. Do not scratch.

Do not worry.

Distinguishing symptoms of the patient	Medicine and potency
A day after Veriloneum. Every four hours until temperature returns to normal.	Antim Tart 200
• Fever with **dry cough.** • Any **movement**, even coughing, talking, hurts.	Bryonia 200
Start with one dose. It cuts short the duration.	Veriloneum 200

CHILDREN

Distinguishing symptoms of the patient	Medicine and potency
• On **exposure to dry cold winds**. Acute • Sudden **congestion of the brain** with high temperature. • Croup of the **frightened** child.	Aconite 30
• **Sudden, intense fever**. • Child's skin hot, face **red. Jumps in sleep** as if going into a spasm. • **Convulsions.** • Cerebral congestion.	Belladonna 200

CHILL

Distinguishing symptoms of the patient	Medicine and potency
• **Entire body ie-cold. Tongue** cold and **trembling**. • Weak pulse.	Camphor 200
• Periodic chill with **clear-cut stages.** • In **malaria**. In **typhoid**. Worse touch.	China 200
• Chill **along spine** in influenza. • **Body pain. Shivering**.	Gelsemium 200
• **Persistent, profuse perspiration**. Foul smell. Skin ever moist. • **Gastric** fever.	Merc Sol 200
• **Periodic chill**. Occurs at 10.30 a.m. • Starts in **extremities which turn blue.** • **Throbbing headache. Teeth chatter. Bones ache. Fingers scorched.** • No thirst during fever. • Otherwise, mucous membranes dry. Great thirst for cold water. • Rolls from side to side.	Nat Mur 200

- Malarial or **any** other **fever with periodicity.**
- Sweating relieves fever and ache.
- Inflammatory or periodic fevers.   Nux Vomica 200
- **Sore throat. Gastric disturbance.**
  Rheumatic inflammation.
- **Spasms** with rigor in the morning. **Finger**
  nails blue.
- Feels chilly on being uncovered but cannot
  stand covering.
- Must be covered in every stage of fever.
- Chill with **extreme coldness and sweat.**   Veratrum Alb 1000
- In cholera. In gastroenteritis. **Rice water stools.**
- **Nausea. Vomiting** uncontrollable.
- **Collapse.**

COLLAPSE

Distinguishing symptoms of the patient	Medicine and potency
• In the **last stages** of collapse in **cholera, in yellow fever**.	Carbo Veg 200
• Cold body. Cold sweat.	
• **Difficulty in breathing. Prostration.** Not taking in enough oxygen.	
• In cholera. **Rice water stools. Nausea**.	Veratrum Alb 1000
• Extreme coldness. **Cold sweat**.	

DIARRHOEA

Distinguishing symptoms of the patient	Medicine and potency
• In cholera, in typhoid, with intense **agony.**	Ars Alb 200
• Total prostration, burning, **restlessness.**	
• Burning thirst. However, body cold as ice.	

- Fever in **chronic diarrhoea**.   Podophyllum 200
- Cholera of infants. During teething.
- Stool green, yellow, watery, gushing, fetid, and profuse.
- **Uncontrollable retching, rice**   Veratrum Alb 1000
  water stools. Cold sweat. Collapse.

EXPOSURE

Distinguishing symptoms of the patient	Medicine and potency
• Inflammatory fever because of **exposure to dry cold.**	Aconite 30
• Fever **sudden**, short, and **high.**	
• Mental anguish. Baseless fear of death.	
• Restlessness.	
• **Cold waves** pass through the body.	
• Pungent, **steaming heat**. High fever because of exposure.	Belladonna 200
• **Flushed face**. Skin red. **Throbbing carotids**. Glaring eyes.	
• **Delirium**. Feet ice-cold.	
• On exposure to **wet air**.	Dulcamara 200

FEVER

Abnormally high body temperature, the normal being 98.4°F, or 37°C.

Any of the various diseases characterized by abnormally high body temperature.

The treatment is decided upon by referring to the accompanying symptoms like periodicity, chill, shivering, digestive complications, body pain, and headache.

Please refer under respective symptoms or names.

HAEMORRHAGE

Distinguishing symptoms of the patient	Medicine and potency
Haemorrhage from bowels in typhoid.	Alumen 30

INFLUENZA

An acute, contagious viral infection involving primarily the respiratory tract.

Symptoms: General weakness. Body pain, sometimes deep in the bones. Sneezing. Coryza. Nasal inflammation with thick mucous. A sensation of coldness going up the spine. High temperature. Sweating and shivering. Headache. Cough. Sore throat.

Influenza can lead to pneumonia if not attended to in time.

The patient is advised complete bed rest. He ought to take plenty of fluids.

For medicines, please refer '*Pain*' below and the chapter, '*The Nose*' under respective symptoms.

However, a quick guide follows.

Distinguishing symptoms of the patient	Medicine and potency
• Acute. On **exposure to dry, cold air**.	Aconite 30
• Useful if taken in the beginning.	
• **High fever** marked by restlessness, physical and mental. Total prostration. **Ice-cold**.	Arsenic Alb 200
• Congestion spreading to **lungs** and turning into **bronchitis.**	Bryonia 200
• **Pain in the centre of ribs on coughing**.	
• Deep seated pain in the **bones**.	Eupatorium Perf 200
• **Body aches** as if someone has beaten it.	Gelsemium 200
• Congestion of the head as if **tied with an iron band.**	Primary medicine.
• **Chill up the spine**.	

One dose to begin with. Later once a day besides other chosen medicine.	Influenzim 30
• General body pain. **Temporarily less on movement.**	Rhus Tox 200
• Tormenting dry cough before and during the chill.	

INTERMITTENT/PERIODIC

Distinguishing symptoms of the patient	Medicine and potency
• High temperature. **Marked periodicity.**	Arsenic Alb 200
• Lack or loss of vital powers. **Total prostration.**	
• Restlessness mental and physical.	
• Malarial fevers. Typhoid.	
• **Always freezing** though temperature is high.	
• Unquenchable thirst but sips a little at a time.	
• Burning relieved by hot application, by hot drinks. Cold food disagrees.	
• Intermittent. **All stages well defined.**	China 200
• Malarial. Typhoid.	
• **Chill in the afternoon.**	
• Intermittent, unyielding fever.	Natrum Mur 200
• **Chronic malaria.** Loss of appetite. Constipation.	
• Chill at 10.30 a.m.	
• **Extremities affected. Turn blue.**	

MALARIA

An infectious disease, an intermittent fever caused by a single celled, microscopic organism of the genus Plasmodium in red blood cells. It is transmitted to humans by the bite of an infected female anopheles mosquito.

Symptoms: An intermittent high fever with sweating, headache, body pain, and attacks of shivering. Confusion. Extreme fatigue between attacks. For medicines, refer '*Intermittent/Periodic*' above.

The most effective medicines are *Natrum Mur, Arsenic Alb, China, and Eupatorium Perf* depending on the predominant symptoms.

MEASLES

A highly contagious, serious viral infection, occurring mostly in childhood. A common disease from which most of the sufferers recover completely.

Symptoms: The patient develops a high fever, running nose, and cough. About four days later a pink rash is visible inside of the cheeks. Later a red, non-itchy rash starts on the head and spreads downwards. Separate flat spots merge to give a blotchy appearance. The eyes turn red and painful. The nose is stuffed or running. The patient has hacking cough.
There can be complications. Consult your physician.

Distinguishing symptoms of the patient	Medicine and potency
• **Debility. Restlessness.**	Arsenic Alb 200
• Thirst for sips of water at short intervals.	
• Midnight aggravation.	
• Hacking **bronchial cough**. Pain in the centre of the rib cage.	Bryonia 200
• Aggravation on movement	
• **Takes care of lung problems. Avoids bronchitis. Cuts short the duration of sickness**.	
• **Eyes, nose and mucous membranes inflamed.**	Euphrasia 200
• Sneezing. **Bloody discharge** from the nose.	
• Relieves cough. Alleviates the distress of fever.	
• For cough, for fever developing **after measles**.	Silicea 200

NIGHT SWEATS

Distinguishing symptoms of the patient	Medicine and potency
• **Sudden**, high temperature with profuse, **cold night sweats**.	Acetic Acid 30
• In **children** with night sweat on the **head**.	Calc Carb 30
• Profuse perspiration. **Debilitating.**	China 200
• In malaria, in typhoid	
• **Fevers with marked periodicity**.	
• **Copious perspiration without relief.**	Merc Sol 200
• **Creeping chilliness.**	
• Gastric or bilious fevers.	
• With snoring respiration.	Opium 200
• **Twitching of limbs**.	
• **Stupor**.	

NAUSEA

Distinguishing symptoms of the patient	Medicine and potency
• Slight chill with much heat.	Ipecac 200
• Nausea, vomiting, and breathlessness.	

PAIN

Distinguishing symptoms of the patient	Medicine and potency
• **Severe aching, deep in the bones,** in influenza, malaria, or bronchitis.	Eupatorium Perf 200
• Bruised feeling in back, arms, wrists, calves.	
• Morning fever preceded by pain in bones and vomiting.	

• **Congestion in head as if it is being tightened by a steel band.**	Gelsemium 200
• Muscular soreness and weakness. Pain all over. **Pain in the eyes** with itching.	
• **Chill creeping up the spine.** Sensation as if ice being rubbed up the back.	
• Nose blocked or running.	
• Influenza.	
• Influenza with **pain in the thighs.**	Rhus Tox 200
• The **entire body aches.**	
• Tormenting, **dry cough** before and during chill.	
• Temporary relief on motion.	

PNEUMONIA

Please refer the chapter, '*The Respiratory System*'.

SCARLET FEVER

An acute contagious disease caused by a haemolytic streptococcus, occurring prominently among children.

Symptoms: Scarlet skin eruption and sudden high fever. The rash of tiny spots has the feel of sandpaper. Fever is accompanied by headache, sore throat, body pain, and fatigue. Vomiting. The tongue has red patches with white coating.

Distinguishing symptoms of the patient	Medicine and potency
• Swelling and **kidney problems** prominent.	Apis 200
• **Swelling in throat** with stinging pain.	
• No thirst.	
• **Smooth, shiny, red eruptions.**	Belladonna 200
• **Throat hot,** dry, **red.**	**Primary remedy.**

• **Nausea**. Retching. Irritated stomach.	
• Temperature high.	
• Body pain, better temporarily on motion.	Rhus Tox 200
• **Muttering delirium**. Drowsiness.	
• Vesicular eruptions.	
On dose per day in addition to the other chosen remedy.	Scarlatinum 200

TYPHOID

An infectious disease of the intestines. The bacteria are carried in human stool.

Symptoms: The symptoms come slowly. There can be a relapse. Periodicity in fever. Constipation and diarrhoea alternate. Pain in the abdomen. Headache and mental confusion. Dry cough. Rash of rose-coloured spots appear on the chest, abdomen, and back.

There can be complications like intestinal bleeding and perforation of the intestines.

Consult a doctor at the earliest.

Distinguishing symptoms of the patient	Medicine and potency
• **High fever**. Periodicity well defined.	Arsenic Alb 200
• Restlessness. **Total exhaustion.**	
• Delirium worse after midnight. **Nightly aggravation**.	
• Nausea. Retching. Cannot bear sight or smell of food.	
• **Abdomen painful,** raw, irritable.	
• In later stages of typhoid, give Rhus Tox first. Then Arsenic alb.	
• Typhoid **with diarrhoea**. Stool smells foul.	Baptisia 30
• Early stages. Stupor.	
• **Unconsciousness** in typhoid.	Cuprum Met 200
• Pulse feeble. Great prostration.	

- Nervous excitability.
- **Urine scanty**.
- Typhoid **complicated with pneumonia**.   Phosphorus 200
- **Loose bowls**.   Rhus Tox 200
- Marked periodicity.
- Tongue dry, brown. **Dry cough**.
- Restlessness
- Headache. **Brain cloudy**.
- One dose early morning in lukewarm   Sulphur 200
  water, **in case fever does not abate**.
  No other medicine that day.

SLEEP

"To all, to each, a fair good night,
And pleasing dreams, and slumbers light,"
Sir Walter Scott, in 'Marmion'.

There is no greater blessing than sound sleep. None of us can do without it. An infant sleeps 14 to 18 hours a day. An adult requires 7 to 8 hours. A lack of enough sleep makes a person sick. In old age, sleep becomes fitful.

All mammals sleep because sleep has a purpose. It recharges our mental and physical batteries. We experience a diminution of efficiency and concentration in case we have not slept well. William Shakespeare, writing in 'Macbeth', inimitably summed up the benefits of sleep thus:

"Sleep that knits up the ravell'd sleeve of care,
The death of each day's life, sore labour's bath,
Balm of hurt minds, great nature's second course,
Chief nourisher in life's feast."

It is beneficial to regulate one's sleeping hours. Go to bed at a fixed time. In the twenty-four hours cycle of the human body, our temperature rises and falls at fixed times. In the afternoon, it reaches its maximum. At midnight, it comes down. It is comfortable to be asleep when the body temperature is at its minimum. Otherwise, one does not feel physically and mentally at one's best. On the other hand, the human body and mind perform at their peak when the body temperature is at the highest level.

For the same reasons, a traveller by air, flying over time zones, requires adjustment of body rhythm.

According to a report published in *India Today*, recent research reveals that, 'sleep fights cancer, protects the heart, boosts memory, and inspires lateral thinking'. It adds that 'sleep deprivation' can batter the heart. A 10-year study of more than 70000 volunteers, published in the *Archives of internal Medicine*, showed that those sleeping five hours or less show a 39 per cent increased risk of heart disease compared with those sleeping eight hours.' [*India today*, dated February 9, 2004.]

The story of Samuel Taylor Coleridge writing a truncated poem, '*Kublai Khan*', after dreaming about it, is well known. The poem remained incomplete because some visitor called him to the door in between. The rest of the dream was lost. However, this anecdote shows that our sleep helps in creative thinking.

In sleep, we dream in the later part of the night. Everyone knows the complicated webs woven during dreams. Alas, it is all forgotten soon after waking up although the brain benefits from this exercise.

Sleeping pills disturb this period of dreams, also known as the period of rapid eye movement. Further, the effect of drugs may last beyond the normal time for waking up and thus affect efficiency and concentration. Avoid them.

Homoeopathy provides harmless medicines for insomnia.

However, a few simple steps can be taken.

Do not take stimulants like coffee or tea late in the evening.

Do not overload your stomach at dinner. A heavy meal disturbs sleep. Eat your last meal at least two hours before going to bed.

Cut on consumption of alcohol. Rather, avoid it altogether. A hangover is not a pleasant experience.

Do not smoke.

Late nights affect health because your sleep pattern is disturbed.

Switch off the television an hour before bedtime.

A bath before going to bed has a positive effect on sleep. So does listening to soothing music. If possible, take a long walk. It is helpful in bringing you a good night's rest. A cup of warm milk at bedtime comforts the body.

Make your sleeping environment as comfortable as possible. It should be neither too hot nor too cold. Sleeping on a very soft bed is not healthy. A bed should be firm, hard and of a proper size. A double bed should have enough room for two to turn comfortably without coming in each other's way.

Sleep well. In sleep, we dream. And dreams can be romantic, at times.

COMA

Distinguishing symptoms of the patient	Medicine and potency
• Profound coma.	Opium 200

DEEP SLEEP

Distinguishing symptoms of the patient	Medicine and potency
• Deep slumber. General drowsiness.	Antim Tart 200

INSOMNIA

Inability to go to sleep or to get sleep for a period sufficient for the needs of an individual. Chronic inability to sleep. It leads to excessive fatigue.

The most common cause of insomnia is worry. The other is depression. Loud noise and other environmental disturbances can also cause a disturbance in sleep. So do taking excessive coffee, alcohol, or colas in the evening.

Avoid sleeping pills.

Use relaxation techniques. Practice yoga. Meditate. Listen to soothing music. Switch off television at least an hour before you go to bed.

Distinguishing symptoms of the patient	Medicine and potency
• Of the **aged**.	Aconite Nap 30
• **Worry** takes away sleep.	Ambra Grisea 30
• Restless and **tired**.	Arnica 200
• Mental and physical **restlessness**.	Arsenic Alb 200
• Insomnia with **cold limbs**.	Camphor 30

- **Obstinate,** intractable insomnia.   Cannabis Indica 30
  Sleepy but cannot sleep.
- **Unbearable pain** takes away **sleep.**   Chamomilla 200
- **Rheumatic** or abdominal pains.
- Uneasiness and anxiety.
- Insomnia after **copious menstrual flow**. China 200
- Mental activity. Of thinkers. Of **men**   Coffea 200
  of ideas.   **A dose an hour before**
- **Inability to go to sleep at the right hour.** **going to bed helps**.
- **Lack of sleep after 3.00 a.m.** Problems Nux Vomica 200
  gather like clouds. Falls asleep early morning,
  only to wake up feeling wretched.
- Of women with **excessive desire.**   Raphanus 30
- Copious, prolonged menstruation.

Further, refer '*Nightmares*' below.

MOANING

Distinguishing symptoms of the patient	Medicine and potency
• During sleep. Sleepy but cannot sleep owing to discomfort.	Belladonna 200

NIGHTMARES

Distinguishing symptoms of the patient	Medicine and potency
• Fear of death. **Irrational fear and agony.** • Ravings.	Aconite Nap 30
• **Disagreeable ideas** disturb.	Calc Carb 200
• Starts up **frightened.** • Insomnia in **delirium**.	Hyoscymus 200
• Wakes up in fright of being **suffocated.**	Spongia 30

NIGHT WALK

Distinguishing symptoms of the patient	Medicine and potency
• Walks in sleep. Has **horrible dreams**.	Kali Bromatum 30
• Walks in sleep. **Rush of blood** in the head with heat.	Silicea 200

SENSITIVE

Distinguishing symptoms of the patient	Medicine and potency
• Catnap. Slightest noise awakens.	Sulphur 200

TWITCHING

Distinguishing symptoms of the patient	Medicine and potency
• Startles. Twitches and wakes up often.	Agaricus 200

YAWNING

Distinguishing symptoms of the patient	Medicine and potency
• **Paroxysms** of yawning.	Agaricus 200
• Sleepy during day. Yawning when walking in **open air**.	Euphrasia 200

CHILDREN

Happy babies bring joy to their parents and to others who are near them. Their smile is infectious and coveted. However, the same children cause concern when they are sick. In their infancy, they cannot even describe what is wrong with them.

All the same, there are indications of a baby's plight. Be attentive to his signals of distress. The symptoms described in the pages that follow are quite exhaustive.

Most of the problems babies suffer from, relate to adults as well. They have been discussed in respective chapters. In this chapter, however, the discussion focuses on a baby's suffering.

I have deliberately reduced the potency of remedies to 30 in most cases. If 30 potency doses are not available, administer 200. Reduce the frequency of the dose to two instead of four.

My preference is for pills, size 20. The baby will love the sweet pills. Let him roll them over his tongue.

Normal dosage is 4-8 pills on dry tongue, 4 times a day.

As the disease is cured and the adverse symptoms disappear, reduce the dose to nil over two days. Homoeopathic remedies are not meant to be taken long except in chronic cases.

BED-WETTING

Symptoms: Unconscious wetting of bed during sleep.
Assure the child that it is not his fault.

Distinguishing symptoms of the patient	Medicine and potency
• **Foul smelling urine**. Colour does not come off easily.	Benzoic Acid 30
• Bed-wetting in **deep slumber**.	Belladonna 30
• Bed-wetting in **first sleep.**	Causticum 30
• Worse in dry, clear weather.	

BOILS/ULCERS IN THE MOUTH

Symptoms: Painful blisters in the mouth, on gums, on the tongue, inside the cheeks. Foul breath. Sometimes pus forms in the blisters.

Keeping a few pills of the chosen remedy inside the lips, near the gums, letting them dissolve slowly, relieves pain and heals the ulcers or blisters. Repeat six times a day.

Distinguishing symptoms of the patient	Medicine and potency
• **Blisters** on the tongue, inside the lips.	Borax 30
• Painful **gumboils**.	
• **Bleeding** ulcers.	
• Painful boils on **gums which are spongy**, purple. Full of **pus**.	Merc Sol 30
• **Fetid smell** from the breath.	
• Painful, **easily bleeding ulcers** in the mouth. Open wounds.	Nitric Acid 30

BRONCHITIS

Chronic or acute inflammation of the mucous membranes of the bronchial tubes.

Symptoms: 'Cold' in the chest. Hacking cough with pain in the centre of the ribs. Begins with common cold. Feverishness, throbbing headache, pain in the eyes, running nose, languor.

Oppressed and hurried breathing. Wheezing. Little expectoration. In chronic cases, green, yellow mucous. Urine scanty.

Cold perspiration, pale cheeks, cold limbs, drowsiness are bad signs. So are convulsions. Call a doctor.

Distinguishing symptoms of the patient	Medicine and potency
• **Fever with frontal headache.**	Aconite 30
• Hacking cough with cold and oppressed breathing.	Acute case. Give every one hour, at least six
• Onset.	doses.
• **Hacking, oppressive pain in the centre of the ribs** on coughing.	Bryonia 200 **Primary medicine.**
• Pain worse on movement.	Alternate with another
• Little expectoration or green, yellow mucous.	chosen remedy.
• **Wheezing**.	Ipecac 30
• Upper respiratory tract infection. The child pants. **Cannot breathe.**	
• Mucous comes out.	
• **Nausea. Vomiting**.	
• Mucous stuck in the lungs. **Cannot take it out**	Antim Tart 30, 200
• Rattling audible outside the room.	
• Ropy, stringy, green mucous **going down the throat**. Futile effort to take it out.	Kali Bi 30
• With green, bland mucous **running out** easily through the nose.	Pulsatilla 30

CHICKEN POX

Please refer under the chapter on '*Fevers.*'

CHOREA/ST. VITUS'S DANCE

A disorder of the nervous system.

Symptoms: Involuntary, convulsive, muscular movements involving face and limbs. Ludicrous gestures. Can neither stand nor walk. Cessation of movement in sleep except in rare cases. Consult a physician.

Distinguishing symptoms of the patient	Medicine and potency
• Twitching of **eyeballs and eyelids.**	Agaricus 30
• Upper parts on one side and lower parts on the other are affected.	
• Right side worse than the left.	Causticum 30
• **Clumsy gait**. Falls easily.	
• Muscles of face, tongue, **arms, and legs** affected.	
• **Starts in fingers, toes** and extends to limbs.	Cup Met 30
• Terrible contortions while awake. Restful in sleep.	
• Due to **fright**, threat of punishment or bad news. After grief or **emotional upset**. In hysterical persons.	Ignatia 30
• Tingling in limbs. Pain in joints.	
• Spinal chorea. **Unsteady gait**.	Nux Vomica 30
• **Rotates arms**. Clasps hands over head.	Stramonium 30
• **Moves feet** continuously, even during night.	Zincum Met 30
• With **vertigo**.	Viscum Alb 30

COLD/CORYZA

Symptoms: Starts as an abnormal secretion from the nose that interferes with breathing and suckling. Itching in the palate. Sneezing. A rise in temperature in cases of exposure or infection.

A chill crawling along the spine. Congestion and pain in the head. Body pain.

Eyes water, turn red and itch. Nose is partially or fully blocked. The child breathes through the mouth.

Distinguishing symptoms of the patient	Medicine and potency
• On **exposure** to dry cold air. Fever.	Aconite 30
• Bouts of **sneezing**.	In the early stages.
• Watery, copious, **excoriating** discharge with sneezing.	Arsenic Alb 30
• Cold in the chest. **Painful** hacking **cough.**	Bryonia 30, 200
• Bronchitis.	
• On exposure to **damp weather**.	Dulcamara 30
• Copious **discharge from the eyes**.	Euphrasia 30
• **Body pain. Congestion in the head**. Pain at its base. Senggish.	Gelsemium 30
• **Chill up the spine.**	
• Eyes heavy, burning.	
• Running nose. Sore throat.	
• Thick, ropy mucous **going inwards.**	Kali Bi 30
• **Pain in the orbits** of the eyes, behind the ears, in sinuses.	
• **Stuffy** cold. Breathes through the mouth.	Nux Vomica 30
• Bland, greenish yellow, **free flowing mucous**. Fetid.	Pulsatilla 30

COLIC

Symptoms: Spasmodic pain in the stomach. Baby cries and doubles up in pain.

Wind colic. Flatulence. Abdomen distended like a drum.

Distinguishing symptoms of the patient	Medicine and potency
• Pain because of **constipation**. Dry stool. Worse on movement, on touch. Thirsty.	Bryonia 200
• Child **peevish** with acute pain.	Chamomilla 200
• Severe. Child **bends double** with pain.	Colocynthis 200
• Flatulence. Stomach **distended like a drum**.	China 200

CONJUNCTIVITIS

Please refer the chapter '*the Eyes*', as well as '*Eyes-catarrhal inflammation of*' below.

CONSTIPATION

Symptoms: Frequent but ineffective urge to stool. Child cries. Feverishness. Restlessness. Headache. Sometimes, vomiting.

Distinguishing symptoms of the patient	Medicine and potency
• Difficult passage of **soft yet sticky stool**. No urge for days.	Alumina 30
• **Large, dry stool. Dark as if burnt.**	Bryonia 30
• Thirst for cold water. Headache.	
• Stool of round **balls** stuck together with **mucous**.	Graphites 30
• Wind **passing downwards** but constipated.	Lycopodium 30
• Hard stool **crumbling** at anus.	Magnesia Mur 30
• With **mucous** in stool.	Merc. Sol 30
• With **blood** in stool.	Merc Cor 30
• Hard, crumbling stool. **Rectal bleeding**.	Natrum Mur 30
• Frequent, ineffectual urging.	Nux Vomica 30
• **Pressure** at the anus.	
• Stool **comes out and slides back**. Rectum weak.	Silicea 30
• Anus sore and oozing mucous.	
Start treatment with one dose early morning.	Sulphur 30

COUGH

Distinguishing symptoms of the patient	Medicine and potency
• On exposure to **dry cold. Sudden**. Sneezing. Sometimes, fever.	Aconite 30
• **Face turns red, hot**. Eyes stare.	Belladonna 30
• Violent, sudden onset.	
• Inflamed **tonsils, red, glistening, hard, painful**.	
• Cold in the chest. Painful **cough coming out from the centre of the ribs**. Thirst for cold drinks.	Bryonia 30
• With **rattling** accumulation of **mucous** in lungs which is difficult to take out.	Antim Tart 30
• **Wheezing**. Oppressive respiration.	Ipecac 30
• **Nausea**. Vomiting.	
• Coughing spasm **strangles**. Yellow, thick mucous.	Hepar Sulph 30
• **Pus in tonsils**. Shooting, piercing pain.	
• Cough loose, rattling, and croupy.	
• Thick, ropy, green mucous **flowing inwards**. Difficult to take out and clear the throat.	Kali Bi 30
• **Brassy, hacking cough.**	
• Old colds.	
• **Dry cough. Larynx sore**.	Nux Vomica 30
• Loose cough. **Yellow, green mucous coming out.**	Pulsatilla 30
• Old colds.	

CROUP

An inflammation of the larynx characterized by respiratory difficulty and a hoarse, brassy cough.

Symptoms: Sudden onset, usually during night. Frequent spasms. Child awakens with a dry, barking ringing cough. Difficulty in breathing because of congestion and swelling of the lining of the larynx.

Crowing respiration. Voice hoarse or lost. Skin hot, dry.
If the face and lips turn blue, contact a doctor immediately.
Meanwhile keep the room humid and warm. Give steam inhalation.

Distinguishing symptoms of the patient	Medicine and potency
• Give every 15 minutes till under control.	Aconite 30 **First medicine.**
• Lungs **choked with phlegm**. Rattling. Inability to take out the phlegm.	Antim Tart 200
• **Nausea**.	
• **Loose metallic cough.**	Hepar Sulph 30
• After fever has subsided	
• Rattling in chest. Difficult expectoration.	
Once a day, early morning, for seven days, during convalescence.	Sulphur 30

CRYING

A child is a bundle of joy. When it cries, it is a matter of concern for the parent.

The cry of a baby is a signal to indicate that it is in distress.

A child's cry is expressive and varies in character.

A normal baby signals hunger, anger, pain, loneliness, or discomfort through a cry.

Cries of loneliness stop when the baby has company.

We somehow do not think of a baby's thirst. Hot weather or peevishness lead to more thirst. Give it a sip of water.

When a baby is tired, it moans softly. Put it to sleep with a lullaby.

A hungry baby cries as a matter of right. A mother normally never lets this happen. Still it is good to think of this possibility and feed the child, if need be.

A sudden shriek indicates that the baby has wet its nappies. Change the wet nappy.

The colic cry can be guessed by the baby drawing up legs, passing wind and showing restlessness. It is a sudden cry that alternates with relaxation.

When the pain is severe, unbearable, the baby cries severely. It is not comforted easily.

When there is no apparent cause, investigate the person of the baby for symptoms of sickness like a skin-bite, earache, stuffed nose, or blue skin caused by an injury or otherwise. The infant should be fully undressed in a warm, comfortable room and looked at. Note the form and movement of its chest and abdomen. See whether its skin is hot, cool, moist, or dry. Look for eruptions.

If the baby is very sick, loses colour, draws up legs, call a doctor.

Distinguishing symptoms of the patient	Medicine and potency
• **Sudden fever. Sudden cold.**	Aconite 30
• On exposure to dry cold air.	
• Restlessness. Anguish.	
• **Insect bites.**	Apis 30
• **Swelling** for any reason. Swollen, red patches.	
• **Injury**. Bleeding due to injury.	Arnica 30
• The child is **tired**.	
• **Head hot, eyes glistening, face flushed.**	Belladonna 200
• Red predominates.	
• Red swollen tonsils.	
• Child **touches the ear** that is aching.	Bryonia 200
• **Dry, hacking cough.**	
• Constipation. **Dry, burnt stool**.	
• Cries when **passing urine**. Feverish.	Cantharis 30
• **Peevish**. Wants to be carried.	Chamomilla 30
• **Dentition pain**.	
• Colic. Draws up legs. Loose bowels.	
• **Cannot go to sleep**. Rolls restless.	Coffea 30
• Severe colic. **Bends over double**. Presses the abdomen.	Colocynthis 30
• Least food intake results in jelly-like, fetid, **dysenteric stool**.	

DECAYING TEETH

Decay in teeth can be prevented by proper oral hygiene.

Symptoms: Teeth black, crumbling. Unhealthy, itching gums.
Consult a dental surgeon for advice and treatment.

Distinguishing symptoms of the patient	Medicine and potency
• **Teeth decay as soon as they appear**. Gums are sore.	Kreosote 30
• **Loose teeth. Bleeding gums.**	Merc Sol 30
• Copious saliva. Fetid breath.	
• **Teeth black and loose.**	Staphysagria 30
• Gums pale, sore, swollen, eroded.	

DENTITION PROBLEMS

Symptoms: The child is peevish, restless. His sleep is disturbed. An upset stomach. Spasms, convulsions. Temperature.

Distinguishing symptoms of the patient	Medicine and potency
• **Suddenly inflamed** gums with fever and restlessness.	Aconite 30
• **Peevish, restless**, irascible. Wants to be carried.	Chamomilla 30
• Stomach upset. Diarrhoea. Colic.	**Continue one dose a day during dentition.**
• Teeth **decay** as soon as they appear. Inflamed gums.	Kreosote 30
• **Constipation**.	
• Dentition diarrhoea. **Green, watery, profuse, gushing stool**.	Podophyllum 30
• Cheeks hot, glowing.	

DIARRHOEA, INFANTILE

Symptoms: Severe loss of body fluids through stool. Life threatening. **Get medical aid immediately**.

The stool can be rice water thin and gushing or green and gushing. At times, there can be blood or mucous in the stool.

Distinguishing symptoms of the patient	Medicine and potency
• **Uncontrollable** motion. Stool passes while passing urine.	Aloe 30
• Mucous.	
• **Green spinach like shreds in the stool**.	Arg. Nit 30
• Results of **food poisoning.**	Ars Alb 30
• **Chronic** cases. Comes and goes. Pale, sunken face.	
• **Dentition diarrhoea**. Stool greenish, frothy, copious, fetid.	Chamomilla 30
• Unbearable colic.	
• Child restless, peevish.	
• Severe colic. **Bends double with pain**.	Colocynthis 30
• **Blood** in stool.	Merc Cor 30
• **Mucous** in stool.	Merc Sol 30
• **Painless, copious** stool, gushing without control as if from a hydrant.	Phosphorus 30
• Sudden, copious, **fetid, yellow stool.**	Podophyllum 30
• **Undigested food** in stool.	
• Frequent retching, but no vomit.	
• Rolling and perspiration of the head.	
• Copious **rice water** stools with vomiting.	Veratrum Alb 200
• Profuse sweating.	One dose will suffice.
• Collapse. Cholera. Gastroenteritis.	Simultaneously start giving the patient boiled and colled water to which a spoonful of sugar and a pinch of salt have been added.

DIGESTIVE UPSETS

Symptoms: Sudden indigestion. Loose motions. Nausea, vomiting. Coated tongue.

Distinguishing symptoms of the patient	Medicine and potency
• **Fetid eructation. Fetid wind.**.	Antim Crud 300
• Furry, white tongue.	
• Results of **overeating.**	
• **No appetite. Acidity**.	Carbo Veg 30
• **Nausea. Vomiting.**	Ipecac 30
• Breast milk disagrees.	
• **Constipation.**	Nux Vomica 30
• Aversion to food or drink.	
• Upset on taking **heavy food**.	Pulsatilla 30
• **Rice white, watery, copious stool with vomiting**. Cold sweat. Collapse.	Veratrum Alb 200

DIPHTHERIA

Please refer the chapter, '*The Throat*.'

EARACHE

Earache can be caused by cold, by acute tonsillitis, by a foreign body.

Symptoms: The infant gives a shrill, piercing cry. Beats or pulls at the ear which hurts. Tosses his head back and forth. Face flushed. Stuffed feeling in the ear. At times, deafness. Rise in temperature with aggravation at night.

Inflammation in the middle ear may be accompanied by vomiting, convulsions.

Consult a doctor.

Of course, the following medicines are of great help.

Distinguishing symptoms of the patient	Medicine and potency
• **Acute ache and throbbing** in the ear, on exposure to dry cold. **Fever**.	Aconite 30
• Red, shining swelling inside.	
• Sudden onset. **Face flushed**.	Belladonna 30
• Worse right side.	
• **Disproportionate** pain. Child **peevish**.	Chamomilla 30
• One cheek red, hot. The other cold and pale.	
• In sinusitis. **Tough mucous going inwards**.	Kali Bi 30
• **Pus** in the ear.	Merc Cor 30
• Chronic cold. Mucous **flowing outwards**.	Pulsatilla 30
• Inflammation of the **middle ear.**	Plantago
• **With toothache.**	Mother tincture diluted
• Pain travels from one ear to the other through the head.	with warm water, in equal parts, to be dropped into the aching ear for relief.

EAR DISCHARGE

Symptoms: Discharge of blood, mucous. Thick, bloody, offensive. Painful. Often, it becomes chronic.

Distinguishing symptoms of the patient	Medicine and potency
• **Pus and blood** with **piercing** pain.	Hepar Sulph 30
• **Bloody, offensive**. Glands swollen.	Merc Cor 30
• Stabbing pain.	
• Green, bland.	Pulsatilla 30
• **After measles or mumps**.	
• Chronic, **unyielding cases**.	Silicea 30

ECZEMA

Please refer under the chapter, '*The Skin.*'

EPILEPSY

Symptoms: Petit Mal: A milder form that occurs between age four and adolescence. The child suddenly stops playing and stands stupefied for a moment. His face turns pale. He returns to normal activity as if nothing had happened.

Grand Mal: A sudden and complete loss of consciousness. Spasmodic contraction of muscles followed by exhaustion and deep sleep.

The patient may utter a terrifying, loud shriek before convulsion. There is a violent movement of neck and head. Jaws clenched. Frothing at the mouth. The epileptic bites his tongue. His eyes are fixed in a stare, or rolling. He clenches his hands firmly over the fingers.

The veins of the forehead are distended. The face turns pale.

Urine and stool pass involuntarily.

After one to three minutes, the child relaxes and goes into deep sleep.

Distinguishing symptoms of the patient	Medicine and potency
• Sudden convulsions with **intense heat, flushed face and throbbing**. Cerebral congestion.	Belladonna 30
• Foam at the mouth. Jumps in sleep.	
• Involuntary movement of bowels and bladder.	
• Caused by **worms**. Throws arms from side to side.	Cina 30
• Distortion of limbs.	
• Inward jerking of the fingers of **right hand**.	
• Aura **begins at knee**. Spasm in **fingers, palms and toes.**	Cuprum Met 30
• Face distorted. Turns blue. Jaws contracted.	
• Foaming. Unconsciousness.	
• In stammerers. Caused by fright.	Stramonium 30

EYES-CATARRHAL INFLAMMATION OF

Symptoms: Redness and swelling of the inflamed mucous membrane inside the eyelids or around the corners. Watering eyes. Sensation of sand under the lids. Fever.

Common cold can be one of the causes.

Mucous under the lids in the morning.

Conjunctivitis.

Trachoma.

Wash with cold water. Do not rub. Avoid glaring light and exposure to cold.

Distinguishing symptoms of the patient	Medicine and potency
• Acute attack. Discharge of **mucous**.	Arg Nit 30
• Acute or chronic, severe cases.	Apis 30
• Sensation of **sand in the eyes**. Trachoma.	**Great remedy.**
• With **fever**. In the initial stages.	Aconite 30
• Caused by **injury**.	Arnica 30
• With **throbbing** in the temples.	Belladonna 30
• Dreads lights. Eyes **red, glistening**.	
• Inflamed conjunctiva. **Running conjunctivitis.**	Euphrasia 30
• From the eyes **persistent**, profuse, excoriating discharge.	
• Bland running nose.	
• **Ulcers** in the inflamed lids.	Merc Cor 30
• Painful discharge. Difficult cases.	
• **Greenish yellow mucous in the eyes. Sties.**	Pulsatilla 30

FEVER

Do not be upset unless the temperature goes high. A fever indicates that the body is building its defences to fight an invader.

Observe the child closely before making the choice of a remedy out of those given below.

If the temperature rises to 39.5°C or higher, sponge the child's body with a cold towel and continue until the fever comes down. Wipe each part dry before sponging it again.

Consult a doctor if the fever still goes high.

Do not lose time. **High temperature can cause irreversible damage to the brain**.

Distinguishing symptoms of the patient	Medicine and potency
• **Sudden chill on exposure** to dry, cold air.	Aconite 30
• Skin hot and dry. Mouth, lips, tongue, dry.	**Start here**. Do not think
• Hurried breathing. Pulse full, hard.	twice. Repeat dose every
• Great thirst.	30 minutes
• With total debility and restlessness.	Ars Alb 30
• **Typhoid.**	
• Thirst for small quantities of water.	
• **Face flushed. Glazed, staring eyes**.	Belladonna 30
• Intense headache.	
• **Inflamed tonsils**. Throat sore and red.	
• Bronchial, **hacking, severe cough**, mainly dry. Oppressed breathing.	Bryonia 30
• **Bronchitis**.	
• Asks for a large sip of water at long intervals.	
• Due to **urinary infection.**	Cantharis 30
• Burning and pain before, during, and after urination.	
• Body pain.	
• Influenza. **Body pain**.	Gelsemium 30
• **Congestion in the head** as if tied by a steel band.	
• Drowsy and **indifferent**. Face puffed, flushed.	
• Running nose. Sore throat. Croupy cough.	
• **Periodic fevers** like malaria.	Natrum Mur 30
• Uncontrollable **shivering**.	
• Fever due to **constipation**.	Nux Vomica 30

FITS/FEBRILE CONVULSIONS

Violent, irregular contraction of muscles followed by relaxation.

Seizures occur during illnesses with fever such as pharyngitis, chicken pox, measles, and mumps. In dentition, during indigestion, from a blow, from worms.

Symptoms: Sudden loss of consciousness. At times rhythmic twitching, shaking of arms and legs. Seizure followed by relaxation.

Recovery is rapid and complete.

Most such cases do not develop into epilepsy in later life.

Lay the child on his side. Clear the mouth of any substance blocking the airway.

Do not try to control the jerking, twitching movements. Loosen clothes. Open the windows. If feverish, sponge with tepid water.

Stay calm. Most of these convulsions do not indicate anything serious unless symptoms of epilepsy [Grand Mal] are present.

If in doubt, get medical help.

Distinguishing symptoms of the patient	Medicine and potency
• **Unconsciousness**.	Camphor Mother tincture. Ten drops on sugar every 15 minutes.
• During fever caused by **exposure** to dry, cold air. Restlessness. **Anguish. Fear**.	Aconite 30
• **Red, shining face**. Staring eyes. Head hot.	Belladonna 30
• **Body rigid.**	
• Startled by the least noise or light.	
• **Teething** problems.	Chamomilla 30
• Twitching of facial muscles.	
• **Worms** causing indigestion and fits.	Cina 30
• Twitching of **different muscles**.	Agaricus 30
• With **nausea**, vomiting.	Ipecac 30
• **Asthma. Wheezing**.	
• Fits caused by **constipation**.	Nux Vomica 30

- **Urine suppressed.**   Opium 30
- **Face** dark, purple, hot, **and puffed.**
- Eyes turned upwards. Insensitive to light.
- Fit caused by **intake of a meal** rich in fats.   Pulsatilla 30

HEADACHE

A child may be too young to complain of a headache. Children under four can hardly describe it.

A headache can be the result of a fall, an injury, exposure to sun, coryza, infected sinuses, indigestion.

Symptoms: Desires to lie down, to have his head supported. Restlessness. The child is peevish.

Distinguishing symptoms of the patient	Medicine and potency
Because of injury. In fever.	Arnica 30
Throbbing pain in the temple.	Belladonna 30
In **colds**. During influenza.	Gelsemium 30
Head feels as if **tightened** with a steel band.	
Body pain. Chill up the spine.	
Sore throat. Congested cold.	
On **exposure to sun**.	Glonoine 30
Sudden fainting. Inability to hold the head erect.	
With **bilious vomiting**.	Iris 30
Because of **indigestion**.	Nux Vomica 30
After taking a **heavy meal**.	Pulsatilla 30

HIP JOINT PAIN

Symptoms: In the beginning, slight limp with pain on walking. Knee joint swollen although the site of disease is hip joint. Limbs shortened. Limp prominent at a later stage. Pain is severe at night. Fever and restless in the evening. During sleep, limbs startle violently. On the buttocks, an abscess forms and bursts.

It is advisable to consult an orthopaedic surgeon at the earliest.

Distinguishing symptoms of the patient	Medicine and potency
• Pus about to form.	Calcarea Carb 30
• **Swelling in knee and hip joints.**	
• **Sharp, sticking, wrenching pain.**	
• In muscles, a tearing pain.	
• **Pus** formed **deep** in bones.	Silicea 30
• **Chronic cases.**	
Start here. Later one dose early morning at 72 hours interval.	Sulphur 30

HYDROCEPHALUS

A rare, abnormal enlargement of the head.

Symptoms: Skull and face disproportionate. Forehead overhangs the face.

Consult a surgeon.

Distinguishing symptoms of the patient	Medicine and potency
• Bulging, soft spots on the skull.	Apis 30
• **After scarlet fever**.	
• **Extraordinarily large head**. Heavy sweating.	Calcarea Carb 30
• Soft spots on the skull not closing.	
• **Bones soft or curved. Joints large.**	
• Teeth delayed or decayed.	
• **Abdomen muscles shrunken**.	
• **After measles and scarlet fever.**	Merc Sol 30
• Copious sweating on the head.	
• **Acute** enlargement.	Helleborus 30
• **Depression of the sensorium,** [the part of the brain that receives and	

coordinates all the stimuli conveyed to various sensory centres].
- **Eyes do not see. Ears do not hear.**
- Frequent and severe convulsions
- The child rolls the head and bores it into the pillow out of uneasiness.

INJURIES

Injury to head can be serious. Consult a doctor.
Take immediate preventive steps to stop bleeding, if any. Use clean bandage to cover the wound.

At times, an injury can cause **internal bleeding**. This **too requires medical attention**.

Distinguishing symptoms of the patient	Medicine and potency
• For **any injury**, administer Arnica immediately.	Arnica 30
• Pain, swelling, **black eye.**	
• **Concussion**. Shock. In tooth extraction. **In surgery**.	
• Apply on a **bruise**, on a **bleeding surface**. On an open wound.	Calendula Mother Tincture or ointment for external application.
• Injury to **nerves. Crushed fingers.**	Hypericum 30
• Injury to **coccyx or on the spine**.	
• **Anti tetanus**. Administer immediately for a **punctured wound.**	Ledum 30
• Continue with Arnica.	
• In injuries of **bones, cartilages, in sprains.**	Ruta 30
• For **tired eyes**.	
• For **internal bleeding**, after Arnica.	Millefolium 30
• Sore bruises. Haemorrhage of **dark clotted blood**.	Hamamelis 30

IMPETIGO

A common, severe, contagious skin inflammation.

Symptoms: Pustules grouped in clusters, run together, forming irregularly shaped, thick, moist, yellowish scales. Intense itching. Skin hot.

Distinguishing symptoms of the patient	Medicine and potency
• Oozing of **corrosive discharge**.	Ars Alb 30
• **Pus** formed. **Stabbing pain**.	Hepar Sulph 30
• **Red spots** turning into blisters which break down.	Mezerium 30
• Eruptions on scalp, on face. Burning, itching.	Viola Tricolour 30
• **Thick scabs** which crack and exude **tenacious yellow pus**.	

INTERTRIGO

Symptoms: Redness and chaffing in folds of the skin. In neck, armpits and groin. In between buttocks. Clear secretions.

Distinguishing symptoms of the patient	Medicine and potency
• Excoriation of **thighs**.	Aethusa 30
• Behind ears. Between the **thighs**.	Causticum 30
• Rawness in bends of limbs, **groin, neck, behind ears**.	Graphites 30

JAUNDICE

Yellow skin, yellow whites of the eye, yellow urine, and yellow stool because of liver derangement.

Symptoms: Whites of the eye, roots of nails, the skin, face, neck, trunk, extremities turn yellow. Urine is deep orange and stains clothes. Faeces shining yellow. Bitter taste. Low fever. Slow pulse. Spirits depressed. Lethargy.

Advised complete bed rest.

Newly born commonly get jaundice on the third or fourth day.
Consult a doctor.

Distinguishing symptoms of the patient	Medicine and potency
• **Jaundiced skin**. Face yellow. Whites of the eye yellow.	Chelidonium 30-
• Tongue yellow. Taste bitter. Nausea. Vomiting.	
• Profuse, foaming, yellow urine. Shining yellow, pasty stool.	
• **Ice-coldness of the finger tips.**	
• **Pain under the inferior angle of the right scapula**.	
• Skin yellow, moist.	Chionanthus 30
• Yellow conjunctiva.	
• **Enlarged liver**.	
• **Dark urine.**	
• **Constipation**. Stool clay coloured, soft and pasty.	
• **Ringing in the ears.**	China 30
• **Great debility** because of loss of liquids from the body for whatever reason.	
• Skull bursting **headache. Dizzy** when walking.	
• **Abdomen bloated. Liver and spleen enlarged**.	

MALARIA

Symptoms: Intermittent fever with headache and devastating shivering. Body pain. Headache.

Distinguishing symptoms of the patient	Medicine and potency
• Chill generally in the **forenoon**.	China 30
• Well defined periodicity and stages.	

- **Distressing shivering.**
- **Vomiting.** Weakness caused by outflow of liquids.
- Unbearable **pain in the bones** besides other malarial symptoms.   Eupatorium Perf 30
- Chill comes at **10.30 a.m.**   Natrum Mur 30
- **Extremities turn blue.**
- **Chronic malarial state** with weakness, constipation, and loss of appetite.

MEASLES

A detailed discussion of the progress of measles and its remedies is available under the chapter, *'Fevers.'*

However, the following further remedies can be looked at according to the developing symptoms.

Distinguishing symptoms of the patient	Medicine and potency
• Severe **body pain. Chill running up the spine.**	Gelsemium 30
• Congestion in the head. A feeling of a **steel band tightening.**	
• Harsh, croupy cough.	
• As the fever declines, **laryngitis** develops. **Hoarse, brassy cough.**	Kali Bich 30
• Earache with nausea.	
• Thick, **ropy, green mucous** flowing down the throat. **Difficult to take out**.	
• Bland, yellow-green, thick mucous **easily flowing out.**	Pulsatilla 30

MUMPS

An acute, inflammatory, contagious disease characterized by the swelling of the salivary glands and sometimes of the pancreas, ovaries, or testes. It can be prevented by vaccination.

Symptoms: Inflammation of salivary glands beneath and in front of the ear. Swelling prominent. First one side, then the other. Discomfort in eating. Terrible pain. Fever. Headache.

Isolate the child for ten days until mumps have subsided.

Distinguishing symptoms of the patient	Medicine and potency
• **Face red,** flushed. Child sensitive to light.	Belladonna 30
• Restlessness.	
• **Soft swelling**. Rose hue. Painful	Apis 30
• **No thirst**.	
• **Hard swelling**.	Bryonia 30
• Irritable. Worse on movement.	
• Lips dry, cracked. **Thirsty** for large quantity of water.	
• When disease has spread to **testes**.	Pulsatilla 30

NAPPY RASH

Distinguishing symptoms of the patient	Medicine and potency
• Abrasions. Sores. Rash.	Calendula.
• Open wounds. Ulcers.	Ointment or mother tincture for local application.

NIGHT TERRORS

Symptoms: Child wakes up suddenly in great fear. Screams. Sobs. Mumbles. Stares into space with a blank look.

Distinguishing symptoms of the patient	Medicine and potency
• Nightmares. **Frightening dreams**. Tossing about. Restless.	Aconite 30
• **Screams in sleep**. Mumbles. Startles to wake up. Stares.	Belladonna 30

NOSEBLEED

Not a serious complaint.

Distinguishing symptoms of the patient	Medicine and potency
• From **excitement**.	Aconite 30
• When injury is the cause.	Arnica 30
• Dark blood oozing drop by drop.	Hamamelis 30
• **Red blood** dripping for no apparent reason.	Millefolium 30

OPHTHALMIA OF THE NEWBORN

Symptoms: Eyelids inflamed. Red. Swollen. Thick, yellow pus. Inside of the eye looks like crimson velvet. Cornea looks sunk.

Appears 3 or 4 days after birth. A serious problem. Can cause irreparable damage.

Consult a doctor.

Distinguishing symptoms of the patient	Medicine and potency
• With fever.	Aconite 30
• **Swelling** most prominent.	Apis 30 **First medicine.**
• Covers all symptoms.	
• One dose every hour until	Arg Nit 30

inflammation reduced.
- Ulcers in the eyelids.   Merc Cor 30

PLEURISY

An acute inflammation, generally one sided, of the sac covering the lungs and the lining of the chest.

Symptoms: Acute onset. Violent chill. Severe, stabbing pain in the chest. The child cannot breathe fully. His cough is short and dry. **Consult a doctor.**

Distinguishing symptoms of the patient	Medicine and potency
• **Fever with dry cough**, restlessness, on exposure to dry cold air.	Aconite 30
• Pain worse on movement. Even breathing hurts.	Bryonia 200 Alternate with Aconite
• Short breaths. **Breathes with abdominal muscles.**	until fever is down. Continue Bryonia until
• Frequent cough but **little expectoration**. Shakes the affected side which hurts.	recovery is complete. Main medicine.
• Once a day during convalescence. Prevents relapse.	Sulphur 30

PNEUMONIA

An acute inflammation of the lungs accompanied by high fever, rapid breathing, dry, persistent cough, pain in the chest and sputum containing blood.

In infants, high fever is accompanied by rapid respiration in which the lower ribs are drawn inwards. Vomiting and convulsions.

For medicines, please refer the entry in the chapter, '*The Respiratory System*'.

POLIOMYELITIS

Symptoms: Paralysis affecting a group of muscles in one or more limbs. The disease starts with fever, sore throat, convulsions, stomach upset. As the fever subsides, the child cannot stand or walk. He has lost the power to use an arm.

Polio vaccine provides complete protection against the disease. Get it in time.

Distinguishing symptoms of the patient	Medicine and potency
Because of exposure to dry cold air. Fever.	Aconite 30
With convulsions, **flushed face, intolerance to light**.	Belladonna 30
Body pain, **congestion in the head, chill creeping up the spine**, fever.	Gelsemium 30

RHEUMATIC FEVER

Inflammation of the heart following an attack of tonsillitis.

Symptoms: Fever. Painful swelling of joints, of fibrous and muscular tissues. Nodules on the exposed bony surfaces like elbow, wrist, vertebrae. Rash on trunk and limbs. Chorea. Involuntary movement of face, arms, and body. Writhing.

Medical consultation is advised.

Distinguishing symptoms of the patient	Medicine and potency
At the outset. Alternate with Bryonia.	Aconite 30
• **Heat and swelling of joints.**	Bryonia 200
• Worse on movement.	
• **Rheumatic heart** case.	Cactus 30
• **Chronic enlargement of tonsils.**	Calc Phos 30
• **Anaemia, stiffness**, pain, and chilliness.	
• Chorea with **muscular rheumatism**.	Cimicifuga
• **Acute rheumatic fever.**	Formic Acid 30
• Relieves pain. Prevents recurrence.	

- **Pain** in ligaments, capsule, and bursa of the **joints, in muscles**.
- **Pain in muscles, tendons, and ligaments.**   Rhus Tox 30
- Temporary **improvement on movement.**
- Worse in damp, cold weather.

RICKETS

A disease of the bones caused by deficiency of Vitamin D.

Symptoms: Bones softened, bent, and deformed. Prominent forehead. Child reaches tenth month without cutting teeth. Starts late to walk.

Chest narrow and prominent. Enlargement of joints of wrists and ankles.

Hunchback. Bones of legs curved.

With early diagnosis, proper treatment, and diet, deformities can be avoided. Talk to your doctor.

Distinguishing symptoms of the patient	Medicine and potency
• **Head and joints enlarged.**	Calc Carb 30
• Delayed teething. Decay of teeth.	
• Spine and limbs curved.	
• Belly swollen	
• Voracious appetite. Diarrhoea.	
• Symptoms as above but **diarrhoea and weakness** more marked.	Calc Phos 30

RUBELLA [GERMAN MEASLES]

Symptoms: Sudden onset. Rash appears on the first day on the face. Rose red spots.

Next day rash extends to body and limbs. It subsides with fever on the third day. Glands on the side of the neck enlarged. Headache. Sore throat. Sharp fever.

No superficial skin is shed. Cold symptoms do not precede Rubella as they do in the case of Measles.

A mild sickness.

Distinguishing symptoms of the patient	Medicine and potency
• Fever with flushed face. **Anguish. Fear. Restlessness**.	Aconite 30 On the first day.
• **Glands enlarged. Throat sore. Fever.**	Belladonna 30
• Alternate with Aconite.	
• On the cheeks, **rosy spots**.	Ferrum Phos 30
• Chill. **Frequent sweats**.	
• Child weepy. Wants company, sympathy.	Pulsatilla 30
• Bland, green mucous flowing free.	

SCARLET FEVER

Normally in the 2nd to 5th year.

Symptoms: Begins with sore throat. Then appear fever symptoms like chills, shivering, hot skin, frontal headache, rapid pulse, nausea, vomiting, thirst.

After 48 hours of the above, rash appears, first on the chest, then on neck, face, body, all over. The tongue takes a strawberry-like colour.

Prevention for others: When scarlet fever is around, administer Belladonna 30, one dose in the morning, another in the evening to all those nearby.

Caution: Diphtheria, laryngitis, pneumonia, bronchitis may develop during scarlet fever. Take appropriate treatment.

Besides the remedies suggested in the chapter on '*Fevers*' under the title, '*Scarlet fever*', the following remedies may also be examined with reference to symptoms.

Distinguishing symptoms of the patient	Medicine and potency
To begin the treatment with. With other chosen remedy, four times a day, until fever subsides.	Aconite 30

- Cold settled in chest. **Dry, hacking cough**.   Bryonia 300
  Pain while coughing. **Bronchitis.**
- Aggravation on movement.
- Copious, **burning discharge** from the **eyes**.   Euphrasia 30
- Lids swollen.
- **Bland, green mucous freely flowing**   Pulsatilla 30
  outwards.
- Gastric upset.
- After eruption has subsided, discontinue   Sulphur 30
  other remedies. Give one dose of Sulphur
  30, for three days early in the morning **to complete recovery**.

SLEEPLESSNESS

Distinguishing symptoms of the patient	Medicine and potency
• From **fright**, agitation or anxiety. **Fever**.	Aconite 30
• **Frightful visions**. Fear. Agitation.	Belladonna 30
• **Cries continuously** for no reason.	
• **Throbbing** temples. Hot head.	
• Due to **pleasant excitement**, laughter, playfulness. Brain overactive.	Coffea 30
• Due to **nervous excitement**. In sensitive children.	Hyoscymus 30
• Due to indigestion, in the **early morning hours, around 3 am.**	Nux Vomica 30
• After a **heavy meal**.	Pulsatilla 30

SORE THROAT/TONSILLITIS

Simple sore throat can be due to congestion.
Tonsillitis is an inflammation of the tonsils.

Symptoms: Sensation of scraping, of heaviness in the throat.

In tonsillitis, tonsils swollen, deep red. White patches on the tonsils with shooting, piercing pain. Fever. Or, purple tonsils. Difficulty in empty swallowing.

You can look at the tonsils easily with a torch beam. Take note of swelling, if any, of the colour of the throat, of patches of pus on the tonsils or other surfaces.

Distinguishing symptoms of the patient	Medicine and potency
• In **initial stages with fever**. On exposure to dry cold air. • **Dry hoarseness**. A scraping sensation.	Aconite 30
• Bright **red**, inflamed tonsils with fever. **Hugely swollen**. Painful.	Belladonna 30
• Sore throat because of taking **very cold drinks or water after a greasy bite**.	Bryonia 200
• **General pain** in the throat. Acute. Chronic.	Baryta Carb 30
• White **pus patches** on the tonsils, in the throat. • **Piercing pain on empty swallowing**. Sensation of a deep cut. • Fever.	Hepar Sulph 30
• Heaviness due to **congestion. Wheezing**. **Gives immediate relief**.	Ipecac 30
• Throat **purple**. • **Difficulty in empty swallowing**. • Worse left.	Lachesis 30

STINGS/INSECT BITES

Distinguishing symptoms of the patient	Medicine and potency
• **Acute** swelling. **Sudden** inflammation. **Fever**.	Aconite 30
• **Insect bites. Stinging pain. Swelling**.	Apis 30 **Primary remedy**.

• In **punctured wounds**. In insect bites. Anti tetanus.	Ledum 30 Alternate with Aconite or Apis.

TOOTHACHE

Symptoms: Pain in a tooth. Pain in the gums. Cavities.

Distinguishing symptoms of the patient	Medicine and potency
• Caused by **exposure to dry cold air**. Fever.	Aconite 30
• **Throbbing pain** extending to **temples**.	Belladonna 30
• Face red, burning hot.	
• **Hot or cold food causes pain**.	Bryonia 30
• Unbearable **spasmodic pain**.	Chamomilla 30
• **Pus** formed. **Itching, stabbing pain.** **Inflammation**. Very **sensitive to touch**.	Hepar Sulph 30
• Pain travels upwards into the ears, eyes, and temple.	
• Pain in **exposed roots**.	Hypericum 30
• In **carious** teeth.	Kreosote 30
• **Gum boil**. Pus formed. Blisters on the gums.	Merc Sol 30
• Pain in roots. **Extends to ears**.	

TWITCHING/TICS

Twitching of the mouth, of eyelids etc.

Distinguishing symptoms of the patient	Medicine and potency
• Out of **anxiety**, baseless **fear**.	Aconite 30
• Twitching of **any muscle**.	Agaricus 30

TYPHOID FEVER

A fever with precise periodicity. Connected with gastric disorders.

Symptoms: Indigestion. Poor appetite. Constipation. Languor. Sleepiness. Delirium at night. Prostration.

Thirst. Dry, red coated, cracked tongue.

Enlargement of abdomen. Sometimes diarrhoea.

Rose coloured dots appear on the 7th day on the abdomen.

Gradual rise in temperature: 2° every night with a fall of 1° every morning in the first week. Decline too is gradual.

Persistent temperature of 40° C is a serious warning.

Complete bed rest is advised. There can be a relapse.

Consult a doctor.

For remedies, refer the entry under the chapter '*Fevers*'.

URTICARIA

Symptoms: Eruptions on the skin. Round or oval wheels, pale in the centre, red at the circumference. Burning, tingling, smarting. Intense itching. A feeling of being stung by nettles.

Distinguishing symptoms of the patient	Medicine and potency
• On exposure to **dry, cold air**.	Aconite 30
• Caused by **almonds, by shellfish**, by overeating.	Ant Crud 30
• **Swelling most prominent** with stinging, burning, and pricking.	Apis 30
• On **excitement**. Rheumatic lameness. Diarrhoea.	Bovista 30
• In **damp** weather.	Dulcamara 30
• **Chronic. Recurring**. Sensitive to the slightest touch.	Hepar Sulph 30
• **Stinging pain** as if someone is inserting a needle.	
• On taking a meal **heavy in fruit or fat**.	Pulsatilla 30

- **Fleabite like spots with purple swelling**   Rhus Tox 30
- Worse on joints.
- Chronic. Take a dose early morning for   Sulphur 30
  a week with other chosen remedy.

WHOOPING COUGH

Affects infants and children.

Symptoms: Violent, spasmodic fits of coughing, ending in a prolonged, shrill, crowing inspiration. Vomiting of thick mucous.

A shrill, crowing inspiration called 'hoop' is a sure indication.

The child turns red, almost black in the face. Appears to be choking.

Between attacks, the child is relaxed, cheerful.

Can lead to convulsions, bronchitis, bronco-pneumonia, and haemorrhage under the skin. Under such circumstances, **seek a doctor's help**.

For remedies, refer under the title '*Cough*' in the chapter '*The Respiratory System*,' particularly, *Aconite, Belladonna, Cuprum Met, Drosera, and Ipecac.*

VOMITING-CHRONIC

Distinguishing symptoms of the patient	Medicine and potency
• Suspected **food poisoning**. Watery diarrhoea.	Arsenic Alb 30
• **Vomits** whatever is eaten.	
• Total **weakness** of limb and of spirit	
• **Colic**. Stomach painful to touch.	
• **Non-stop vomit. Rice water stools.**	Veratrum Alb 30
• **Body cold**. Prostration. Collapse.	
• Cholera.	
• Gastroenteritis.	

WORMS

Threadworms, roundworms, or tapeworms can exist in the digestive system without being suspected unless noticed in evacuation. Caused by drinking impure water, eating vegetables or meat prepared in unhygienic environment.

Symptoms: Picking at the nose. Grinding of the teeth. Impaired appetite. Straining at stool. Itching and irritation about anus. General restlessness and irritability.

For medicine, refer under '*The Digestive system*'.

MISCELLANEOUS

ADDISON'S DISEASE

A rare problem in which the body becomes incapable of responding to physical stress.

Symptoms: Dark spots inside the mouth. Loss of appetite. Nausea. Pain in the abdomen. Low blood pressure.
The skin turns dark, more so on exposure to the sun.
The patient experiences complete exhaustion after even a slight effort.
Slight injury or infection leads to collapse.
Consult a doctor.

Distinguishing symptoms of the patient	Medicine and potency
• **Ulceration** of the mouth. **Tongue** turns **blue.**	Arsenic Alb 200
• **Darkening skin.**	
• **Debility**, exhaustion, restlessness with nightly aggravation.	
• Detests the sight of food. Unquenchable thirst. However, takes little at a time.	
• Nausea, vomiting after a meal.	
• Inside of the stomach burns.	
• **Small wounds bleed a lot**. Heal and break again.	Phosphorus 200
• Spirits low. **Brain tired**.	
• **Vertigo on standing**. Faints.	
• Cutting pain in the abdomen. Relieved by cold food.	
• Worse on physical or mental exertion, in the evening, with warm food or drink.	

ALCOHOLISM

When a social drinker does not know when to stop, he is said to be suffering from *'alcoholism'*.

Symptoms: Does not know when to stop or does not want to cry halt. Drinks alone. Wants to hide the habit from others.

BEWARE

Alcohol dulls the brain and retards its activity. Its euphoric effect is a myth. Alcohol depresses the brain and slows down various centres of control. Under its influence, a person finds it difficult to articulate his thoughts. He stumbles when walking. At times, he may sleep into a coma.

An overdose of alcohol leads to nausea, vomiting, wild gestures, and the uttering of incoherent words.

Most of the alcohol that goes into the human body is oxidised by the liver and converted into acetic acid which can be used by the body. However, the liver has a limited capacity to perform within a period. Beyond this, it cannot handle the intake of alcohol. Perforce, the excess alcohol continues to circulate in the blood stream and affects the brain causing aberration of behaviour and other problems.

The liver cannot process more than a quarter of an ounce of alcohol in an hour. Any dose larger than this, in the end, damages the liver cells and can lead to irreversible cirrhosis of the liver.

"When the wine is in, the wit is out", wrote Thomas Bacon, the English philosopher and essayist. Alcohol damages the centres of thinking and learning in the brain. A drunkard cannot concentrate, cannot perform arithmetical exercises as efficiently as a normal person can. He is no longer alert.

"Wine is a mocker, strong drink is raging: and whosoever is deceived thereby is not wise." [Proverbs 20, 1.] The euphoria generated by alcohol is illusory. The blood is warmed and so is the skin. It is this warmth that makes a drinking person feel uplifted. In reality, the temperature of the body comes down because the heat generated by the skin is soon dissipated by its contact with the air.

Alcohol dulls the brain and thereby kills the desire for sex. In 'Macbeth,' the porter puts it concisely: "It provokes the desire, but it takes away the performance. Therefore much drink may be said to be an equivocator with lechery."

Another after-effect of excessive alcohol intake is passing urine more frequent than normal. It affects that part of the brain which controls discharge of water by kidneys.

An evening of cosy drinking is followed by hangover, a disagreeable physical after-effect of drunkenness, experienced several hours after cessation of drinking. There is fatigue on waking up, severe headache, nausea, and indigestion.

Keep away from alcohol in your own interest.

Distinguishing symptoms of the patient	Medicine and potency
• **Excessive desire** for alcohol.	Arsenic Alb 200
• **Vomiting, diarrhoea** after a bout of drinking.	Administer once a day for quite sometime until there is improvement.
• **Intense craving.**	Capsicum 200
• Excessive peevishness.	
• **Fond of excessive drinking,** stimulating food.	Nux Vomica 200
• Leads a fast life. **Persistent hangover.** Indigestion. Cannot tolerate noise, smells and light.	Remedy for a person who has taken a peg too many.
• Nausea. **Vomiting after** heavy drinking.	
• Chronic alcoholism.	Sulphuric Acid 200

ANAEMIA

A common blood disease where the number of red blood cells in the body is reduced considerably. Further, within the red blood cells, there is a dilution in the red haemoglobin, the pigment that carries oxygen.

In severe anaemia, a patient's life is at risk. Seek medical advice.

Symptoms: Pallor of the skin. Ankles swollen. The patient is easily tired, feels dizzy. Suffers from headache, shortness of breath, palpitation, and lack of sleep.

Look at the patient's diet. Quite a few cases can be redressed by changes in diet. **Talk to a dietician.**

Persistent anaemia is not desirable. Consult a doctor.

Distinguishing symptoms of the patient	Medicine and potency
• **Profound anaemia**. Face and skin **waxen, swollen, and cold. Lips blue.**	Acetic acid 30
• **Cold sweat** on the forehead.	
• **Eyes sunken.** Dark rings around the eyes.	
• In women when there has been an unusual loss of blood after labour.	
• Diabetes. Great thirst. Copious urine. Debility.	
• Total prostration and anxiety.	Arsenic Alb 200
• Cerebral anaemia due **to malaria or excessive use of quinine.**	
• **Violent palpitation**.	
• Swelling.	
• **Stomach easily upset**.	
• **In children**.	Calc Phos 30
• Child peevish. Flabby. Poor digestion.	
• Numbness. Crawling sensation.	
• In women with **excessive menstruation** and violent headache.	
• Caused by **excessive outflow of liquids from the body,** for whatever reason.	China 200
• Abnormal loss of blood in injury, tooth extraction, gastric ulcers, piles, menstruation etc.	
• A weak mind. **Inability to think, to concentrate. Loss of memory.**	
• Splitting headache. **Dizzy when walking.**	
• **Noises in ears.**	
• Face pale, eyes sunken.	
• Sweats easily on motion.	
• Thin, pale weak, **easily exhausted.**	Ferrum Aceticum 1000
• **Shortness of breath.**	**Tackles even stubborn**
• Worse sitting still and lying in bed.	anaemia.
• **After intermittent fevers** like malaria, typhoid.	Ferrum Met 200
• Face pale. At times, face flushed.	

- Skin puffed. Pits on pressure.
  Extremities swollen.
- Cerebral anaemia. **Faints easily**.
- With **throbbing pain in the head**.   Ferrum Phos 200
  Scalp sensitive.
- **Chronic anaemia. Depression. Wants**   Nat Mur 200
  to be left alone to cry.
- Caused by loss of fluids, by irregular
  menstruation, by grief or any other
  sickness of the mind.
- **Numbness and tingling in fingers,** in
  lower extremities. Legs cold. Ankles
  weak. Turn easily.
- **Catches cold easily**. Body weak, emaciated.
  Palms hot and sweating.
- In **pernicious anaemia**. The bone marrow   Picric acid 30
  lacks vitamin B12.
- **Tongue inflamed and sore.**
- Fingers numb.
- Persistent diarrhoea.
- **Nails dry and brittle.**   Silicea 200
- Following pregnancy, copious menstruation
  or any other blood loss.

DEBILITY DUE TO HAEMORRHAGE

Distinguishing symptoms of the patient	Medicine and potency
• Caused by **flow of blood from any part of the body, internal or external.**	China 200
• Faints. Vision weak. Ringing in the ears.	
• Dropsy following loss of blood.	
• Bleeding leucorrhoea.	
• Excessive menstruation.	
• Convulsions in the midst of bleeding in childbirth.	
• Flow of dark, clotted blood. Part turns black.	

FATIGUE/DEBILITY

Distinguishing symptoms of the patient	Medicine and potency
• For **general mental exhilaration** and buoyancy. Physical vigour. All blues dissipated.	Alfa Alfa Mother tincture, 10 drops, four times every day for months.
• With **improved digestion**, body **puts on weight.**	
• Increases quantity and improves quality of milk in **nursing mothers.**	
• **Physical or mental exhaustion.**	Arnica 200
• **Tired. Overworked**. Cannot sleep when tired.	
• Eyes sore due to exertion, studying, and sightseeing.	
• Fatigue due to heavy exercise. Body and muscles sore, bruised.	
• Chronic vertigo. Other objects appear to whirl.	
• Jaded state, mental or physical, due to overwork.	Calc Carb 30
• **Excessive perspiration**.	
• Fatigue due to imperfect **oxygenation, poor digestion.**	Carbo Veg 200
• **Body cold and blue**. Face swollen.	
• Debility after any **acute illness**, from nursing, due to an unending cycle of disease.	
• Caused by **excessive outflow of liquids,** blood, mucous etc., from the body for any reason.	China 200
• Loss of fluids in nursing, in salivation, long continuing diarrhoea, copious pus formation, mucous in influenza, haemorrhages from wounds, lungs, nose, and bowels.	
• **Faints. Loss of vision. Ringing in ears.**	
• Overall weakness of the body.	
• Emaciation. Nervous prostration	Nat Mur 200

- **Throbbing headache**.
- **Palms sore and perspiring.**
- **Numbness and tingling** in fingers, legs, lower extremities.
- **Exhaustion on physical effort**, while climbing stairs.
- Due to **overuse of drugs, alcohol.**   Nux Vom 200
- **Hangover**. Excessive drinking. Late nights.
- Tired as soon as he wakes up. Always out of tune with the world.
- **Nervous exhaustion**. Mental debility first,   Phosphoric Acid 30 physical later.
- Ravages of **acute disease, of excessive grief**, of loss of vital fluids.
- **Hair grey early** in life. Fall out
- Blue rings around ryes.
- **Eyes fatigued after close work** like sewing,   Ruta 200 reading, knitting, typing.

INJURIES

Throughout life, we are never far away from injuries. An injury can be external, internal, or emotional. It can be just a bruise or it may bleed. A bone may break. It can be a sprain or a strain. A surgeon inflicts a controlled injury in the interest of the patient. A mother in childbirth willingly suffers an injury to her body. The newborn unavoidably suffers a hurt.

We can injure ourselves during exercise by overdoing it or by accident.

Insect bites or dog bites are also injuries.

A finger pressed between a door and its frame suffers terribly.

All injuries are painful. A tear in the skin, a fracture of a bone, tearing or crushing of a nerve, the cut of a razor, all add to our suffering.

An injury should be attended to immediately. That will reduce pain and start the healing process.

Bleeding, if any, must be stopped. Otherwise, a human being can bleed to death.

Wounds must be dressed. Open wounds can become septic and cause complications.

In the table that follows, the best of homoeopathic remedies have been discussed for your convenience in case of an accident, an injury, bleeding, concussion, strains, sprains, and during several other situations.

All these remedies are effective to take care of their respective symptoms. In my experience, they have seldom failed.

No home, no office, no factory should be without a supply of Arnica 200. Administer a dose as soon as someone has been injured. Any other selected medicine can follow. Besides relieving pain and healing the tissues, Arnica helps in slowing down bleeding, if any.

For external application, use Calendula, mother tincture. It is available with homoeopathic chemists as a ready to use ointment.

Administer a dose of Ledum 200 to stall tetanus.

It would be advisable to seek medical guidance wherever you feel diffident, where an injury shows no sign of responding to treatment for a day, or so, or where the bleeding cannot be controlled. Hospitalization may be necessary. A fracture must be attended to by a surgeon. No time must be lost.

INJURIES/BRUISES/CUTS/FRACTURES/INSECT BITES/ PUNCTURED WOUNDS/SPRAINS/STRAINS/SURGICAL SHOCK

Distinguishing symptoms of the patient	Medicine and potency
• **Neuralgic pain** following **amputation** or **injury to nerves.**	Allium Cepa 200
• Pain like a fine thread cutting through.	
• **Chronic traumatic neuritis**.	
• **Insect bites.**	Apis 200
• **Swelling**. Red. Burning, stinging pain.	
• **Concussion. Shock**. Traumatic injuries however old.	Arnica 200 First medicine in any
• **Bruised feeling all over**. A bed feels hard. Continuous change gives relief.	injury, mental, physical, in shock, in grief.In acute
• Skin turns **black and blue** on a hit.	stages quick relief.
• Black eye.	Provides long-term
• **Emotional suffering**. Loss of a dear one.	relief.Acts on capillaries,
• Trauma of the **infant in childbirth**. (Use 30 potency.)	relaxes them. **Not sufficient for strains of**
• Administer a few doses before any surgery.	**muscles and tendons.**
• **Haemorrhage** in injuries.	

- **In sprains**.   Bryonia 200
- **In stiffness** with pain anywhere.
- **Joints** red, swollen, stiff, painful.
- Stiffness in the **knee**.
- **Old sprains.**   Calcarea Carb 30
- Injuries to **tendons** and **muscles**.
- After Rhus Tox has been used, some
  weakness might persist. Calcarea Carb
  completes the cure.
- Promotes repairs or reunion of **broken bones**. Calcarea Phos 30
- **Chronic cuts, wounds,** bruises. **Pus** formed.   Calcarea Sulph 30
  Dry, yellow crust.
- **Bruises,** cuts, laceration, razor cuts.   Calendula
- **Any open injury.**   Mother tincture or
- Prevents formation of pus, heals the wound,   ointment for local use.
  smoothens the skin and help to keep the   **A great remedy.**
  wound odourless.
- Relieves local pain and suffering.
- Surgical shock. **Collapse after surgery.**   Carbo Veg 200
- Skin blue. Heart weak.
- Dizziness and weakness from **exhausting**   China 200
  discharge of blood or mucous.
- Intense **throbbing of carotids**. Splitting
  headache. Ringing in ears.
- **Punctured wounds**, painful, bleeding   Ledum 200
  scantily. Swelling at the site.   **Anti tetanus.**
- Wounds with pus.   First to be used if the
- **Insect bites.**   cause of injury is metal
- Black eye from a blow.   or tetanus is feared for
- Shooting pain where **nerves** have been   any other reason.
  injured. Hypericum follows.
- In injury where Arnica has not completed
  the cure, Ledum comes in to finish the job.
- Injury to **spine, coccyx,** sustained by   Hypericum 200
  concussion, fall or in labour.
- Damage to **fibres of the spinal cord.**
- Injury to **nerves,** especially to **fingers, toes,**
  and nails. Crushed fingers. Torn nails.

- **Punctured wounds** from nails, splinters, pins, dog bites, even rat bites.
- After Ledum has been administered, when pain shoots up the nerves from the punctured wound.
- **After tetanus** sets in.
- Internal injury. Stinging, tearing pain.
- Severe haemorrhage. **Bleeding of dark, clotted, and venous blood** from eyeballs, nose, bowels, bladder, and urethra.
- Open, painful wounds.
- Acts more upon **veins which are full, enlarged, and sore.** [Arnica acts on capillaries, causing their relaxation.]
- **Internal haemorrhage.**

Hamamelis 200
Mother tincture for local application.

Millefolium 200
Repeat every half hour until haemorrhage controlled.

- Wounds which **do not heal**.
- **Strains of muscles and tendons.**
- Extreme restlessness. He cannot keep still.
- When **muscles are torn**, use Calcarea Carb 30 after Rhus Tox.
- **Bruises** of the bone, cartilage, tendons, periosteum, about the ear and joints. Wherever **nerves are involved.**
- In **sprains**, Ruta follows Arnica.
- **Eyestrain** from study, artisan's work, sewing etc. Eyes ache, feel sore and strained. Burn like balls of fire.
- **Chronic neuralgia** with stinging, burning, and tearing pain, **especially about eyes.**
- Neuralgia of the face, **of wrist, of lower extremities.**
- Every part of the body **feels bruised if it comes under pressure**.

Nitric Acid 200
Rhus Tox 200

Ruta 200

- Surgical incisions. **Clear-cut wounds** as   Staphysagria 200
  if made with a sharp instrument. With
  burning and stinging pain.
- **Limbs sore**, bruised. **No strength left**.
- **Debility following surgery.**   Strontia 200
- Cold breath. Body cold. Bleeding.
- **Post-surgery shock.**
- Surgical shock.   Veratrum Alb 200
- **Skin blue. Cold sweat**. Collapse.

INTERNAL HAEMORRHAGE

Bleeding ought to be taken seriously, whether the flow of blood is more or less, external or internal.

Parts of the body bleed if a blood vessel, whether a large artery or a narrow capillary, breaks.

External injuries cause external and sometimes internal bleeding as well. Coagulation of blood under the skin makes it look purple. Internal bleeding from an injured muscle or a joint can cause inflammation.

Bleeding inside the body can also be a result of a disease affecting a particular organ.

Haemorrhage in the brain is a life-threatening situation. An artery may burst because of high blood pressure. **Reach for a doctor**.

Internal bleeding can be in the eye, the retina, or conjunctiva.

Bleeding can occur from the ear in an acute middle-ear inflammation.

Bleeding can occur from inflamed gums.

In lung cancer, or cancer of the larynx or in tuberculosis, a patient may throw blood while coughing.

The oesophagus or the stomach can bleed. The patient vomits blood. Bright red colour blood indicates that the bleeding is fresh.

Vomit of dark blood could mean cancer. It also shows that the blood has been in the system for some time.

Blood may also pass through stool which gets darker. In the lower digestive tract, bleeding can be copious and the resultant stool black or like tar.

Blood in urine can mean a simple infection or cancer of the bladder, stones in the kidney or in the bladder.

Piles and anal fissures also bleed bright red.

Bloody dysentery is painful and debilitating.

In women any bleeding other than menstruation, requires medical attention.

For internal bleeding, administer a dose of Millefolium 200 as a first aid. Repeat every four hours.

Seek medical guidance in all but simple, superficial bleeding situations.

Distinguishing symptoms of the patient	Medicine and potency
• Cases of food poisoning.	Arsenic Alb 200
• Vomit of **blood, bile, green mucous.**	
• Cancer of the stomach. **Brown black vomit** mixed with blood.	
• Total prostration. Restlessness. Intense heat.	
• **Blood in urine,** from kidney or bladder.	Cantharis 200
• Constant urge to pass urine. Cutting pain before, during, and after urination.	
• In cases of **persons continually sick:** bleeding from **weak and spongy skin.**	Carbo Veg 200
• From nose, lungs, stomach, bowels, bladder.	
• **Nosebleed.**	Cinnamon 30
• Post delivery haemorrhage.	
• **Bright, red blood in early,** profuse, and prolonged **menstruation**.	
• **Clotted blood. Black and stringy.**	Crocus 30
• Clots with long strings from uterus.	
• In threatened abortion.	
• Bleeding when **blood does not clot.**	Crotalus H 200
• Non-inflammatory retinal haemorrhage.	
• Blood from **ears.**	
• Dark, bloody **urine.**	
• **Intestinal** haemorrhage. Blood dark.	

• Oozing from **rectum** when standing or walking.	
• **Cancer of tongue** with bleeding. Black or ground coffee-coloured vomit.	
• **Cancer of stomach** with bloody, slimy mucous.	
• **Painless flow of dark, clotted,** and venous blood.	Hamamelis 200 Mother tincture for local
• **Does not coagulate.**	application on piles etc.
• **Piles** exuding dark blood.	
• Blood from **anywhere.**	
• Blood and pain in **dysentery**. Stool hot and slimy.	Merc Cor 30
• **Persistent tenesmus.**	
• **Bright red blood** while coughing from lungs, from nose, from bowels, in urine, from urethra, from piles etc.	Millefolium 200
• Early, profuse, and protracted menses.	
• Bright red blood from **bowels.**	Nitric Acid 200
• **Bleeding ulcers.**	
• Haemorrhage in **typhoid.**	Phosphoric Acid 200
• Grows **faint, feels dizzy** while bleeding.	Trillium 30 internally.
• Bright red blood in sputum while coughing, in abortion, in climacteric.	Mother tincture for external application.
• From fibroids.	
• **Chronic uterine bleeding.**	
• Bloody diarrhoea with mucous.	

NAUSEA AND BLEEDING

Distinguishing symptoms of the patient	Medicine and potency
• Wheezing.	Ipecac 200
• **Nausea present.**	
• Copious flow of bright red blood from anywhere with nausea.	

SMOKING

"A custom loathsome to the eye, hateful to the nose, harmful to the brain, dangerous to the lungs, and in the black, stinking fume thereof nearest resembling the horrible stygian smoke of the pit that is bottomless." James 1 of England

Smoking is not a sickness. It is a curse. The only advice I can offer to habitual smokers is to give up the habit. Those who do not smoke should stay away.

According to US Health Authority, smoking is "the largest preventable cause of death in America."

Millions of people die all over the world every year because they smoke cigarettes, pipes, and cigars. Smoking is a risk factor in causing coronary heart disease and is a definite cause of lung cancer and of skin cancer.

Smoking has a direct and adverse effect on the lungs of the smoker. The entire respiratory system is coated with unwelcome soot from the cigarette smoke. The lung alveoli where the gaseous exchange takes place and the airways of the respiratory system are not designed for this sort of over-wrap. Intake of clean air into the respiratory system is thus reduced and the brain gets a diminished supply of oxygen.

The efficiency of heart declines because Nicotine, a highly toxic alkaloid, a by-product of tobacco, increases the heartbeat and thus strains the heart. An average of 20 years of life span is lost to a male smoker who dies of coronary heart disease. A quarter of the deaths because of coronary heart disease can be traced to the ill effects of smoking.

Deaths due to sudden heart failure are more than three times higher in smokers than in non-smokers. The risk factor increases in direct proportion to the number of cigarettes smoked in a day and the duration for which the activity of smoking continues.

A similar situation prevails in case of lung cancer and bronchitis. A heavy smoker runs a risk greater than others who do not smoke or smoke less. However, every smoker can develop chronic bronchitis or lung cancer. Most of the deaths from these two diseases are caused by cigarette smoking.

Available evidence suggests that the damage to the lungs can largely be reversed if the smoker totally gives up smoking. The affected portions of the lungs may heal on their own in due course.

Smokers of pipes and cigars run the risk of developing lip and mouth cancer. So do the users of chewing tobacco and even the betel leaf with lime and tobacco.

No smoker is ever safe. There is no such thing as moderate smoking. Even the unborn child of a smoking pregnant woman runs a risk. It might die during the first few days after birth. If the child survives, it would be physically smaller and its height would be less than that of the children of non-smoking mothers.

Smoking is an acquired habit and not a necessity. It does not overcome fatigue, nor does it provide relaxation. This is an illusion. Nobody makes more friends just because he smokes. In reality, a smoker makes the lives of others, who happen to be in his company by sheer necessity or chance, miserable. They passively smoke his exhalations as well as the smoke of the burning cigarette. It suffocates them. It affects their lungs adversely.

By way of personal hygiene, the smoker is at a disadvantage. His fingers turn yellow, his teeth, and gums stained. No mouthwash can make his mouth feel fresh or deodorize his breath. No non-smoker desires to sit in the company of a smoker.

A smoker loses his smell of smell, of taste.

Use your will power to give up smoking. It is never too late.

For relaxation, listen to music, read a good work of fiction, or meditate.

Go to Mother Nature to look at the flowers of the spring and to listen to the bird song. Count the petals of a flower and feel their softness. Inhale their mild scent. Look long and deep into the designs of different flowers. Take a long walk in a garden.

Climb a mountain.

Stand and stare at the rise and fall of the magnificent waves of the ocean.

Admire the shape and forms of the clouds in the sky, and wonder at the colours and sweep of a rainbow.

Appreciate the phases of the moon and the twinkling stars in the sky.

For relaxation, read Kalidasa. Read Shakespeare. Read Wordsworth. Why smoke and kill yourself?

CANCER

While writing this chapter, I am aware of the limitation of any system of medicine in treating cancer. Research is on in the best of laboratories of the world to find a cure. I hope that some day mankind would overcome this messenger of death.

I have designed this chapter primarily to describe symptoms, palliatives in homoeopathy and prognosis.

I firmly believe that for proper care and treatment of a cancer patient, a consultation with a cncer specialist and hospitalization, if recommended, is necessary.

Our body cells grow in a well-regulated manner. When this control mechanism falters, the cells grow uncontrollably. Solid tumours form in specific sites of the body. From there the disease spreads everywhere through the circulatory and lymphatic systems.

Literally, the word '*cancer*' means a pernicious, spreading evil. This description aptly applies to the disease known as cancer.

Hippocrates, the Greek physician, likened cancer to a crab because its tentacles spread like a claw. The description is quite accurate. A cancerous tumour spreads without inhibition and restraint and destroys its victim.

Cancer is a killer next only to coronary heart disease in advanced countries. Tobacco smoke is one of the main culprits in the spread of cancer.

Not all tumours are cancerous or malignant. These do not spread through the body. Hence, it is necessary to investigate any lump that appears on the body or inside in order to rule out malignancy. **This is not a job for the layman but for a specialist.**

While children rarely suffer from cancer, in adults the chances of developing a cancer at some stage in their life are high. A cancer might be detected while investigation is being carried out for some other disease. Otherwise, certain symptoms develop over a period and manifest in the failing health of the patient. Take notice of the following and consult your physician as soon as possible

Easily noticeable symptoms:

1. Nausea with weight loss and a loss of appetite.
2. Persistent fatigue.
3. Recurring abdominal pain with change in bowel habits. Bleeding from rectum and/or vagina.
4. Blood in urine.
5. Sputum with a sprinkling of blood.
6. Swollen and bleeding jaw that does not heal.
7. A wound that does not heal.
8. A mole that grows and changes shape.
9. Any lump on or under the skin, even if painless. Feels firm to touch.
10. Persistent headaches.
11. Voice becomes hoarse and changes in pitch and tone.
12. Uncomfortable swallowing. Oesophagus feels obstructed.

These symptoms are apparent. They must not be ignored. If a cancer is detected at an early stage, the chances of its cure are good.

THE BRAIN

Any part of the brain can be affected by cancer. The causes are yet not known.

Symptoms: Cancer of a particular part of the brain affects those parts of the body which that part controls. Look out for unusual symptoms.

In children, it can be blindness, double vision, squint. Difficulty in walking properly and steadily. Nausea and vomiting.

In adults, persistent headache, decline in mental faculties, faulty speech, and failure of locomotor system, weak memory, and increasing drowsiness.

Prognosis: Extremely slim in grown ups. Better in the case of children.

Palliatives:

Calcarea Carb 200. Vertigo. Headache on turning the head. Piercing, stitching pain in the head sensation ice-cold in the head.

Conium 200. Scorched feeling on the top. Staggering gait. Limbs give way when walking. Headache. Nausea. Vomiting. Sensation of a foreign body under the scalp.

Thuja 200. Brain tumours with intense migraine and pain.

THE MOUTH, THE TONGUE

Happens on lips, the tongue, or the tissue in the tongue. Quite often on the gums, on the palate, or on the lining of the cheek.

Cancer of the mouth is mainly caused by use of tobacco, particularly chewing tobacco.
Excessive drinking and smoking are the other risk factors.

Symptoms: The tumour is red, hard, and fibrous.

Prognosis: 50 % cure in case a small tumour is detected and treated in time.
Cancer of the mouth does not easily respond to radiation therapy.

THE LIP

Prolonged exposure to sunlight, smoking of cigarettes, pipes, and cigars are some of the known causes.

Symptoms: In the beginning no clear-cut symptoms. Later, blisters on the lip which refuse to heal or which bleed. Ulcers on the lips.

Prognosis: A high rate of cure if detected early and treated.
Give up smoking altogether. Avoid exposure to sunlight.

Surgery and radiation therapy are useful.

Palliatives:

Apis 200. Tongue dry, swollen, cracked, sore, ulcerated. Inability to swallow.

Aurum Ars 200. Bluish discolouration. Pale, coppery eruptions. Red spots.

Condurango 30. Ulceration. Painful cracks in the corner of the lips.

Conium 1000. Distortion of tongue and mouth. Hard tumour of the lip.

Crotalus H 200. Tongue so swollen that the mouth cannot contain it. Haemorrhage. Tongue protrudes, goes to the right.

Phosphorus 1000. Cancer with blood and pus. Open sores. Hole through the tongue. Tearing, burning pain.

THE LARYNX

Once again, the root cause is smoking, and chewing tobacco.

Symptoms: Sound box and the vocal cords are affected. The voice changes its key. The throat is persistently sore. Swallowing is difficult. Blood in cough and sputum. Pain in ears and throat. Breathing becomes noisy and difficult. Weight loss.

Prognosis: Not good in most of the cases.

Palliatives:

Arsenic Alb 200. Dirty looking growth on laryngeal membrane. Burning pain. Short, spasmodic cough.

Kali Bi 200. Benign tumour of the larynx with thick, ropy mucous that is difficult to take out.

Phytolacca 30. Fibrous growth. Glands swollen. Pain at the root of the tongue extending to ears.

Thuja 200. Benign tumour. Chronic laryngitis.

THE LUNGS

It begins with the bronchial tube and then extends to either or both lungs. Cigarette smoking is the main cause of lung cancer. Industrial pollutants, radioactivity, processing metals like chromium, nickel, iron, or substances like arsenic, asbestos, can also lead to lung cancer.
Lung cancer develops usually after 40 years of age.

Symptoms: Persistent, dry, irritating cough. Blood in sputum. Difficult breathing. Pneumonia. Loss of weight. Severe pain in the chest. Difficulty in swallowing.

Prognosis: The survival rate is not even 10 % in spite of excellent treatment.

GIVE UP SMOKING. CHANGE YOUR WORKING ENVIRONMENT.

Palliatives:

Millefolium 200. Coughs pure blood

Phosphorus 200. Streaks of blood in mucous from the lungs.

THE OESOPHAGUS

Caused by excessive use of alcohol, of tobacco.

Symptoms: Initially, no symptoms. Later, difficulty in swallowing. Pain in oesophagus. Sudden weight loss. Even drinking water leads to choking.

Prognosis: If the cancer of the oesophagus has advanced, the chances of recovery are not bright. Surgery is effective in some cases.

THE STOMACH

Specific cause not known. Those who suffer from chronic gastric problems, ulcers that do not heal or pernicious anaemia are more likely to develop cancer of the stomach.

Symptoms: Slow and steady loss of weight. Loss of appetite. Blood in vomit, in stool. Anaemia. Pain in upper abdomen.

Prognosis: Poor.

Palliatives:

A change in dietary habits can keep the cancer of the stomach away. Avoid taking polished and junk food. Take a diet high in fibre, fresh vegetables, and fruit.

THE LIVER

A patient of cirrhosis of the liver may develop cancer of the liver. Liver cancers are often secondary, spreading from a cancer at another site of the body.

Symptoms: No early symptoms. Even later ones are misleading. Rapid loss of weight. Constipation. Pain and distension in the abdomen. Nausea. Vomiting. Jaundice.

Prognosis: The survival rate is nil because early detection is virtually impossible.
Stop consuming alcohol.

THE PANCREAS

Glands situated near the stomach which secrete insulin and digestive juices can become cancerous for unknown causes.

Symptoms: Indigestion. Constipation. Jaundiced skin. Weight-loss. Pain in the abdomen. Dark coloured urine.

Prognosis: Usually fatal.

THE COLON, THE BOWEL, AND THE RECTUM

Statistically more persons who take a diet, low in fibre, rich in carbohydrates and fats, or polished or refined food, suffer from the cancer of the colon and rectum than those who take a diet rich in vegetables, fruit, a diet with high content of fibre and food made with unpolished or whole grain.

Symptoms: Frequent changes in bowel habits whether accompanied by a flow of dark red blood from the rectum or not. Cramping pain in the intestines. Constipation or persistent diarrhoea. Painful anal spasm. Loss of appetite, of weight.

Prognosis: If diagnosed early, the survival rate is 50%. This cancer comes around middle age. **Surgery is of great help**.

Palliatives:

Alumina 200. Cancerous growth in rectum with pain after motions. Constipation.

Arsenic Alb 200. Cancer of the stomach. Of oesophagus which feels blocked. Nothing passes through. Heat as if fire is burning inside the stomach. Of palliative help even in malignancy. Unquenchable thirst. Restlessness and anguish.

Carbo Veg 200. Severe acidity. General debility. Burning and flatulence in the upper stomach region. Continue for a long time.

Cardus Marianus, mother tincture. Rectal cancer resulting in profuse diarrhoea.

Crotalus H 200. Vomit of bloody, slimy mucous. Black or coffee-coloured vomit.

Nitric Acid 200. Palliative in painful cancer of the rectum. Vomits blood and slime. Ulcers in the stomach.

Ruta 200. Carcinoma affecting lower bowel and rectum. Prolapse of anus every time the bowels move, particularly after confinement. Tearing, cutting pain in the rectum.

THE KIDNEY

Cancer of the kidney affects more men than women. Often after the onset of middle age.

Symptoms: Pain while passing urine. Pain in the back in the region of the kidneys. Blood in urine.

Prognosis: Once the cancer has spread beyond kidneys to the lymph nodes, the chances of recovery are not bright. Otherwise too, the survival rate is hardly 50% after a prolonged treatment.

THE BLADDER

The site is the inner lining of the bladder. Smokers and workers in dyes and chemical factories are more prone.

Symptoms: Deep red or brown urine. Increased frequency. Discomfort while passing urine. Mostly old persons get this cancer.

Prognosis: Good chances of recovery unless the cancer has spread to lymph nodes. Get the best possible medical advice.

THE BREAST

Develops as a hard lump. It spreads to the lymph glands in the armpits and then throughout the body.

Women who have had children are more prone to develop breast cancer than those who have not.

Around menopause, women run a greater risk of developing breast cancer

Symptoms: A hard lump forms. Abnormal change in colour. A retracted nipple. Discharge from the nipples. Skin ulcerates.

Prognosis: If detected early, the rate of cure is more than 80%. However, the incidence of this cancer is so high that a large number of women die of breast cancer all over the world every year. A regular check-up in a proper hospital facility is essential. Fortunately, most lumps in the breast are not cancerous.

Palliatives:

Arsenic Alb 200. Palliative in cancer of the breast with restlessness and severe burning.

Asterias Rubens 30. Acute stabbing pain. Ulceration. Armpit glands swollen, hard, knotted.

Conium 200. Strong, hard tumours.

THE UTERUS

Women between 40 and 70 sometimes suffer from uterine cancer. This is different from the cancer of the cervix and is more common after menopause.

Women who have not borne children, whose menstruation cycles have been irregular, whose climacteric comes late, run a greater risk of uterine cancer than others do. So do diabetics and patients of high blood pressure.

Symptoms: Bleeding from vagina after coitus. Unusually heavy periods. Bleeding between periods.

In women whose menopause has set in, any bleeding from the vagina can be a symptom of cancer of the uterus.

Prognosis: The survival rate is as high as 80 % if the cancer is detected and treated at the earliest. It is not good if the cancer has spread to the surrounding areas.

Palliatives:

Aurum Arsenic 200. Eruptions and itching on the vulva. Heightened sexual desire. Irregular menstruation.

Carbo Animalis 30. Cancer of the uterus with burning, stabbing pain down thighs.

Kali Carb 30. Cancer of the uterus with severe pain from hip to knees. Worse right side.

Lapis Albus 30. Uterine carcinoma. Fibroid tumours. Intense burning pain with copious haemorrhage.

THE CERVIX

Malignant growth forms on the neck of the uterus. Promiscuous women are more prone to the cancer of the cervix.
Women who conceive frequently are at a greater risk than others who do not.

Symptoms: Bleeding from vagina after sexual intercourse. Pain during coitus. Bleeding between periods. Copious flow of menstrual blood.
Any unusual bleeding from vagina requires medical advice.

Prognosis: If diagnosed early, chances of cure are good.
Once it spreads to the surrounding areas, such as the bladder, the urethra, or even the rectum, recovery is difficult.

THE OVARY

Cancer in ovaries develops from unknown causes.

Symptoms: Unfortunately, no symptoms appear until cancer has advanced substantially. There is pain low in the back. Unusual vaginal discharges. A growth can be felt in the pelvis. Abdominal swelling and pain.

Prognosis: Not good once cancer has advanced and spread beyond ovaries. Otherwise, too the relief is not permanent.

THE PROSTATE

In males, prostate is a frequent site for cancer. A simple blood test [PSA], conducted periodically can reveal its absence or presence. Enlargement of prostate occurs in old age in most males.

Symptoms: Difficulty in passing urine. Frequency increased. Blood in urine. Pain in the back.

Prognosis: Good. Early detection and treatment can be helpful.

Palliatives:

Arsenic Alb 1000. Patient restless because of pain.

Crotalus H 200. Cancer of prostate with haematuria.

THE SKIN

An existing mole or pigmented spot on the skin may become cancerous. It is called *malignant melanoma.*

Another type of skin cancer may be a painless lump which ulcerates. It can be caused by excessive exposure to sunlight, radiation or certain chemicals over years. Its site is the face, the neck, the head, the ears, the hands etc.

Rodent ulcer may grow on the face, the eyelids, the neck, the nose or the ears.

Symptoms: Sudden increase in the size of an existing mole. Darkening of the colour. Ulceration. Bleeding of the mole. Warts on face, hands, ears, lips, neck or other parts of old persons enlarge and ulcerate.
At times, a round pimple forms which later changes into a shiny nodule which ulcerates.

Prognosis: An early detection can lead to a cure in 70% of the cases. With the spread of cancer to lymph nodes, the survival rate declines. **Malignant melanoma spreads rapidly and can lead to death. Immediate attention is required.**
Rodent ulcer does not spread to other parts of the body.

Palliatives:

Anthracinum 30. Malignancy with terrible burning.

Condurango 30. Painful cancer of the skin. Ulcers. Fissures. Cracks in the corner of the mouth.

THE BLOOD [LEUKAEMIA]

Production of abnormal white blood cells overpowering the normal white cells, the red cells, and platelets.

Symptoms: Anaemia. Loss of weight. Easy bleeding. Susceptibility to infection. Swelling of spleen, liver, and lymph nodes. Persistent low fever.

Prognosis: Chances are not bright.

THE BONE MARROW

Atomic radiation, X-rays are suspected to be some of the causes. Yet no specific cause is known.

Symptoms: Continuous, sharp pain in the bone. Loss of consciousness because of the severity of the pain. Rapid loss of weight. Bones become brittle and break on their own.

Prognosis: Extremely slim in grown ups. Better in the case of children. Not many patients survive.

MATERIA MEDICA

MATERIA MEDICA

Homoeopathic system of cure does not use any drug that has not been proved on healthy human beings. By 'proving', we imply that a pure substance is administered to healthy volunteers and its effect on their mind and body is noted in minute detail. The volunteers' descriptions of the effects are analyzed by doctors. When a particular result is noted in most of the cases, that manifestation is considered a proved symptom/malady for which that substance can be used as a drug in pure or potencized form. A common example of this fact is the use of Arsenic to cure the results of food poisoning. Use of pure Arsenic, otherwise, can lead to fatal consequences.

Homoeopathic Materia Medica uses almost a thousand herbal and mineral substances, poisons extracted from plants, animals and insects, roots, flowers and essences, metallic compounds and other scientific combinations.

The foundation of the Homoeopathic Materia Medica was laid in the principles enunciated by Dr. Samuel Hahnemann. He wrote, *"in all careful trials, pure experience, the sole and infallible oracle of the healing art, teaches us that actually that medicine which, in its action on the healthy human body, has demonstrated its power of producing the greatest number of symptoms similar to those observable in the case of a disease under treatment, does also, in doses of suitable potency and attenuation, rapidly, radically and permanently remove the totality of the symptoms of this morbid state, that is to say the whole disease present, and change it into health: and that medicines cure, without exception, those diseases whose symptoms most nearly resemble their own, and leave none of them uncured."*

This was the basic principle of homoeopathy: 'Like cures like' or 'Similia Similibus Curentur'.

Next to the principle of *like cures like* is the theory of 'potencization' which was applied to reduce the possibility of an adverse effect of any substance used for a cure. The quantity of drug is reduced to infinitesimal proportions through a process of dynamic dilution. On conducting thousands of experiments Dr. Hahnemann and his associates discovered that *dilution* done in the prescribed manner, achieved three benefits.

Firstly, it eliminated the possibility of adverse reaction in the human body.

Secondly, and this was sheer inspiration, greater the dilution, the more beneficial a drug changed to cure. *Potencization* brought out the inherent healing powers of a substance in direct proportion to its dilution.

Thirdly, this sublimation process increased the shelf life of a homoeopathic drug.

"In homoeopathic cures experience teaches us that from the uncommonly small doses of medicine required in this method of treatment, which are just sufficient, by the similarity of their symptoms, to overpower and remove from the sensation of life principle the similar natural disease, there certainly remains, after the destruction of the latter, at first a certain amount of medicinal disease alone in the organism, but on account of the extraordinary minuteness of the dose, it is so transient, so slight, and disappears rapidly of its own accord, that the vital force has no need to employ, against this small artificial derangement of its health, any more considerable reaction than will suffice—to complete recovery."

Paragraph 68, 'Organon of Medicine.' Dr. Samuel Hahnemann.

For the convenience of the reader, I have selected 47 often-used drugs based on my study and experience, for discussion in the chapters which follow. I have noted other medicines too in the chapters on various parts of the human body to indicate the symptoms that those can take care of.

A study of individual drugs reveals fascinating aspects of their effects because of the stress on *leading symptoms* in the system of homoeopathic cure. I recommend a repeated reading of Materia Medica. Some excellent books have been listed in the Bibliography that follows.

Throughout this book, I have tried to differentiate the drugs that apparently deal with almost similar symptoms. Invariably, there is a pointer, a distinguishing symptom that separates the drugs leading to a correct choice. If Bryonia is indicated in muscular pains aggravating on movement, Rhus Tox is required in similar pains temporarily reducing on movement. In sinusitis, Kali Bichrome benefits cases where thick, green or yellow mucous goes into the throat. When such a mucous comes out easy, outwards through the nose, the medicine indicated is Pulsatilla.

With experience, you learn to identify these differences.

Every drug chapter begins with a summary of the *leading indications* for the use of a particular drug. Although these indications cannot be decisive in the choice and prescription of a drug, yet their value for setting the sights cannot be underestimated.

For instance, a leading indication for the use of Aconite is fear without basis, fear of death in the mind of the patient. Another leading indication is inflammation, fever, cold, resulting from exposure to dry, cold winds. A third indication for Aconite is acute, sudden, and violent onset of disease. If these indications are kept in mind, a dose of Aconite can be given to a child who comes from the playfield, where he might have been exposed to dry cold winds, screaming with pain in his face or in his ear. In acute cases of croup, bronchitis, pneumonia, etc., Aconite is the first choice because the malady comes suddenly, becomes severe, and is generally violent. Exposure to dry, cold winds, [as opposed to exposure to cold, wet winds], is often the cause of the sickness.

Repeated reading and experience will enrich your mind and enable it to react fast to a situation. Think of Antimony Tart when a rattling sound is produced because of an accumulation of mucous in the lungs and when the patient cannot expel it Use Ipecac if mucous can be coughed out easily. An uncomfortable and sudden irritation and heaviness in the throat requires a dose of Ipecac. If you see a swelling anywhere with burning, stinging pain, use Apis. The swelling could have been caused by any one of several reasons.

I think of Veratrum Alb, when I hear of loose, watery, white stools with or without nausea. On the other hand, uncontrollable stools, though loose and watery, require Aloe. Yellow loose motions require Podophyllum. Thus, for different types of gastroenteritis, varying symptoms indicate different medicines.

A thorough study of the Materia Medica is of great help in the choice of the best remedy for symptoms exhibited in the mind and body of the patient. Yet it cannot be anybody's case that all the symptoms as produced in a healthy human being in 'provings' with a particular drug would be present at the same time in a patient. Dr. Hahnemann was aware of this situation. In Para 153, of the *Organon of Medicine*, he observed that the *"more striking, singular, uncommon and peculiar [characteristic] signs and symptoms of the case of disease are chiefly and most likely to be kept in view."* These, in particular, ought to correspond with similar ones in the list of symptoms of the selected medicine. *"The more general and undefined symptoms: loss of appetite, headache, debility, restless sleep, discomfort and so forth, demand but little attention when these are of vague and indefinite character"*.

It has been my experience that by carefully focusing on the most prominent symptoms of a patient, we can select a suitable remedy and achieve a cure. Please encourage the patient to describe his symptoms as exhaustively as possible. Help him by asking probing questions, and only thereafter, ferret out aspects of his suffering he may not have thought of. Classified symptoms in the Materia Medica and the chapters on different maladies will help you to ask leading questions as a last resort so that you do not overlook any uncommon and definitive symptom.

There has been a debate whether we can use homoeopathic medicines in combinations or mixtures. The orthodox view has been against this procedure. However, in my personal experience I have found that if two or more drugs are compatible, a mixture is of great convenience and is equally effective. For instance, I have found a mixture of Bryonia and Cimicifuga, efficacious in taking care of cervical spondylosis whenever the symptoms are present. These days many drug companies, in India as well as abroad, are marketing mixtures for specific ailments. The convenience of handling a number of drugs required simultaneously is justification enough for the use of combinations, unless otherwise warranted. Yet, there is no denying the magic of a single dose in Homoeopathy. It works.

"It is next to impossible that medicine and disease cover one another symptomatically as exactly as two triangles with equal sides and equal angles."

Dr. Samuel Hahnemann.

ABIES NIGRA

Leading Indications

1. **Indigestion of old people.**
2. **Constriction in the oesophagus.**
3. **Abnormal, rapid heart beat.**

Abies Nigra eases a sensation of constriction in the oesophagus. The patient feels as if a hard-boiled egg is lodged at the cardiac end of the stomach. Sensation of a lump that hurts, just above the pit of the stomach.

Abies Nigra can be used beneficially in the following circumstances as well:

- Typical symptoms of indigestion are present. No appetite in the morning. Offensive breath. Frequent eructation. Constipation. Pain in the stomach after eating.
- The patient experiences constriction of the lungs. On lying down, he loses breath. The heart beats heavy, slow, or abnormally rapid.

Mental state: The patient lacks cheer. His spirits are low. He keeps awake at night.

Abies Nigra is an underrated remedy. Its effect is quick and lasting.

The patient is worse: After eating.

Recommended potency: 200

ACONITUM NAPELLUS

Leading Indications

1. **Exposure to dry cold winds.**
2. **Acute, sudden, violent onset of disease.**
3. **Fear, without reason. Restlessness.**

4. **Numbness, tingling.**
5. **Skin dry, hot feverish.**
6. **Screaming, stabbing pain.**

Whenever a malady has been caused by exposure to dry, cold weather, or by fright or both, Aconite helps. Think of it, in inflammation, inflammatory fevers, when an attack is acute, sudden, and violent. Restlessness, physical and mental, is present.

Aconite can be used beneficially in the following circumstances as well:

- Sudden attacks of croup, bronchitis, pleurisy, rheumatism, and tachycardia. It is a short acting remedy, required at the first stage. Other selected medicines follow.
  The patient has an unfounded fear of death, of crossing a street, of social interaction, of impending disaster.
  The pain is intolerable, worse as the evening progresses.
- Numbness, tingling, and a sensation of crawling insects, whatever the cause.
- Acute, sudden, high fever with thirst. The pulse is hard, full, and fast. The patient is implacable, tosses in agony. His skin is bright red. Evening chill and cold waves pass through his body. [While Aconite fever is characterized by dry, hot skin, no sweat, restless tossing, irrational fear, Belladonna fever has the patient sweating on covered parts, greater surface heat than Aconite, semi stupor, jerking of the limbs, delirium.]
- Croup, when the child awakens frightened, and has a dry, hoarse, croupy cough, Aconite gives relief.
- In a newborn child, Aconite relieves retention of urine caused by shock of birth.
- Neuralgia of the face, sudden, violent, caused by exposure to dry, cold winds. Intense pain like hot wires running along either side of the face. Numbness. Tingling.
- Terrible toothache caused by such exposure.
- Coryza sudden, violent, with severe headache.
- Coryza of rosy and chubby babies.

- Inflammation of the eye, lids swollen rapidly, difficult to open, a feeling of foreign body under the lids; intense cutting pain in the ear, children returning from playfields. Caused by exposure to dry, cold winds.
- Inflamed, dry throat with violent cough, acute asthmatic attacks. Sciatica with sensation of ice-water poured along the nerves, shooting rheumatic pains with a tingling sensation and loss of sensibility in hands and feet, joints red, shining, and swollen.
- Vertigo because of fright. In terrible allergic urticaria.
- Pneumonia, where it is a supreme remedy. Sudden inflammation of the viscera, of the pleura, of the lungs. Shortness of breath. Oppressed breathing on least motion. Mucous streaked with bright red blood. [Iron rust mucous needs Bryonia or Rhus Tox depending on other symptoms. Aconite mucous is cherry red.]
- Acute urethral pain. Stoppage of urine.

The patient is better: By uncovering, in open air.
The patient is worse: In the evening during chest problems, lying on left side, in a warm room with warm covers, listening to music, inhaling tobacco smoke.

Recommended potency: 30, 200. Repeat 30 in acute cases. Aconite is a rapid worker.

ALLIUM CEPA

Leading Indications

1. *Copious, bland watering from eyes.*
2. *Corroding, continuous discharge from the nose.*
3. *Colds in cold, damp weather.*

Allium Cepa is the remedy in acute coryza and allied respiratory problems. Violent sneezing. The nasal discharge corrodes the upper lip and the nose.

Allium Cepa can be used beneficially in the following circumstances as well:

- Eyes running, bland, and profuse. Yet, they burn and smart. [Use Euphrasia when the eye discharge is acrid, burning.]
- Respiratory problems when there is tickling in the larynx. The latter develops violent, rapid inflammation. The patient is hoarse. He has a hacking cough on breathing in cold air. He has pain in the ear.
- Whooping cough, with indigestion, vomiting, and flatulence.
- Neuralgic pain following an amputation or an injury to nerves. It feels like a fine thread cutting into the body.

The patient is better: In open air, in a cold room.
The patient is worse: In the evening, in a warm room

Recommended potency: 200

ALOE

Leading Indications

1. **Insecurity in the rectum. It feels full of heavy fluid that wants to get out.**
2. **Abdomen bloated like a tent. Thundering rumble.**
3. **Involuntary stool while passing urine or flatus.**
4. **Prolapsed rectum.**

Aloe is the remedy when one has lost control over passing the stool. The patient feels that his rectum would fall out if he does not clear immediately. There is a feeling of urgency and total helplessness. This, even when making water or expelling wind.

Aloe stool can be solid, passing in large balls or liquid. It can be yellow, or bloody, or transparent or full of mucous. The leading indication is 'involuntary'.

There is a rumbling in the stomach, loud, noisy. Burning flatus. Bloated abdomen. Pulsating pain near the navel, in the rectum.

Aloe can be used beneficially in the following circumstances as well:

- In prolapse where the rectum protrudes like a bunch of grapes. The haemorrhoids are blue, itch intensely. Burning in anus disturbs sleep. Cold water soothes.
- In dysentery with a feeling of violent tenesmus, a never-done feeling, heat in the rectum, profuse sweat, debility, profuse jelly like mucous.

In my experience, Aloe has never failed.

[Podophyllum is another remedy for gushing stools. However, here the patient does not feel a loss of control. Prolapse of the rectum is common but it is not always present. In Podophyllum, there is empty retching while in Aloe no nausea is present.]

The patient is better: In cold, open air, by cold-water application on piles, by uncovering in the bed.

The patient is worse: In hot, dry weather, in summer, early morning, after intake of food or drink, while walking or standing.

Recommended potency: 200

AMMONIUM CARBONICUM

Leading Indications

1. **Nose ever blocked. Dry, stuffed coryza. Has to breathe with mouth open. Chronic cases.**
2. **Unclean habits. Dislike of open air, of bathing.**
3. **Snuffles of children.**
4. **Very sensitive to cold air.**

The Ammonia Carb patient is sensitive to cold air. His nose is blocked at night. He is compelled to breathe through an open mouth. A child cannot breathe through his nose because the nostrils are stuffed with mucous.

Ammonia Carb can be used beneficially in the following circumstances as well:

- In diphtheria when the nose is stuffed.
- For acrid saliva, acrid tears, acrid stool, and acrid leucorrhoea. The acrid nature of the discharges causes cracks in lips, in eyelids, in female genitals.
- Women with bleeding piles that aggravate during menstruation. The menstruation is frequent, is accompanied by profuse, clotted and black blood. The discharge is acrid. There is pain in the thighs. Violent, tearing pain in vagina. Genitals swollen. Clitoris irritated. Aversion to sex.
- Big toe is swollen and painful. The heel pains on standing. There is tearing pain in ankles and the bones of the feet.
- Teeth, jawbones ache violently.

The patient is better: Lying on painful side, on stomach.
The patient is worse: From cold, wet weather, in the evenings, from washing, during menstruation.

Recommended potency: 200

ANTIMONIUM CRUDUM

Leading Indications

1. **Digestive disorders due to overeating. Milky, coated tongue.**
2. **Foul wind. Stinking eructation.**
3. **Warts on hand, nails, finger ends.**
4. **Shoe corns.**

Antim Crud is a remedy for gluttons. With an overloaded stomach, they experience nausea, fullness, and discomfort. However, sometimes these symptoms appear without overloading the stomach. Even then, the remedy is the same if the flatus or the eructation stinks. Continuous belching requires Antim Crud.

Antim Crud can be used beneficially in the following circumstances as well:

- A milky coating on the tongue in indigestion.
- A person with bad eating habits is peevish. Stomach disorder gives him a headache, sometimes vertigo.
- Piles with a continuous oozing of mucous. Itch in the anus. Linen soiled often.
- Old persons who eat indiscriminately suffer from diarrhoea and constipation alternately.
- For warts, hard and horny and for painful excrescences under the nails, and from ends of fingers. For split and crushed nails. For toenails growing out of shape, brittle. For callosities, painful and tender, on the feet. Thickening skin.
- Toothache in a hollow tooth.

The patient is better: In open air, taking rest, in moist warmth.
The patient is worse: In the evenings, at night, from cold washing, taking acids, pickles, wine, liquor, overeating, from exposure to hot sun, from exertion, near open fire, in damp weather.

Recommended Potency: 200. 1000 for warts etc.

ANTIMONIUM TARTARICUM

Leading Indications

1. **Difficulty in expectoration.**
2. **Large accumulation of mucous in the lungs.**
3. **Failing lungs. Sleepiness, nearing coma.**
4. **Face blue from lack of oxygen. Pale, sickly.**

Use Antim Tart beneficially in the following circumstances:

- When there is accumulation of mucous in the air passages with coarse rattling and an inability to expectorate. An impending paralysis of lungs.
- In infants, young children dying of bronchitis, of bronco-pneumonia, blue for lack of oxygen, and old persons with chest

full of rattles and wheezes, with lungs filling up fast, and no power to raise the phlegm. Such a situation can occur during bronchitis, pneumonia, whooping cough, or asthma. Use 1000 potency.

(Ipecac rattling has the power to cough out the mucous. Not so in an Antim Tart case.)

- Cases of intense nausea. Ipecac has failed. Think of Antim Tart. In Ipecac, nausea is persistent and is not relieved by vomiting. In Antim Tart, there is relief on vomiting. Cold sweat is present.
- Violent pain in sacro-lumbar region. A sensation of heavy weight at the coccyx. A feeling of being dragged down all the time.

The patient is better: Sitting erect, from eructation, from expectoration. *The patient is worse:* Lying down at night, in the evening, in damp cold weather, from warmth, taking milk, sour things.

Recommended potency: 200, 1000.

APIS MELLIFICA

Leading Indications

1. **Swelling anywhere. Pits on pressure.**
2. **Insect bites. Burning, stinging pain.**
3. **Shrill, sudden, piercing screams.**
4. **Scanty Urine. Not flowing**
5. **Dropsy.**
6. **Conjunctivitis. Trachoma.**

Apis Mel acts fast on swelling, oedema, virtually anywhere on the body. The pain is burning and stinging like the sting of a honeybee. [The medicine is made from honeybee poison.]

Think of Apis first in insect bites.

Apis Mel can be used beneficially in the following circumstances as well:

- Oedema anywhere, on the face, ears, and eyelids, throat as in diphtheria, breasts, and genitals, on skin as in erysipelas, carbuncles and urticaria, on anus, in haemorrhoids. Almost invariably, the characteristic burning and stinging pain is present. A pit forms on pressure.
- The skin is puffed. It pits on pressure. A swollen face, eyelids looking like bags, uvula hanging like a balloon full of water. [Swelling of upper lids responds to Kali Carb.]
- Thick, rosy, rough rash on the skin.
- Conjunctivitis. [The medicine has never failed me]. The lids are swollen, rough inside, and red. Tears are hot. Stinging, burning pain. Chronic granular lids. In trachoma, use a high potency and notice a marked difference.
- Complaints that appear with rapidity, with violence. Acute diphtheria, swollen throat, swollen uvula, swollen tongue. Absence of thirst. Imminent danger of death due to suffocation, by closure of throat and larynx.
- Swollen labia. Cold-water application helps. Stinging, burning pain.
- Inflammation of kidneys, of knees, of feet. Dropsy in hands with numbness. Swelling of fingertips.
- Urticaria, erysipelas of the eyes and of the side of the face, extending from right to left, with rosy colour and stinging swelling.

Apis and Rhus Tox are inimical. Do not use both at the same time.

The Patient is better: In cold room, in cold air, by cold application, cold bath.
The patient is worse: After sleep, on touch, from heat, in a warm room and late in the afternoon.

Recommended potency: 200, 1000

ARGENTUM NITRICUM

Leading Indications

1. **Painful acidity. Hiatus hernia.**
2. **Pus, inflammation, sand sensation in the eye.**
3. **Pessimism. Fear of failure.**

Argentum Nitricum is recommended in the following circumstances:

- Think of Arg Nit in ophthalmia and other eye problems for optimum results. Pus has formed. Conjunctiva is swollen. There is profuse, purulent discharge. Swollen lids. Acute, sudden, granular conjunctivitis. Chronic ulceration of the margins of the eyelids. Canthi red as blood. Stinging, burning pain.
- Painful acidity, hiatus hernia, two interconnected problems. Unbearable, shooting, gnawing and ulcerating pain in the centre of the ribs, near the diaphragm. An unfailing remedy.
- Severe, painful distension of the abdomen caused by flatus. Ulcers in the stomach when pain radiates in all directions.
- In diarrhoea when the stool is green like chopped spinach, has shreds of mucous, when there is severe flatulence, loss of appetite.
- Terrors of anticipation, of an examination, interview, or a conference. The patient is irrational.
- Hemicrania. Pain in the frontal eminence. The eye feels enlarged.
- Debility or rigidity of calves.

The patient is better: From eructation, from cold milk, in cool, fresh air and from pressure.
The patient is worse: From sweets, from cold food, lying on left side, at night, from heat, warmth in any form.

Recommended potency: 200

ARNICA MONTANA

Leading Indications

1. **Any injury. Trauma, physical, emotional, acute, or chronic.**
2. **Black or blue skin due to an injury.**
3. **Angina Pectoris.**
4. **Fatigue. Bruised, sore feeling.**

We recommend Arnica in the following circumstances:

- For injuries, however remote in time, physical or mental. Results of blow, of contusion. Body feels sore, for whatever reason. Limbs ache as if beaten.
- Concussion, fracture of the skull with compression of the brain. For trauma occasioned by drilling and extraction of the teeth. Sore and bruised eye. Blue, beaten skin.
- Fatigue after strenuous work, long hours. Sleeplessness after continuous hard work.
- Pain in injured joints, in injured back. An infant's trauma in childbirth. Trauma of surgery.
- Trauma of grief, of sudden loss, financial or otherwise.
- The patient wants to be left alone. He is morose. He is irritable. His body feels sore.
- As first aid in cerebral haemorrhage, and in bleeding from nose due to injury.
- To prevent formation of pus after injury. Use it before and after surgery to prevent pus formation.
- When a patient suffers angina pectoris. There is spasmodic choking and a suffocating pain in the region of the heart. Pain travels to the elbow of the left arm. There is constriction in the chest. **This is an emergency. Make the patient sit immobile and seek medical help.** Meanwhile administer Arnica 1000.
  An angina patient must always carry Arnica.
- Hoarseness of voice after overuse.

Arnica is useful both in acute and chronic ailments.

For external use in case of injury, use Calendula ointment. Arnica is meant for internal consumption. The former will keep the wound odourless, reduce pus formation, and favour granulation.

The patient is better: Lying down, lying head low.
The patient is worse: On motion, by least touch, in damp cold, in heat.

Recommended potency: 200, 1000.

ARSENICUM ALBUM

Leading Indications

1. **Food poisoning.**
2. **Debility. Sudden prostration.**
3. **Excoriating discharges.**
4. **Restlessness, mental or physical.**
5. **Gradual loss of weight from impaired nutrition.**

We recommend Arsenic Alb in the following circumstances:

- In cases of food poisoning, of indigestion, along with other remedies according to symptoms. The stomach pain is unbearable. It worsens by the least intake of cold food or cold drink. There can be diarrhoea with black, bloody, and offensive stools. The stomach burns inside. The burning is relieved by hot drinks.
- Cases of total debility, of restlessness, mental or physical, sleeplessness due to being restless. The patient is irritable, sad, wants to commit suicide.
- Acute burning sensation whether in the brain, in the inner head, in the stomach, in the bladder, vagina. Nightly aggravation.
- Intense photophobia with burning, acrid discharge, copious flow, ulcerated, red, granulated lids.
- In fevers of a typhoid character. [Here Arsenic is one of the finest of remedies. It follows Rhus Tox and ought to be administered in later stages of typhoid].

- In intermittent fevers like malaria, if the headache is periodic, the burning sensation is relieved by hot application, the lips are parched and dry, and the patient has an unquenchable thirst. The patient is restless and feels debilitated. Cold food disagrees.
- Burning anus. Piles burn like live coals.
- When a profuse discharge of mucous excoriates the lips, the wings of the nose, when a patient is always sneezing with every change in weather. [In such cases, first try Arundo, then Arsenic. Failing these, use Nat Mur.]
- Eruptions on the genitals with burning ulcers, herpes of the foreskin and of labia, with offensive discharge. There is all round swelling, stinging, burning pain.
- Cases of suppressed chronic eczema. The skin is dry and scaly, but usually burning. Arsenic helps in ulcers with an offensive discharge, in oozing pit holes on the skin.
- A tendency to shrivel is noticed on the skin surface. The skin turns black, wrinkled, and prematurely old.
- In diabetic gangrene in extremities and in taking care of the ulcers on the heels.

The Arsenic patient is always freezing. He is oversensitive. He is a fastidious person.

The patient is better: From heat, from warm drinks, sweating.
The patient is worse: After midnight, from cold, from cold food, cold drinks, from movement.

Recommended potency: 200, 1000.

ARUNDO

Leading Indications

1. **Unbearable itching of the palate, of the gums, of the eyes**
2. **Onset of severe cold. Acute discomfort in the eyes, nose, ears, and the throat.**

Arundo is an excellent remedy for

- The onset of acute, distressing cold, for annoying itching in the nostrils and the roof of the mouth. The patient starts sneezing. His eyes water. There is an overall feeling of extreme discomfort.
- Burning and itching in the ears, in the auditory canals and in the gums. At times, the gums bleed.

Take a dose or two of Arundo and feel comfortable. Other medicines can follow as indicated.

Recommended potency: 200.1000

AURUM MET

Leading Indications

1. **High blood pressure with despondency.**
2. **Decaying bones with pain. Syphilis.**

We recommend Aur Met in the following circumstances:

- For high blood pressure which brings violent headache, congestion in the head, sometimes double vision, and sleeplessness. Pulse is rapid, irregular, and feeble.
- In enlarged liver accompanied by cardiac afflictions.
- Pain in bone decay and because of destruction of bones in secondary syphilis. Caries of nasal, palatine, and mastoid bones require Aurum Met. The nose is obstructed with feted discharge. It is painful and ulcerated. Lumps under the scalp.

The Aurum Met patient exhibits despair and hopelessness.

The patient is better: In open air, by cold application, washing.
The patient is worse: In winter, during night.

Recommended potency: 30,200. For high blood pressure, begin with 30.

BARYTA CARB

Leading Indications

1. Frequent tonsillitis on exposure to cold. Stinging pain in tonsils.
2. Child with retarded growth. Catches cold easily.
3. Difficulty in swallowing.

Use Baryta Carb beneficially under the following circumstances:

- In ailments of the throat where tonsils are inflamed with pus. Swallowing is difficult, is accompanied by stinging pain. Baryta Carb counteracts the tendency to suppurate in the throat if a high potency dose is given at intervals of 24 hours.
  (Baryta Carb tonsillitis develops slowly. Belladonna cases develop rapidly. Hepar Sulph cases suppurate and develop with speed.)
- Chronic cough with enlarged tonsils.
- For paralysis of the tongue. The tip of the tongue burns and smarts.
- When the glands around the ears are swollen and painful.
- A weak spine and stiff sacrum.

It is useful for children with a weak body and a weak mind. The child does not grow normally.

The Baryta Carb patient is bashful, averse to strangers, irresolute and mentally weak.

This remedy is slow in action.

The patient is better: Walking in open air.
The patient is worse: Washing, lying on painful side, on exposure to cold.

Recommended potency: 30, 200.

BELLADONNA

Leading Indications

1. **Red surface, anywhere.**
2. **Sudden, violent, throbbing inflammation. Swelling.**
3. **Throbbing pain. Intense heat. Burning. Dry.**
4. **Sudden onset. Sudden relief.**
5. **Turmoil in brain.**

Think of Belladonna if you notice a shining red surface, red, bloodshot eyes, red, puffed face, red, swollen throat, red skin that radiates heat. Most of the time, acute inflammation.

Belladonna maladies come suddenly, violently, run their course and disappear suddenly.

We recommend Belladonna in the following circumstances as well:

- For localized inflammation, like a carbuncle in the head, breast or throat, or anywhere, red, painful, and throbbing, Belladonna is the remedy in the first stage.
  Intense heat is present in such cases. A sore throat feels like coals on fire. The patient wants water in small quantities, often.
- Inflammation that is sensitive to touch. Invariably, there is throbbing and pain. The head throbs. The carotids throb. There is delirium, spasm, jerks, and twitching. All with great violence.
- In delirium, wild and terrible, wherein the patient imagines that he sees ghosts, hideous faces, animals and insects. He is violent. For acute, destructive mania.
- The Belladonna patient suffers from hallucinations, a host of visual illusions. He lives in a world of his own.
- For abnormal surging of blood into the head. The patient's face is bloody red, hot, shining, and swollen. The upper lip, the pupils, and the eyelids swell.
- In sunstroke and in congestive headache, Belladonna and Glonoine run neck to neck. However, Belladonna cases are sensitive to cold and the Glonoine patients are worse by heat.

- Congestive and neuralgic headaches. Throbbing pain. Worse on bending forward, lying down. Pulsation as if hammers are hitting the inside of the skull. The head is bursting outwards. Can be a result of exposure to cold air, or because of suppressed catarrh, or sunstroke. The last is an emergency. Get a doctor.
- Violent, throbbing pain in the face, throbbing carotids, worse on the right side, worse from movement, after exposure to cold wind. [Administer Causticum if the patient has suffered paralysis of the face from exposure.]
- Erysipelas of the face, with intolerable itching, face bright red, changing to purple, with or without fever.
- In conjunctivitis, eyes red, swollen, protruding, dry, burning, and fiery. Intense photophobia. Orbital neuralgia. Inflammation of the optic nerve, of the retina.
- Swollen, violent red tonsils, painful and burning. Difficult swallowing.
- Acute laryngitis. Sudden hoarseness. The throat is raw, scraping. Dry cough. Key of the voice changed. Spasm in the larynx.
- Intolerable pain in the middle and external ear. Throbbing pain in the teeth. Use 1000 or 10000 potency, one dose.
- Belladonna is a remedy for a child whose problem appears suddenly, with intense heat and fever. His skin is hot, his face red. He jumps in sleep.
- Violently painful haemorrhoids, intensely red, swollen, burning, sensitive to touch.
- In menstruation which is too early, profuse, with bright, red, hot, foul smelling blood. The patient suffers pain like that of being in labour. The remedy is also used in a sensation of bearing down through the vulva.
- Pain of inflammatory rheumatism, caused by sudden exposure to cold winds. Violent cramps.

The patient is better: By pressure on head.
The patient is worse: From motion, from being shaken.

Recommended potency: 200, 1000, 10000. In acute cases, use 200 frequently.

BRYONIA ALBA

Leading Indications

1. **Stiffness anywhere. Aggravation on movement.**
2. **Stitching, tearing pain in muscles, in chest, in head.**
3. **Rheumatic pain with increasing severity. Bronchitis.**
4. **Splitting headache associated with indigestion or constipation.**

Bryonia provides relief in the following situations:

- Muscular pain that aggravates on motion.
  Whatever is the name of sickness, if movement results in increased discomfort, think of Bryonia. The pain is stitching, tearing. The patient feels better when pressure is applied.
- When knees are stiff and painful. The joints are red, swollen, and hot. Inflammation in rheumatism.
- Stiffness and pain in the small of the back, worse on movement.
- Stiff neck in spondylosis or otherwise.
  [Bryonia pain comes gradually. Aconite pain comes with violence. Belladonna pain is sudden.]
- Bronchitis. Infection in the lungs and trachea. Severe, stitching pain in the ribs when the patient coughs. The cough is dry and suffocating. [Add Pulsatilla if green, yellow or grey mucous is thrown out. Use Natrum Sulphuricum, besides Bryonia, when there is loose cough with soreness.]
- The mucous surfaces of the Bryonia patient are excessively dry. His lips are parched, dry, and cracked. His stool is hard. He needs large quantities of water to quench his thirst.
- Headache that comes early morning. It could be a constipation headache or congestive. So severe, as if the skull would split open. The pain is worse from motion. The patient looks imbecile. There is relief on tying a band around the head.
- For women whose breasts pain during menstruation. Intermenstrual pain with abdominal and pelvic soreness. Menses come early and are worse on motion. Copious flow of blood.

The patient is better: At rest, lying on painful side, from pressure, from cold air, cool application.

The patient is worse: Any motion, in warm weather, eating, in the morning, on even slight touch, if visitors come.

Recommended potency: 200, 1000. The higher potency is useful in bronchitis and stiffness of the neck or of limbs.

CALCAREA CARBONICA

Leading Indications

1. **Frequent relapse of sickness. Interrupted convalescence.**
2. **Pernicious anaemia.**
3. **Lack of stamina. Hopelessness.**
4. **Icy coldness, general or specific.**
5. **Deep abscess.**
6. **Irregular bone development. Deformed extremities.**

Calcarea Carb comes handy in the following conditions:

- Cases of deficient and irregular bone development. A crooked spine. A softening of the bone. Deformed extremities.
- The patient experiences icy coldness of internal and external parts of the head, of the feet, of the legs. There is a general feeling of coldness. [In Sulphur cases, the sensation is exactly the opposite. It is burning all over]
- The Calcarea patient is forgetful, obstinate, is unable to perform sustained mental operations, and is interested in trivia alone.
- In cases of profuse sweating, particularly on the head. This sweating occurs in cases of debilitating illnesses. The lower extremities feel cold. Cramps in calves. Knees swollen and cold. Sharp, twisting, tearing rheumatic pain.
- Cases of pernicious anaemia.
- Polyps in the nose, ear, bladder, urethra. An offensive odour emanates from the nose. The nostrils are sore and ulcerated.

Lingering nasal catarrh. Large, black, bloody lumps come out in the morning from the nose.

- Abscess deep in muscles, in the neck, in the thighs, or in the abdomen.
- In treatment of spots and ulcers on the cornea, swollen thyroid in goitre, thick, yellow, or bloody mucous flowing in cases of chest infection and prolonged cough.
- In menstruation with vertigo, too early, profuse, lingering, with cold feet. Milky leucorrhoea. Heavy sweat on genitals.

Bryonia and Calcarea Carb do not go together.

The patient is better: Lying on painful side, in dry climate, sneezing.
The patient is worse: In water, washing, in wet weather, from mental exertion, ascending.

Recommended potency: 200.

CALCAREA FLUORICA

Leading Indications

1. **Hard, stony glands.**
2. **Calcaneal spur. Heel bone enlargement.**
3. **Varicose, enlarged veins.**
4. **Bony formations. Hard knots in female breast.**

Indurations, hardening, are the key word leading to the use of Calcarea Fluorica. Indurations of skin, bones, or glands.
We recommend Calcarea Fluorica for the following situations as well:

- Ulcers on the scalp with hard edges, hard excrescences on the scalp, hard swelling on the cheek, on the jaw, unnatural looseness of the teeth and for gumboils.
- Ulceration of the cornea with hard edges, chronic suppuration of the middle year with deafness, ringing and roaring noises.

- For dilated blood vessels with vascular tumours, in varicose veins of the vulva, uterine fibroids, hard nodules in the female breast, and hardness of testicles.
- Congenital syphilis, where the mouth and the throat are ulcerated, where there is decay of the bones, of the teeth, with heat and pain in the affected parts.
- In gout with copious, pale urine and loose stools. In chronic swelling of the knee joint, for fibroids in the hollow of the knee.
- In chronic lumbago.
- In tumours at the back of the wrist, gouty enlargements of the finger joints and for defective bone formation. For cracks, fissures in the palms and for ulcers with hard, elevated edges, when the skin around is purple and swollen. Scar tissues, adhesions after surgery.

The patient is better: By heat, by warm application.
The patient is worse: During rest, by change of weather, on exposure to cold, to drafts, to damp weather.

Recommended potency: 200, 1000. The medicine takes time. Do not repeat it often.

CANTHARIS

Leading Indications

1. **Burning, scalds, blisters. Burns, by fire, by sunlight, by boiling water.**
2. **Difficult, burning, frequent urine. Intolerable tenesmus.**
3. **Frenzied delirium.**
4. **Sexual mania.**

Cantharis is made from Spanish fly.
Cantharis is most suitable for the following maladies and symptoms:

- Severe, cutting pain is experienced before, during and after passing urine. There is a 'never get done' feeling. Pain in the bladder violent,

burning, and cutting. Traces of blood. Violent paroxysms of burning and cutting pain in the kidney region.
- Burning anywhere with the above symptoms.
- Take care of burns, scalds and blisters with Cantharis Mother Tincture diluted in water. Apply with a soft cloth to the site as many times as you can. Great results in healing and reduction of pain.
- In burning in soles of the feet at night, erysipelas with burning and urinary symptoms, severe itching of the vulva with inflammation.
- For acute mania, particularly sexual. An unquenchable sexual desire. The patient sings lewd songs and talks nothing but porn.
- Excessive desire for sex in men as well as women.

Repeat frequently. In burns and scalds, apply diluted Mother Tincture on the site as well as administer potencized medicine internally.

The patient is better: Rubbing.
The patient is worse: From touch, while passing urine, drinking cold water or cold coffee.

Recommended potency: 200, 1000. Mother tincture for local application.

CARBO VEGETABILIS

Leading Indications

1. **Acidity. Stomach disorders. Indigestion. Ulcers. Pain.**
2. **Collapse. Imperfect oxygenation. Blueness.**
3. **Surgical shock.**
4. **Cold sweat, cold breath, cold tongue, voice lost. Beginning of the end.**
5. **Pneumonia, 3rd stage.**
6. **Partial recovery from successive illnesses.**

All disorders of the stomach respond to Carbo Veg. For acidity, without severe pain, this medicine is unrivalled.
Use Carbo Veg, with tremendous relief, in the following circumstances:

- For flatulence with eructation, a feeling of heaviness; ulceration pain in the stomach like burning from glowing coals, slow digestion, aversion to milk, fats, meats. [After a heavy meal, use Pulsatilla. Failing this, use Carbo Veg]. In patients who need Carbo Veg, 'the simplest of foods distresses.'
- Bleeding retracted gums.
- Septic condition after surgery, after shock.
- Old asthmatic turning blue.
- In the 3rd stage of Pneumonia.
- For varicose veins in pregnancy. Carbo veg helps relieve nausea during pregnancy. It restores health to women grown weak from nursing.
- Internal burning and external coldness. Massive haemorrhage internally, from lungs, from uterus, from bladder or from other mucous surfaces.

Carbo Veg is a saviour of life. A patient has been transiting from sickness to sickness. He lies motionless as if dead. His breath is cold, his pulse intermittent, and his sweat is cold. Yet he needs a strong fan. He cannot get enough of oxygen. His face turns blue, his skin pale, and his digestion weak. It may be a state of collapse in cholera or typhoid. Revive him with Carbo Veg.

Carbo Veg is the *Amrit* of Homoeopathy. A pinch of a divine's *vibhuti*. We make it from charcoal ash.

The patient is better: From eructation, fanning cold air.
The patient is worse: In the evening, at night, in open air, taking fats, butter, coffee, milk; in warm weather.

Recommended potency: 200.

CAUSTICUM

Leading Indications

1. **Chronic arthritic and paralytic afflictions.**
2. **Deformities in arthritis.**

3. **Old warts.**
4. **Chronic burns.**
5. **Gradually appearing paralysis.**

We recommend Causticum in the treatment of the following maladies:

- Chronic arthritis of joints, of muscles, and paralysis accompanying it. Excessive deformity of joints. Joints enlarged and soft. Tearing pain worse in cold weather. Benumbing. Progressive loss of muscular strength. Restlessness.
- Stiffness and pain in the neck and the throat. The muscles feel as if tied with a rope.
- Right side paralysis. [Left side needs Lachesis]. Paralysis appears gradually, a local paralysis of the vocal cords with loss of voice, of muscles in the oesophagus, of the tongue, of the eyelids, face, bladder, extremities.
- Left side sciatica. Contracted tendons, temporary or permanent.
- Old warts on eyelids, eyebrows, nose, on the face. Warts are large, jagged, easily bleeding and on the nose or fingertips. Causticum comes next to Thuja in the treatment of warts.
- Soreness in the folds of the skin, between the thighs and at the back of the ears.
- Chronic burns.
- Swollen haemorrhoids. Itching, burning, stinging, smarting, rawness, and moist. Piles worse on walking. Severe constipation. The patient's face turns red while straining.

Causticum is a chronic remedy, useful in diseases that have come over a period.

The patient is better: In damp, cold weather, in warmth, in the heat of the bed.

The patient is worse: In dry cold winds, in clear, fine weather, from motion in a carriage.

Recommended potency: 200, 1000. In a chronic case use high potency infrequently.

CHELIDONIUM MAJUS

Leading Indications

1. **Jaundiced skin. Yellow eyes, face, hands, stool. Tongue thickly coated yellow, with red edges. Urine yellow. Liver affected.**
2. **Constant pain under the lower inner angle of the right shoulder blade.**
3. **Right side neuralgia, top to bottom, with liver symptoms.**
4. **Vertigo in liver upsets.**
5. **Gall stone pain.**

Chelidonium is primarily a liver remedy. Other symptoms are secondary. In most such cases there is a dull or sharp but fixed pain under the lower angle of the right shoulder blade. It can be in jaundice, in diarrhoea, pneumonia, menstruation, or while coughing.

Nevertheless, this pain may be absent in many cases of liver disorder.

Chelidonium alleviates suffering in the following circumstances:

- Pain in the region of the liver, enlargement, sensitivity of the liver to pressure. Thickly coated, yellow tongue with red margins showing imprints of the teeth, and a bitter taste in the mouth. The stools are grey, yellow, or gold. Urine is yellow or dark brown. The patient loses appetite. Has nausea. Vomits bilious matter. Retains nothing but hot drinks.
- Gall bladder stones colic. Shooting, stabbing, tearing pain. It extends through to the back. Spasm of the gall bladder.
- Vertigo in liver disorders. Pain in the occiput, and in the nape of the neck. Ice-cold occiput. Head as heavy as lead. At times neuralgia of the right eye, right cheekbone, and right ear. Eyes water.
- Ailments affecting the right side of the body: right shoulder pain, shooting pain in the right hip, right thigh, right leg or right foot. The right foot may be cold as ice while the left foot is normal.

The patient is better: After dinner, from pressure.
The patient is worse: Right side, by motion, touch, change of weather, early morning.

Recommended potency: 200.

CIMICIFUGA

Leading Indications

1. **Vertigo in cervical spondylosis.**
2. **Nausea caused by cervical or spinal pain.**
3. **Migraine.**
4. **Muscular pain. Cramps of neurotic origin.**
5. **Rheumatic pain in the muscles of back and neck.**

I have found Cimicifuga extremely useful in cervical spondylosis and vertigo caused by it. It gives welcome relief in a short while.

Cimicifuga is an excellent remedy for the following ailments:

• Many problems of neck, back and extremities. Upper spine sensitive. Neck and back stiff, feel contracted. Muscular pain in these regions. Pain in the lumbar and sacral regions, down the thighs and through the hips. Stiffness in tendo-achilles. Heaviness in lower extremities.

• Migraine which has the sensation of a cloud enveloping the mind. In the brain, a waving sensation. Feels too large. Shooting, throbbing pain in the head that feels like bursting. The pain is like electric shocks being administered. Deep shooting pain in the eyes. Aversion to artificial light. Pain travels from the eye sockets into the head.

• Nausea and vomit caused by pressure in the spine and cervical region.

• Ovarian neuralgia.

• Pain across pelvis.

The patient is better: By warmth.
The patient is worse: In the morning, during menstruation with suffering increasing with the quantity of the flow.

Recommended potency: 200, 1000.

CINCHONA OFFICINALIS/CHINA

Leading Indications

1. **Debility caused by excessive discharge of blood, mucous, saliva, or by night sweats.**
2. **Flatulence all over. Stomach distended like a tent.**
3. **Periodic diseases. Typhoid. Malaria.**
4. **Easy bleeding followed by dropsy.**

We recommend China under the following circumstances:

- Debility caused by excessive flows out of the body. It can be the loss of blood on injury or otherwise, loss of fluids because of nursing, leucorrhoea, menstruation, or prolonged diarrhoea. Haemorrhages from wounds, from the lungs, from the nose, a sudden depletion leading to fainting at times.
- Debility makes a person apathetic, low-spirited, lose memory, disinclined to think. He faints easily, sees darkness before his eyes, and hears ringing sounds. His face is pale, sallow, his eyes are sunken, and he sweats on least motion.
- Periodicity in the onset of disease is a clear indication. It happens in malaria, typhoid and many other maladies. Intermittent fevers coming at a fixed time and intervals with well-marked stages, increasing sharply at midnight. Thirst precedes the chill, which generally comes in the afternoon. Profuse night sweats.
- Where a patient bleeds easily. Bleeding from any surface of the body, from nose, throat, lungs, uterus, etc. The affected area turns black. There could be convulsions amidst bleeding such as in confinement.
- Anaemia with pallor and weakness. Blue circles around eyes.
- Flatulence where the stomach is distended like a tent. Colic. Slow digestion, although hunger is acute
- Chronic lever problems with pain in the right side. Liver is enlarged, hard, and sensitive to touch. Spleen is swollen. The pain increases periodically.

- Children's diarrhoea with undigested food in stools, painless, with rumbles in the stomach.
- For women with painful, excessive menstruation. Abdominal distension. Bloody leucorrhoea. Early menses.

The patient is better: From hard pressure on the suffering part, in open air, by warmth, bending double.
The patient is worse: From touch, from drought, chill, exposure, motion, at night, loss of fluids, after eating, eating fruit, sour things.

Recommended potency: 200.

COLOCYNTHIS

Leading Indications

1. **Colic, terrible.**
2. **Dysentery like diarrhoea with colic.**
3. **Pain and cramps in sciatica, from hip down the posterior of the thigh.**

Use Colocynthis beneficially in the following conditions:

- In cases of terrible colic where the patient feels compelled to bend double or press his stomach with a hard object. The colic is neuralgic in character and is often accompanied by vomiting and/or diarrhoea. The pain is clutching, digging and cramping. Colocynthis colic is often accompanied by anger, impatience, or indignation. Violent neuralgia in the head, eyes, down the spine and in the intestines.
- Facial and sciatic neuralgia. The sciatic pain extends from hip down the back of the thigh, is better from pressure and heat, and is worse from gentle touch.
- Joints are stiff, muscles contracted.
- Pain in the left knee joint.

The patient is better: Doubling up, by hard pressure, warmth.
The patient is worse: From anger, indignation, annoyance.

Recommended potency: 200.

CUPRUM MET

Leading Indications

1. **Epilepsy.**
2. **Spasms. Cramps.**
3. **Convulsions in children in whooping cough.**

We recommend Cuprum Met in the following circumstances:

* 'Spasm' is the most characteristic symptom of cases which require Cuprum Met. It can occur in epileptic convulsions, in meningitis, cholera, whooping cough. The spasm begins with a twitching in the fingers and toes and spreads to other parts of the body.
* Cramps in calves, legs, and palms.
* Spasmodic asthma alternating with spasmodic vomiting. In whooping cough attacks ending in convulsions. Here the face turns blue, the eyes turn up, the fingers, and nails lose colour. Clenched thumbs and cramped fingers.
* Epileptic fits. The aura begins at the knees, ascends to the pubic region, and above. Unconsciousness follows. Foaming and falling. Contracted jaws. The face and lips turn blue. The tongue may be paralyzed or may protrude like that of a snake. The thumbs are drawn into the palms and then the fingers close over them with great violence. Hands cold. Stammering.

The patient is better: Drinking cold water, perspiring.
The patient is worse: Vomiting, before menses, from contact.

Recommended potency: 30, repeatedly, in epilepsy, in an acute attack. 200, 1000

GELSEMIUM

Leading Indications

1. **Sluggishness. Deep seated muscular pain. Onset of influenza.**
2. **Nervous chill. Chill up the spine.**
3. **Dizziness, drowsiness, dullness, trembling.**
4. **Congestive head. Congestive cold. Pain in occiput. Head feels tightened with a band of steel.**

We suggest the use of Gelsemium when the following symptoms are present:

- General body pain, sluggishness, congestive pain in the head. Normally, in such cases coryza and throat infection are present. Other symptoms are, a chill up the spine, burning and itching in the eyes, sneezing, a feeling of coolness at the root of the nose, and fever. There is nothing like Gelsemium in the treatment of influenza.
- Tickling in the soft palate, in the throat and nasopharynx. The throat is rough. It burns. Pain radiates into ears from temples and from throat. The feeling of congestion is like someone tightening a band of steel around the head. Pain at the base of the skull.
- Vertigo spreads from occiput.
- Orbital neuralgia with contraction and twitching of the muscles.
- The patient experiences a chill along the spine upwards. He trembles as if someone is running ice up his back.
- Loss of muscular co-ordination. A sort of motor paralysis in the eye, throat, chest, larynx, sphincter, or the urethra.
- Writer's cramp in the muscles of the forearm.
- Fever that runs in waves from sacrum to occiput. The chill is without thirst. The eyelids feel heavy. Fingers do not write. Legs tremble.

A feeling of sleepiness comes a few days in advance. The patient feels dull and wants to be left alone in peace. He cannot concentrate. Use Arundo and Influenzim with Gelsemium for fast relief.

The patient is better: Bending forward, passing urine, in open air, by continuous motion, using stimulants.

The patient is worse: In damp weather, in the early hours, due to emotional shock.

Recommended potency: 200, 1000.

GLONOINE

Leading Indications

1. **Sunstroke. Exposure to the sun. Meningitis**
2. **Heatstroke. Sudden and severe congestion of the head.**
3. **Surging of blood to the heart leading to fainting, palpitation, and dyspnoea.**

Glonoine is an emergency drug for sunstroke or heatstroke.
Use Glonoine with benefit under the following circumstances:

- Violent congestion of the brain and of the spinal cord. Any surging of the blood to the brain. The patient may come down with cerebro-spinal meningitis. The neck is drawn back. The face is intensely hot, red, and shiny. The eyes are congested. The head and upper parts of the body are warm. Lower extremities are cold and covered with cold sweat. The patient may experience severe convulsions through all the limbs, in the neck. He may lose consciousness. His body is drawn back.

- In headache with a sensation of continuous hammering. Unimaginable severity. Visible throbbing in carotid arteries. High blood pressure with these symptoms.

- In angina pectoris, asthma or heart failure. Here Glonoine is a first aid remedy. It should be administered in diluted Mother Tincture [that is, pure medicine drops,] doses. The patient's pulse is weak. Pallor, collapse, arterial spasm.

- In women, after menopause, when the climacteric flushes are most felt in the head.

Glonoine maladies have a sudden onset. Heat and brightness are the cause.

The patient is worse: In the sun, on exposure to bright light, near a bonfire, from wine, stimulants, from warm bed, from mental application.

Recommended potency: In emergency, Mother Tincture. Dissolve fifteen drops in five table spoons of mildly-warm water and administer in sips every few minutes. Otherwise, 200.

GRAPHITES

Leading Indications

1. **Oozing skin eruptions; offensive, sticky, thick fluid.**
2. **Fissures with numbness.**

Homoeopathy uses Graphites for the following symptoms:

- Skin problems like eruptions, oozing a thick, sticky, and offensive fluid. On any part of the body, ears, nose, vagina, on the skin, in perspiration.
- Eczema of the legs with sticky oozing.
- Eczema of the eyelids, moist eruptions, and fissured lids.
- In eczema of the anus, in anal fissures.
- In constipation where stools are large lumps united by mucous.
- A woman has cracks in her nipples. Cracks around mouth, in the ends of fingers, on the labia and between toes. Burning pain. A feeling of tearing, stitching. Numbness.
- On the skin, every little injury suppurates. Glutinous discharge. Crusty ulcers.
- Finger and toe nails growing thick and out of shape.

The patient is mentally depressed.
Graphites is a chronic, deep acting remedy.

The patient is better: In warm clothing, in the dark, waking up.
The patient is worse: From cold in winter, from heat in summer, in a warm room, in a warm bed, morning, evening.

Recommended potency: 200, 1000. On sore nipples, use diluted Mother Tincture.

HEPAR SULPH

Leading Indications

1. **Abscess. Tendency to pus formation.**
2. **Stinging pain in the pus filled area.**
3. **Sweats day and night without relief.**

Use Hepar Sulph with immense benefit in the following circumstances:

- Suppuration with shooting, needling pain. Every little injury suppurates. This medicine can abort pus formation, if administered at an early stage. Later it will hasten the ripening of the pit, discharge and help in healing the wound.
  The Hepar Sulph patient is chilly, sensitive to cold, and wants heavy clothing. He wants a warm room. He is sensitive to touch, to pain, to cold air.
- Unhealthy skin. Deep cracks on the hands, on the feet. Bleeding ulcers on the skin. Shooting, piercing pain.
- Chronic, recurring urticaria.
- In profuse sweat, offensive, sour, day and night.
- Abscess in the ear. Foul smelling pus. Pus in auditory canal, in the middle ear. Rupture in the eardrum. Bloody discharge with piercing pain.
- Suppurating throat. The skin of tonsils has white, pus-filled pockets. When swallowing, it feels as if someone is trying to force a knife into the skin. [In Lachesis, the pain is general and the skin is dark purple. In Belladonna, the throat is shining red].
- Swollen glands in the neck, the axilla, the groin, or the female

breast. Shooting, splinter pain. Inflammation with redness all over. Followed by suppuration.
- Abscess in the labia, leucorrhoea with offensive smell of old cheese.
- Discharge from the roots of the nails.

Silicea does most of the jobs that Hepar Sulph does. However, there are differences. A Silicea patient has profuse head sweats at night. His foot sweats are offensive. Glandular suppuration is slow. He lacks self-confidence. On the other hand, the Hepar Sulph patient has general sweats night and day. He is better in dry, warm weather. Gland suppuration is rapid.

Hepar Sulph precedes Silicea in the treatment of suppuration.

The patient is better: In damp weather, by wrapping his head up, from warmth, after eating.
The patient is worse: From dry, cold winds, from the least draught, touch, lying on painful side, early morning.

Recommended potency: 200, 1000.

HYPERICUM

Leading Indications

1. **Crushed nerves. Crushed fingertips.**
2. **Threatened tetanus.**
3. **Punctured wounds.**
4. **Injury to coccyx.**

We recommend Hypericum under the following circumstances:

- An injury to sensitive nerves. (Arnica, to be followed by Hypericum.) Inflammatory symptoms in injured nerves. A bruised, crushed fingernail or toe.
- In fractured skull with bone splinters.
- To prevent tetanus.
- In neuritis of toes, fingers, fingertips, with tingling and burning pain.

- Puncture wounds caused by insect bites. Ledum comes at a stage before Hypericum. If Ledum fails, switch over to Hypericum.
- Injuries to spine. Injury in the coccyx. Colour of the skin black. Abscess. Excruciating pain. For the fibres of the injured spinal cord, and of meninges.
- In bleeding piles, externally and internally because the anus is rich in nerves.

The patient is worse: In cold, in dampness, in a closed room, by touch, by exposure.

Recommended potency: 200. For local application: Mother Tincture.

IPECAC

Leading Indications

1. **Persistent nausea.**
2. **Nausea in any sickness.**
3. **Wheezing. Bronchitis.**
4. **Asthma, chronic or acute.**
5. **Amoebic dysentery.**
6. **Chest infections of infants.**
7. **Congested throat.**

Ipecac yields excellent results in the following situations:

- Nausea in any sickness, whether connected with a digestive upset or not. There is no relief from vomit.
- Women vomiting during pregnancy.
- Unyielding cases of gastritis where even a drop of water is not retained. Sharp pain in the stomach, going from left to right, and pain in the back. Bile comes out as vomit.
- After taking food like raisins, fats and cakes, in case digestion is a problem.

- Cholera in infants. Colic pain from left to right. Fermented stools. Mucous. Stool of grass green colour. Sometimes bloody.
- A first medicine in wheezing. [In cases of rattling mucous, Antim Tart is the choice.]
- In asthma with constriction in the chest. Incessant, violent cough. Little mucous. Loss of voice. At times, bleeding from the lungs. A violent degree of dyspnoea, of difficulty in breathing.
  In asthma, alternate Ipecac 30 and Aconite 30 at 15 minutes interval when an attack occurs. Continue until the patient is comfortable.
- Bronchitis with similar symptoms.
- Congested throat, with dry cough. A sensation of heaviness in the throat. Mild pain.
- In bad colds of children, in bronchitis, in dry cough, in coarse, loud rattling. Acute attack. The child looks pale and sick. Ipecac is a friend of the infants.
- For whooping cough when there is nausea, violent cough, convulsions, red face and vomit.
- Bright red haemorrhage from anywhere in the body, from nose, lungs, stomach, womb, kidney, bladder or rectum, accompanied by vomit or nausea.
- In amoebic dysentery with tenesmus. Nausea when the patient tries to pass stool. Cutting pain, worse around navel. A little slime, a little blood in frequent motions.
- Headache with nausea. Crushing pain in the skull bone, extending to the teeth and to the root of the tongue.

The patient is worse: In moist, warm weather, lying down, intermittently.

Recommended potency: 200, 1000.

KALI BICHROMICUM

Leading Indications

1. **Tough, ropy, green discharge inwards from the nose.**
2. **Chronic cold. Severe sinus pain running into ears.**
3. **Pain at the root of the nose, in the centre of the eye, in the bones on the rim of the eyes.**
4. **Round, deep, punched out ulcers.**

Kali Bichrome is a remedy in the following situations:

- In the treatment of chronic sinusitis, in diphtheric croup, in old colds. The discharge of mucous is tough, sticky, green, or yellow, going inwards. It is very difficult to take out. The patient makes an unsuccessful effort to clear his throat all the time, particularly early morning. Kali Bich loosens this mucous. [If mucous is flowing easy, outwards, Pulsatilla is the remedy.]
- Sinusitis: Pain in the sinuses, neuralgia in the orbits of the eyes, snuffed nose, violent sneezing at times, and chronic inflammation of the front sinuses.
- Thick, ropy, and stringy discharge can occur from any orifice in the body: nose, mouth, pharynx, larynx, trachea, bronchia, navel, or vagina, in leucorrhoea with intense itching in the vulva.
- Chronic cold with similar symptoms.
- Inflamed tonsils, with uvula bloated like a balloon but hanging, with intense pain at the root of the tongue.
- Chronic intestinal ulceration with cutting pain in the stomach soon after eating.
- Left-side severe sciatica, better by motion, worse in hot weather, with tearing pain in the tibia.
- Wandering rheumatic pain in joints with swelling, heat, and redness.
- In eczema of the scalp, with thick, heavy crusts oozing a glutinous substance.

The patient is better: From heat.

The patient is worse: In the morning, in hot weather, while undressing. He is sensitive to cold.

Recommended potency: 200.

LACHESIS

Leading Indications

1. **Purple surfaces. Coagulation of blood below the skin.**
2. **Purple, inflamed throat, tonsils.**
3. **Constriction. Feels tight in any dress. High blood pressure.**
4. **Left-sided paralysis.**

Lachesis provides relief in the following situations:

- Purple face. [While red inflammation leads us to Belladonna, purple hints at the use of Lachesis]. The eyes are engorged. Inflamed glands are purple. Throat is purple and there is difficulty in swallowing. In diphtheric paralysis.
- Lachesis helps in high blood pressure with constriction and in heart disease when the face is purple and bloated.
- In haemorrhages with persistent bleeding, easily started. [Lachesis is a product of snake poison. In pure form, it decomposes the blood and makes it flow easy].
- A tendency to chronic sore throat. Red and grey ulcers. Red patches full of pus.
- Diphtheria that commences on the left side and spreads to right. Thick, white, ropy mucous in the morning.
- Paralysis of the vocal cords. Voice lost.
- In an attack of asthma, where there is a sudden flush of heat, orgasm of blood, threatened paralysis of lungs or heart, where the patient wants to loosen clothes to prevent suffocation.
- Troublesome menopause. Flushes of heat. Uterine haemorrhage, palpitation, fainting spells, and a feeling of suffocation in a warm room.

- In varicose veins during pregnancy. Blue, purple, sensitive to touch. Relieved by pressure.
- In facial neuralgia on the left side, heat running into the head. Tearing pain in the jawbones. The face is purple, swollen and looks jaundiced.
- Paralysis of the left side of the body, later extending to the right side.
- In erysipelas where the skin is purple, boils are malignant, swollen. Skin turning black.

The patient is better: Loosening clothes, warm application, by onset of discharge, menses, and nasal flow.
The patient is worse: In spring, on taking a warm bath, during sleep, by touch, in a warm room, on even a slight exertion of the mind.

Recommended potency: 200 and higher. Not to be repeated frequently.

LYCOPODIUM

Leading Indications

1. **Chronic liver trouble with flatulence.**
2. **Flatulence pressing downwards.**
3. **Dry catarrh.**
4. **Indigestion on taking food that ferments.**

Lycopodium helps in the following situations:

- Indigestion where food ferments inside the system. It relieves a bloated and full abdomen wherein the wind is pressing downwards. Even a small intake of food causes flatulence. Food tastes sour. Burning eructation. [Flatulence upwards is relieved by Carbo Veg. Overall flatulence responds to China.]
- Patients of chronic liver trouble suffering from flatulence. Pain shoots in lower abdomen from right to left. The liver is sensitive. Swelling. Brown spots on the abdomen.

- Piles which are painful to touch and formed in case of chronic liver patients.
- The patient has been constipated for several days. No desire to pass stools. Insides are full. When the motion occurs, the first stool is hard, then soft and gushing.
- In chronic dry catarrh of the nose. At night, the patient has to breathe through the mouth.
- In cases of impotency. High potency, say 1000, dose once in two days.
- In cases of dry vagina, painful coitus, varicose veins on the vulva.
- Eczema associated with liver, urinary, and gastric problems. Eruptions behind the ears. On smooth, hairless patches on the skull. Patches of copper colour.

The Lycopodium patient is melancholy, apprehensive, and confused. He has lost self-confidence. He is irritable and peevish.

The patient is better: After midnight, in motion, in cool, open air, from being uncovered, by warm drinks in throat and abdomen.
The patient is worse: After eating, in the afternoon, in a warm room, in bed, from heat.

Recommended potency: 200. Higher in case of impotency but infrequently.

MERCURIUS CORROSIVUS

Leading Indications

1. **Tenesmus. A 'never get done' feeling.**
2. **Bloody dysentery, acute, violent.**
3. **Iritis. Pain as if the eyeball is being forced out.**
4. **Violent sore throat. Sore eyes. Sore nose.**

If there is one word which leads us to the use of Merc Cor, it is 'tenesmus', a 'never get done' feeling. It so occurs in blood dysentery, in bladder, in problems of the throat.

Use Merc Cor under the following circumstances:

- For dysentery which is violent, bloody and when the patient can hardly leave the commode. Burning in the rectum. Acute start. Rapid spread. The patient needs full bed rest.
- The tenesmus of the bladder and the rectum occurs at the same time. Urine is passed in drops and with a lot of pain.
- In both trachoma and conjunctivitis when inflammation is acute, violent, painful, and red. Corrosive discharge. It feels as if the eyes are being forced out. Iritis. Iris muddy in colour. Eyelids swollen, red, and excoriated.
- When the throat is red, intensely inflamed, burning, and painful and when there is a sharp tearing pain into the ears. Uvula is swollen.
- For dry, bloody scraps in the nose.
- When penis or the testes are swollen. In the second stage of gonorrhoea where the opening of urethra is swollen and red. Greenish, thick discharge. Burning and persistent tenesmus.

Merc Cor goes deeper than Merc Sol does.

The patient is better: At rest.
The patient is worse: In the evening, at night, taking acids, pickles, fried food.

Recommended potency: 30, 200.

MERCURIUS SOLUBILIS

Leading Indications

1. **Tendency to pus formation.**
2. **Mucous dysentery. Cutting colic.**
3. **Tendency to ulcerate.**
4. **Perspiration, without relief.**
5. **Indurating glandular inflammation.**
6. **Fetid odour in saliva, in suppurating throat, mouth, gums, ear discharge.**

We recommend the use of Merc Sol for the following symptoms:

- Pus formation anywhere in the body, particularly in tonsils.
- Painful ulcers in the mouth.
- Uncomfortable running nose.
- When an offensive odour emanates from urine, stool, or sweat. Nasal as well as mouth diseases have a foul odour.
- If a patient has a tendency to suppurate. The pus is thin, green, foul smelling, at times streaked with thin blood.
- In purulent ophthalmia, with swollen lids.
- Inflammation of the cornea. Iritis.
- Cold in the eye of rheumatic and gout patients.
- Throat ulcers. Foul smelling and painful, ulcerated, swollen tongue, and fetid saliva.
- Blisters on gums. The gums are sensitive to touch. Foul smell. Itching, spongy, and bleeding gums. Purple or blue in colour. Abscess in the roots of the teeth or gums
- In tonsils where pus has formed, although there is no shooting pain. [In case of shooting pain, use Hepar Sulph. In purple tonsils, use Lachesis. In red, shining ones take Belladonna]. The patient has fever, chill and sweat, is worse during the night.
- In fetid discharge from the ears. Stinging pain. Otitis media and a ruptured drum.
- A thick, green, yellow, corrosive discharge from the nose.
- Non-stop, thin running nose.
- Mucous dysentery, acute or chronic. Stools are frequent, quantity small. Colic and rumbling distension. A sure cure.
- Glandular inflammation with hardness. Inflammation in the breasts, near the ear, beneath the tongue, lymphatic glands of the neck, groin, and axilla, even the liver, skin inflammations when hard.
- Creeping chilliness in fever.

A Mercurius patient is sensitive to heat, to cold, to a warm room, a warm bed. His troubles are worse at night. He perspires without relief. Night sweats.

The Merc Sol patient is intensely thirsty. He is always hungry.

The patient is better: from cold drinks.
The patient is worse: In wet, damp weather, in cold, open air, at night, lying on the right side, perspiring, in warm room, in warm bed.

Recommended potency: 200.

NATRUM MURIATICUM

Leading Indications

1. **Anaemia. Great debility. Palpitation.**
2. **Intermittent fever.**
3. **Numbness of lips, tongue, fingers, knees, legs, feet.**
4. **Dropsy. Oedema.**

Natrum Mur is an effective remedy for the following symptoms:

- Anaemia, caused by loss of fluids, by menstrual irregularities, by grief or mental distress. The patient eats well. Yet, she is pale, emaciated, and anaemic. She has a throbbing headache, feels exhausted on climbing steps and by exertion. In case of some women, the menses flow is scanty.
- Anaemia with palpitation, fluttering of heart, abnormally rapid beat, and sensations of coldness and constriction.
- Cases of violent and fluent running nose, stuffed nose, breathing difficulty, with loss of smell and taste.
- Chronic malaria. Unyielding cases of intermittent fever. Weakness, constipation, loss of appetite. Blisters in the mouth.
- Periodic chills. The chill sets in early morning, around 10.30 a. m. It begins in the extremities which turn blue. Throbbing headache. Thirst for cold water. No thirst during fever later on. Chattering teeth. Aching bones. Scorching fingers in high fever. Fever relieved by sweating. Malaria or any other fever with these symptoms.
- In intermittent fevers, sometimes the patient suffers from a blinding headache. This headache comes after menstruation and

lasts from sunrise to sunset. Other chronic headaches can also be of the same duration. All these will respond to Nat. Mur. Nausea and vomit sometimes. Face pale.

- Mental depression because of chronic illness. The patient does not like to be consoled.
- In acute spinal meningitis with chronic jerking of the head and in dropsy of the brain.
- In oedema of the lower extremities, in numbness and tingling of knees, legs, feet, in the lips or tongue, in weak ankles.
- Obstinate constipation, inactive rectum, bleeding and torn anus.

The patient is better: By pressure against back, taking cold bath, in open air, lying on right side.
The patient is worse: About 10 a.m., by heat, in a warm room, from noise, from music, from mental exertion, from consolation.

Recommended potency: 200.

NITRIC ACID

Leading Indications

1. **Anal fissure, fistula, haemorrhoids.**
2. **Cracks, splinter pain in mucous outlets, anywhere.**
3. **Ever catching cold.**
4. **Ulcers in mouth, in throat.**
5. **Foul smelling faeces, urine, sweat.**

Any pain in the outlets in the body where mucous membranes and the skin meet, responds to Nitric Acid. It is a sticking pain as if a splinter is piercing.

We recommend the use of Nitric Acid when the following symptoms are present:

- Problems at the corners of the mouth, in the nose, gums, canthi, anus. Splitting pain, swelling, and pus formation.

- The patient is sensitive to cold. Always feels chilly. He is ever catching cold, one cold following another. Coryza every winter. Nasal catarrh with offensive discharge. Nose stuffed at night. A feeling of splinters in the nose. Green crusts are blown out in the morning. Discharge yellow or green. The Nitric Acid patient has given up after suffering too much.
- Ulcers in the mouth with splinter pain. Same for white patches in the throat with similar pain. Swallowing uncomfortable and painful.
- Tearing toothache. Gums bleed. Pulsation. Tooth decay.
- In prolonged suppuration in glands with no tendency to repair, with sticking pains.
- For anal fissures with splinter pain. Severe pain after passage of stool, even soft stool. Exhaustion afterwards. Prolapse of the anus. Fistula. Carbuncles. Haemorrhoids. Even cancer of the rectum. In all cases, sensitivity to touch, splinter pain, sometimes bleeding, internal as well as external. Copious discharge of pus and blood. Tenesmus. Foul odour. [It is a great remedy here. In Ratanhia fissures, there is a burning sensation which is absent in Nitric Acid. There are sudden knifing stitches. Rectum feels as if full of broken glass.]
- In cases of dark, offensive, burning urination with sticking pain. In small ulcers on the prepuce. Herpes thereon. Gonorrhoea cases.
- Tender, splintered nipples.

The patient is better: Riding in a carriage.
The patient is worse: In the evening, in the night, in cold climate, hot weather, from hot and cold drinks.

Recommended potency: 200.

NUX VOMICA

Leading Indications

1. **Early morning insomnia.**
2. **Hangover. Life of a jet setter.**
3. **Blocked nose. Snuffles.**
4. **Headaches with dyspepsia.**
5. **Constipation. Dysentery. Blind piles. Colic.**
6. **Overlapping menstruation cycles.**

For the jet setter Nux is a remedy of great use. He is fond of late nights, hard drinks, rich food, leading otherwise a sedentary life, followed by a hangover. A dose before going to bed will take care of sleeplessness and the morning hangover.

The patient is sensitive to noise, to medicine. He does not like to be contradicted. He scolds others unnecessarily.

We recommend the use of Nux Vomica in the following further circumstances:

• Gastric symptoms followed by haemorrhoids and headache.
• Sunshine headaches. Headaches increasing on mental exertion, from fresh air.
• Vertigo after dinner or on waking up in the morning, with a momentary loss of consciousness.
• Stuffy, dry cold caused by exposure to cold, dry atmosphere. The child can hardly breathe. Worse in fresh air and at night.
• The patient wakes up at three a.m. He cannot go to sleep. Give him a dose of Nux. He will sleep well.
• In constipation, with a frequent desire to pass stool but with little to show. In dysentery, in colic, in blind piles, [no bleeding], in backache occurring with piles. Constant uneasiness in the rectum, feeling of ineffectual pressure. Nux has a soothing effect on the digestive system.
• In menstrual disorders when one cycle runs into another. Menses start early, last long, have black blood, pain in the sacrum, and a constant urge to pass stool.

- Elevated red patches of urticaria, burning, respond to Nux. The patient is chilly but hates a covering. He is irascible.

Nux performs best when administered at night.

The patient is better: In damp, wet weather, from undisturbed sleep, in the evening while at rest, by strong pressure.
The patient is worse: By mental exertion, by touch, waking up in the morning, after meals, intoxicants, spices, narcotics, in dry, cold weather.

Recommended potency: 200.

PULSATILLA

Leading Indications

1. Old colds. Chronic. Smell lost.
2. Thick, bland, yellow, green mucous flowing easy, from anywhere.
3. Ever changing, shifting pains. Changing symptoms of the same disease.
4. Dyspepsia due to intake of fatty food. Loss of taste.
5. Sties.
6. Late menstruation. Scanty flow.
7. Lack of thirst.

Pulsatilla is of great use in the following situations:

- Chronic cold. A thick, bland, greenish yellow or grey discharge. The mucous flows freely. [In Kali Bich, it is sticky, tough, does not come out easily.] The sense of smell is lost.
- Thick, bland, green, yellow, or grey discharge anywhere in the body, from the nose, eyes, ears, lungs, in leucorrhoea, or in gonorrhoea. In vagina, however, the discharge excoriates.
- Where pain travels from one part of the body to another, from one joint to another. The patient passes different types of stool.
- Where the digestive system gets upset easily because of intake

of heavy food. Flatulence, pain in the stomach an hour or so after taking food. In such cases, there is a loss of taste, a foul smell from the mouth. A lack of thirst.

- In cases of chronic constipation, where the stool is large, hard and difficult to excrete. Blind haemorrhoids may be present, with violent, stitching pain.
- Sties on the eyelids.
- Varicose veins. Ulcers surrounding such veins bleed black blood, which coagulates easily.
- In suppressed or scanty, late and painful menstruation. The patient is restless, gets no relief even tossing in the bed. The menses start, stop, start, and flow again. She is of a mild, sweet, and gentle temperament. Cases of abnormally delayed menstruation.
- Headaches accompanying menstruation. Throbbing and congestive.
- In women, nymphomania, a limitless desire.
- Thick, yellow, green, and excoriating leucorrhoea.
- In men, orchitis, inflammation and swelling of the testicles from mumps and from catching cold. Strong sexual desire.
- Gonorrhoea with thick, yellow, or green discharge requires Pulsatilla.

Mentally a Pulsatilla patient is mild, of yielding disposition, does not feel thirsty, and is peevish and chilly.

The patient is better: Taking cold foods and drinks, though not thirsty, by cold application, by slow walking, in open, cool, and fresh air, with head raised on a pillow.

The patient is worse: Taking rich food, after eating, towards evening, in a warm room, by warm baths, lying on left or painless side.

Recommended potency: 30, 200.

RHUS TOX

Leading Indications

1. **Muscular pain, temporarily relieved on movement.**
2. **Pain caused by exposure to wet cold, on suppression of perspiration due to exposure.**
3. **Strain. Muscular stiffness, temporarily better on movement.**
4. **Old, chronic arthritis.**
5. **Backache. Lumbago. Sciatica.**
6. **Eczema of face, of genitals.**

Think of Rhus Tox if the following symptoms are present:

• Any muscular pain where the cutting pain is temporarily relieved by movement. [In Bryonia, pain increases on movement.] The patient is restless, internally uneasy, wants to be on the move. His is a tearing-asunder pain, a bruised pain, often accompanied by numbness and paralysis of the limbs, with loss of sensation.

• Muscular lameness and stiffness, whether it is of a rheumatic character or whether caused by a strain such as the lifting of a heavy article or unguided exercise.

• In sprains where Arnica has reduced pain and swelling, complete the cure with Rhus Tox.

• In chronic rheumatism, when limbs are stiff and paralyzed, when there is a tearing pain in the tendons, ligaments, and numbness of joints. The joints are hot, painful, and swollen.

• Rheumatic pain in the nape of the neck, in the thighs, tenderness in the knee joints. In all such cases the patient gets relief by movement, although temporarily.

• In lumbago, Rhus Tox comes first. Temporary improvement on movement. The patient feels better lying on a hard surface. Exposure in cold and damp weather, lying in wet sheets, from suppression of sweat.

• In left side sciatica, with tearing pain in the lower limbs, worse during rest, better temporarily on movement. High potencies furnish quick relief.

- In dysentery when there is pain in the thighs and legs.
- In eczema of the face and the genitals. The scrotum gets thick and hard. Swelling in the genitals. Severe itching.
- In facial eczema with chronic suppuration and eruption.
- Erysipelas with large, burning splinters, inflammation, pitting on pressure. Urticaria. Every time restlessness and intense itching.

In muscular pain, if need be, alternate Bryonia and Rhus Tox, in 200 potency, three times a day each for a few days, if the symptoms are not clear.

Rhus Tox is inimical to Apis. The two should not be taken during the same treatment.

The patient is better: From motion, walking, in warm, dry weather, by change of position, by warm application, bath, rubbing, on stretching limbs.
The patient is worse: In cold, wet weather, during sleep, on being drenched while perspiring, in cold, fresh air, which hurts the skin.

Recommended potency: 200, 1000.

SEPIA

Leading Indications

1. **Bearing down sensation in vulva. Labour like pain.**
2. **Pain in the small of the back in women.**
3. **Climacteric flushes.**
4. **A sensation of ball in vagina, rectum.**
5. **Uterine and vaginal prolapse.**
6. **Excoriating milky discharge. Curd like leucorrhoea.**

Sepia gives excellent results in the following maladies:

- Uterine maladies. A sensation as if all the internal organs will come out of the pelvis. Pelvic displacement, with inflammation, ulceration, leucorrhoea, sometimes even a malignant growth.

- Pain in vagina, especially during intercourse.
- Pain extending from pelvis into the small of the back.
- Yellow, greenish leucorrhoea with intense itching, irregular menstruation, either too early and profuse, or too late and scanty.
- Ulceration of the cervix.
- Menopause flushes. A feeling of bearing down in pelvis.
- Headache on one side when the previously mentioned symptoms exist.
- Prolapse of the rectum along with pelvic congestion.
- Excoriating and milky discharge whether in leucorrhoea, in throat, from nasal passages, or the vagina.
- Yellow blotches on the face of the patient.

Emotionally the sepia patient is not affectionate. She cannot stand a difference of opinion.

It is a remedy for the exhausted homemaker, overburdened with work and children. She has no stamina for work.

Sepia is a chronic remedy.

Lachesis is inimical to Sepia.

The patient is better: By exercise, by pressure, in the warmth of the bed, by hot application, sitting cross-legged, loosening clothes, after sleep.
The patient is worse: In the afternoon, in the evenings, by washing, laundry, exertion, walking, in damp cold air, at climacteric, taking milk, left side.

Recommended potency: 200.

SILICEA

Leading Indications

1. **Chronic inflammation with deep-seated pus.**
2. **Glandular or bony ulceration.**
3. **Unyielding cold.**
4. **Children with defective assimilation.**

Silicea is of great benefit in chronic cases of inflammation with pus, even in tendons and ligaments. It helps

- In the expulsion of foreign bodies from tissues. It can take out deep-rooted abscess.
- In boils, old fistulas, ulcers, scar tissues.
- In patients who can never get rid of their cold. Violent cough when lying down. Sputum full of mucous, offensive, thick, yellow, and lumpy. [Think of Silicea as a chronic of Pulsatilla].
- Old cases of the catarrh of the ear with offensive, green mucous. Pain like a pinprick.
- Constipation in which the stool protrudes but slips back. Spasm of the sphincter.
- Serous cysts in the vagina, projecting out or upwards, the size of a pea.
- Warty growths on the skin, moist eruptions, pimples, pustules, suppurating cavities.
- Weak children whose assimilation is defective. Shrunken limbs, big belly, pinched face.

The Silicea patient lacks stamina. He has a pale face. He is nervous and irritable. He sweats profusely on the head. His foot sweat is offensive.

In cases, where Hepar Sulph has discharged the pus, Silicea will heal the wound.

Mercury and Silicea do not go together.

The patient is better: In wet and humid weather, in summer, by warmth, wrapping up head.

The patient is worse: Taking milk, lying down, getting feet wet, uncovering the head, washing, in damp cold weather.

Recommended potency: 200.

SULPHUR

Leading Indications

1. **Burning sensation, anywhere. Chronic cases.**
2. **Itching, scratching leading to burning on skin.**
3. **Dirty, unclean habits. Ragged philosopher.**
4. **Selected medicines not helping. Relapses.**

Sulphur brings a patient back from the fires of hell. Burning sensation anywhere, inside the head, on the scalp, burning mucous from nose, burning in the face, on the mouth, on the tongue, burning and itching in the piles coming in bunches, burning urine, burning vagina, nipples on fire, burning skin, palms, soles.

Use Arsenic Alb in acute cases of burning and Sulphur in chronic case. We recommend Sulphur for the following further symptoms:

- In skin maladies where scratching is followed by burning. Itching eruptions on the skin anywhere. Dry, scaly skin. Patients habitually unclean. Washing aggravates. Sweating excoriation in armpits, and leg pits.
- Body orifices like the mouth, ears, eyelids, urethra, anus etc., turning red, vermillion. Itching. Burning.
- Indurations from pressure, like corns, callosities on the soles.
- A susceptibility to catch cold, with change of weather, on movement from a warm into a cold room, on taking bath or on over-exertion.
- Menstruation too late, scanty, and painful. Blood thick, black, excoriating. In between acrid and burning leucorrhoea.
- Chronic constipation as an intermittent remedy.
- If an infant does not develop properly. His bones do not grow. Use Calcarea Carb followed by Sulphur.
- Complaints which relapse.

Sulphur revives the effect of remedies already administered. Give one dose per week early morning. Dissolve 15 pills in lukewarm water and sip over thirty minutes.

In acute problems, Sulphur follows Aconite well.

Merc Sol and Calcarea Carb are effective after starting the treatment with a dose of Sulphur in chronic cases.

Use Sulphur in the beginning in a chronic case. In acute cases, give Sulphur to complete the treatment.

The patient is better: From dry, cold weather, lying on the right side, from open windows when respiration is difficult.

The patient is worse: In the morning, eleven a.m., washing, bathing, at rest, standing, at night, from alcoholic drinks, periodically.

Recommended potency: 200.

THUJA OCCIDENTALIS

Leading Indications

1. **Warts. Polyps. Elevated lesions of the skin. Cauliflower excrescences.**
2. **Carbuncles, ulcers.**
3. **Spongy tumours.**

Thuja is indicated in the following circumstances:

- Spongy tumours. Carbuncles. Ulcers near the genitals.
- Warts on the vulva and on the pelvic floor. Warts, fig warts, polyps, and elevated lesions of the skin, mostly on the genitals, the anus, or other mucous membranes.
- Inflammation of the foreskin and glans penis.
- Cauliflower excrescences in the vagina, on the cervix, about the anus.
- White, scaly dandruff. Hair dry, falling.
- Persistent insomnia.

The patient is better: Left side, drawing up limbs.

The patient is worse: In cold, damp air, stretching limbs, at night, from the heat of the bed, after breakfast, taking tea or coffee.

Recommended potency: 200. In warts, 1000, or higher.

VERATRUM ALB

Leading Indications

1. **Collapse with cold sweat on forehead. Ice-cold. Total prostration.**
2. **Cholera. Rice water stools. Retching. Cramps in calves.**
3. **Violent mania. Lascivious.**
4. **Surgical shock.**

Veratrum Alb is a remedy for severe gastroenteritis, for collapse, for cholera where the patient is throwing upwards as well as passing frequent stool.

We recommend Veratrum Alb when the following symptoms are present:

- Cold sweat on the forehead. [This can happen in heart attack as well. However, there the pain will be unremitting, spreading from centre of the chest in all directions, particularly along the left arm, a constriction. There will not be any gastro symptoms. However, do administer a dose till hospitalization.]
- In gastroenteritis, where the stool is like rice white water. It flows copiously. Cramps in the legs. Cold sweat. Vomit. Nausea. Aggravation by drinking cold water. Use 1000 potency. In such cases, there is a sinking, empty, and cold feeling in the stomach. The abdomen is swollen. Terrible colic.
- Total collapse. Complete prostration. Cold breath. Cold sweat. Skin blue, purple. Body ice-cold. All this can happen in cholera of the infants, in bronchitis, pneumonia, typhoid, and intermittent fevers.
- Irregular and feeble pulse. Palpitation and anxiety. Audible and rapid respiration.
- Surgical shock.
- Delirium. Patient curses day and night. Talks lewd, tears clothes, and is religious and amorous by turns.
- Cramps in calves. Sciatica pain coming like electric flashes.
- Menstruation with cold sweat and prostration.

The patient is better: On walking, in warmth.
The patient is worse: At night, in wet, cold weather.

Recommended potency: 200. In acute cholera, 1000.

REMEDIES WHICH ARE INIMICAL TO ONE ANOTHER

Pease do not use inimical remedies simultaneously or in immediate succession.

Remedy	Inimical	Remedy	Inimical
Acid Acetic	Borax Causticum Nux Vom Ranunculus B Sarsaparilla	Digitalis	China
Acid Lactic	Coffea	Dulcamara	Acid Acetic Belladonna Lachesis
Acid Nitric	Lachesis	Ferrum Met	Acid Acetic
Allium Cepa	Allium Sativum. Aloe	Ignatia	Coffea Nux Vomica Tabaccum
Ammonium Carb	Lachesis	Kali Bi	Does not follow Calcarea.
Apis	Rhus Tox	Kali Nitricum	Camphor does not follow.
Arum Triphyllum	Caladium Senguinum	Kreosotum	Not to follow Carbo Veg
Asterias Rubens	Coffea Nux Vomica	Lachesis	Acid Acetic Acid Carbolic Acid Nitric Dulcamara Ammonia Carb Psorinum
Aurum Muriaticum	Coffea	Ledum	China
Baryta Carb	Does not follow Calcarea.	Lycopodium	Sulphur follows but Lycopodium does not follow Sulphur.
Belladonna	Acid Acetic	Mercurious	Acid Acetic

Remedy	Inimical	Remedy	Inimical
	Dulcamara		Silicea.
Borax	Acid Acetic	Millefolium	Coffea
Bovista	Coffea	Nux Vomica	Acid Acetic.
			Ignatia.
			Zincum Met
Caladium	Arum Triphyllum	Phosphorus	Causticum
Calcarea Carb	Acid Nitric	Ranunculus	Acid Acetic
			Staphysagria
			Sulphur
Calendula	Camphor	Rhus Tox	Apis
Camphor	Calendula. Kali Nit.	Sarsaparilla	Acid Acetic
Cantharis	Coffea	Selenium	China
Carbo Veg	Kreosotum	Sepia	Bryonia
			Lachesis
Caulophyllum	Coffea	Silicea	Mercurious
Causticum	Acid Acetic	Squilla	Allium Sativa
	Coffea		
	Phosphorus		
Chamomilla	Zincum Met	Staphysagria	Ranunculus
China	After Digitalis or Selenium	Stramonium	Coffea
Cistus Can	Coffea	Sulphur	Sulphur follows Lycopodium and not vice versa.
Cocculus	Coffea	Zinc	Chamomilla
			Nux Vomica
Coffea	Cantharis		
	Causticum		
	Cocculus		
	Ignatia		

Extract from a chart prepared by R. Gibson Miller. Reproduced from POCKET BOOK OF HOMOEOPATHIC MATERIA MEDICA by Dr. William Boerick, M. D.

BIBLIOGRAPHY

Any one interested in going deep into the study of Homoeopathy would benefit immensely from a study of. the following books.

A few other books of general interest have been added for being used for reference to health related information.

1. *Organon of Medicine and Materia Medica Pura* by Dr. Samuel Hahnemann.
2. Samuel Hahnemann: *His life and Works* by Richard Haehl.
3. *Lectures on Homoeopathic Materia Medica* by James Tyler Kent.
4. *Boericke's Materia Medica with Repertory* by William Boericke, M. D.
5. *The Guiding Symptoms of our Materia Medica* by C. Hering, M. D.
6. *The Encyclopaedia of Pure Materia Medica* by T. F. Allen, M. D.
7. *Leaders in Homoeopathic Therapeutics* by E. B. Nash.
8. *Homoeopathic Guide to Family Health* by R. K. Tandon and Dr. V. R. Bajaj. English, Hindi and Urdu editions.
   [All these books are available in Indian prints published by B. Jain Publishers Pvt. Ltd, New Delhi, 110055.]
9. *Family Medical Adviser-An A-Z Guide to Everyday Ailments, Their Symptoms, Causes, and Treatment.* Published by the Reader's Digest Association Ltd.
10. *Foods That Harm Foods That Heal, an A-Z Guide to Safe and Healthy Eating.* Published by The Reader's Digest Association Limited, London.
11. American College of Physicians, *Complete Home Medical Guide*, Published by D K Publishing, Inc, New York.

12. *The Incredible Machine*. Published by the National Geographic Society, Washington D. C.

13. *Love and Survival. The scientific Basis for the Healing Power of Intimacy* by Dean Ornish, M. D., Harper Collins Publishers.

14. Dr. Dean Ornish's *Program for Reversing Heart Disease*. Ballantine Books, New York.

15. *Light on Life. The Journey to Wholeness, Inner Peace and Ultimate Freedom* by B. K. S. Iyengar. Published by Rodale International Ltd., London.

16. *The Complete Book of Cancer Prevention*. Rodale Press Inc., USA.

17. *The Doctor's Book of Home Remedies*. Published by Rodale Press, USA.

18. *The Complete Guide to Your Emotions and Health*. Published by Rodale Press, USA.

19. *New Atlas of Human Anatomy*. Published by Constable, London.

A SHORT CIRCUIT TO SELECTION OF REMEDIES

A repertory for instant reference, in home, office and for travellers

Keep a copy of these pages handy in office or during travel. They provide you with an excellent 'Quick Prescription Guide.'

Sickness and symptoms	Remedy
Abscess	
• With piercing pain.	Hepar Sulph 200
• Chronic abscess. Deep rooted in any part.	Silicea 200
Acidity	
• Hyperacidity with shooting pain in the centre of ribs radiating in all directions. Painful ulcers in the stomach.	Argentum Nitricum 200
• Acute or chronic acidity with or without foul eructation. Flatulence. No appetite. Slow digestion.	Carbo Veg 200
Anal irritation	
• Pressure. Irritation. Constipation.	Nux Vomica 200
• Irritation with burning.	Sulphur 200

Angina Pectoris
- First aid for severe pain in left shoulder, elbow of the left arm with stitching pain in the region of the heart.   Arnica 200
- Acute pain with suffocation and a feeling of constriction.   Cactus, Mother tincture, 10 drops in water every 30 minutes until condition stabilises.

Appetite-loss of
- Due to overeating. Foul eructation. Stinking flatus.   Antim Crud 200
- Slow digestion. Acidity, Aversion to milk, meats, fats.   Carbo Veg 200

Aphthae/Blisters in the mouth
- Painful blisters in the mouth, on the gums.   Borax 200
- In the mouth with foul breath and pus, wounds. Ulcers of gums, inside cheeks.   Merc Sol 200
- In the mouth, ulcers, not responding to Borax or Merc Sol. Painful.   Nitric Acid 200

Arthritis
- Inflammatory rheumatism. Pain worse on movement. Joints inflamed red-hot. Stiffness. Knee pain for any reason.   Bryonia 200
- Rheumatic pain, pain in muscles. Strains. Pain temporarily better on movement.   Rhus Tox 200

Asthma-bronchial
- Sudden, violent attack.   Aconite 30 and Ipecac 30 to be alternated every 15 minutes until the condition stabilises.
- With severe wheezing. Incessant and violent cough.   Ipecac 200

Backache
- Caused by an injury.   Arnica 200

- With stiffness. Pain in the neck. Worse on movement. Bryonia 200
- Rheumatic pain in the back, shoulder blades, lumbar, sacral regions, down thighs and through hips. Cervical spondylosis. Cimicifuga 200
- Caused by exposure. Temporary relief on motion. Rhus Tox 200

Bad breath Merc Sol 200

Black eye
- Caused by injury. Arnica 200
- From blow or contusion when nerves have been injured. Ledum 200

Bleeding-external
- First remedy when bleeding has been caused by an injury. Arnica 200.
For local application Calendula ointment or mother tincture.

Bleeding-internal
- Bleeding of dark, clotted blood. Hamamelis 200.
Mother tincture for applying on bleeding piles.
- Bleeding from lungs, bowels or any other internal surface, of bright, red blood. Blood in sputum. Millefolium 200

Bleeding gums
- After tooth extraction. Arnica 200
- Gums spongy, swollen, and bleeding. Pulsation in gums and their roots. Merc Sol 200

Bleeding nose
- Persistent nosebleed. Millefolium 200

Blisters
- Blisters caused by insect bites. Apis 200
- By sunburn, fire, scalding liquids or by Cantharis 200.

excessive walking.

Mother tincture, diluted in water for local application.

Blood pressure-high
- With violent headache and double vision.
- Surging of blood to head and heart. Confusion. Dizziness. Breathlessness.

Aurum Met 200
Glonoine 200

Blood pressure-low
- Low pulse rate. Feeble heart muscle.
- In a person who is always sick. Has a weak digestion.
- Caused by exhaustive discharges from any part of the body.

Caffeine 200
Carbo Veg 200

China 200

Bronchitis
- With rattling of mucous, that is difficult to take out.
- Dry hacking cough. Stitching pain in the centre of the ribs. Little expectoration.
- Terrible wheezing. Acute bronchitis of the infants with rattling of coarse mucous.
- With green sputum.

Antim Tart 200

Bryonia 200

Ipecac 200

Pulsatilla 30. To be taken with Bryonia.

Bruise
- Caused by injury.

Arnica 200
Calendula ointment for local application.

Burning in the eyes
- Burning, smarting eyes with bland discharge.
- Burning in the eyes with acrid discharge.
- With body pain. Congestion in head. Shivering up the spine.

Allium Cepa 200
Arsenic Alb 200
Gelsemium 200

Burns/scalds
- First aid as well as a cure.

Cantharis 200.
Apply mother tincture

diluted in water as often
as possible to soothe, heal,
and leave no scar.

Cholera
- Yellow, greenish, and offensive stool   Podophyllum 200
- Uncontrollable retching with profuse, rice   Veratrum Alb 1000
  water motions. Cold sweat. Collapse.

Give continuous sips of water [boiled and cooled],
in which a little salt and some sugar has been
dissolved. This takes care of dehydration.

Chronic cold
- Sinusitis with or without thick, tough,   Kali Bichrome 200
  greenish discharge of mucous into the throat.
  Needle pain in the eye, in the bones above
  the eyes and in sinuses.
- Old cold with yellow, green, grey, bland   Pulsatilla 30
  discharge running outwards. Repeated attacks
  of cold. Running nose alternating with
  stuffed nose.
- Chronic cases, unyielding   Silicea 200

Colic
- Food poisoning. Burning in stomach.   Arsenic Alb 200
- Burning cutting pain with distension.   Belladonna 200
- Colic with acidity and ulcers.   Carbo Veg 200
- Agonising, cutting pain in abdomen.   Colocynthis 200
- Colic after several hours of eating.   Nux Vomica 200
  Cutting pain in persons with irregular
  eating habits or with fondness for alcohol.
- Colic during cholera.   Veratrum Alb 1000

Collapse
- For emergency, before you can call a doctor.   Camphor, mother tincture,
  to smell. 10 drops on sugar
  dose every 15 minutes.

- In cholera. Rice water, copious stool.   Veratrum Alb 1000
  Cold sweat. Unstoppable retching.

Common cold
- Corrosive, thin discharge from the nose, with sneezing, burning, and restlessness.   Arsenic Alb 200
- With bronchitis.   Bryonia 200
- With body-ache. Steel band grip around the head.   Gelsemium 200
- Violent, fluent discharge from the nose. Difficult to stop.   Natrum Mur 200
- Yellow, green, bland mucous coming out from the nose.   Pulsatilla 30

Concussion
- Injury to head, loss of consciousness.   Arnica 200

Conjunctivitis
- Swollen, red, and granular lids.   Apis 200
- Acute granular, swollen conjunctivitis. Profuse discharge.   Arg Nit 200
- Conjunctivitis with cold. Burning discharge from eyes. Sticky mucous.   Euphrasia 200
- Green, flowing or sticky mucous.   Pulsatilla 30

Constipation
- No desire. No ability. Intestinal tract dry.   Alumina 200
- Dry stool. Hard as if burnt. No desire.   Bryonia 200
- Obstinate constipation although inside is full.   Lycopodium 200
- In persons leading a fast and irregular life.   Nux Vomica 200

Coronary thrombosis
- With tightness and constriction in the chest.   Arnica 200
- Constriction as if the heart was squeezed by a band.   Cactus 30.
  In emergency, mother tincture, 10 drops in water every half an hour until condition stabilises.
- Acute coronary thrombosis with numbness in the left arm. Left side paralysis.   Lachesis 200

Hospitalize immediately.

Cough

- Dry, violent cough on exposure to dry cold air or otherwise. Acute — Aconite 30
- Bronchitis. Dry hacking cough from upper trachea, little expectoration, with pain in the bottom centre of the rib cage. — Bryonia 200
- With nausea, wheezing. — Ipecac 200
- With irritation in the throat. Green, stingy mucous difficult to take out. Violent sneezing early morning. Compulsion to clear throat early morning. Pain in ears on coughing. Pain in sinuses, in the eyes, in bones above the eyes. — Kali Bi 200

Cuts

- By sharp instruments. — Staphysagria 200
Calendula ointment for local application.

Diarrhoea

- Profuse. Loss of control. Mucous. — Aloe 200
- Dentition diarrhoea. — Chamomilla 30
- Yellow, greenish stool. Painlessly gushing out. — Podophyllum 200
- Severe with copious rice water, thin stool gushing out. Cholera. Cold sweat. Collapse. Uncontrollable retching. — Veratrum Alb 1000

Dysentery

- Large quantity of mucous with loss of control over anal muscles. Pain in rectum after stool. — Aloe 200
- Painful amoebic dysentery. — Ipecac 200
- Violent blood dysentery. A never get well feeling. Pain. — Merc Cor 30
- Mucous dysentery. Pain. — Merc Sol 200
- With pain in the thighs and legs. — Rhus Tox 200

Earache

- Throbbing, intense pain, on exposure to dry cold wind. — Aconite Nap 30

- Shooting pain in Eustachian tubes with water flowing from eyes and nose.   Allium Cepa 200
- Terrible pain in middle and external ear.   Belladonna 200
- Sharp, stitching pain in the ear with sinusitis. Severe pain during a flight take off or landing.   Kali Bi 200

Ear discharge

- Discharge of pus. Skin irritated, inflamed.   Calendula ointment for local application.
- Stinking pus. Shooting pain.   Hepar Sulph 200
- Pain in the ear with green mucous flowing easy.   Pulsatilla 30

Eructation

- Foul. Tasting of food recently taken.   Antim Crud 200
- Rancid. Sour. Putrid. Acidity.   Carbo Veg 200
- After taking fruit, green vegetables, cakes or heavy food.   Pulsatilla 30

Exposure

- Inflammatory fever because of exposure to dry, cold wind.   Aconite 30
- High fever with delirium on exposure.   Belladonna 200
- Exposure to wet air.   Dulcamara 200

Fainting

- Out of fear, anguish, and sudden loss.   Aconite 30
- Due to concussion.   Arnica 200
- Because of shock. Body ice-cold.   Camphor, mother tincture, 10 drops on sugar every 15 minutes. Smell on a clean cloth.
- Caused by exhausting discharges from the body in haemorrhages, menstruation, in childbirth, or in fevers.   China 200
- In epileptic fits.   Cuprum Met 200
- Because of sunstroke or heatstroke. Heart attack.   Glonoine 200

Fetid stool

• Stinking flatus. Result of overeating.	Antim Crud 200

Fever

• On exposure to dry, cold air.	Aconite 30
• Because of injury.	Arnica 200
• With severe running nose. In intermittent or periodic fevers with restlessness. In typhoid at a later stage.	Arsenic Alb 200
• Tonsils swollen, red, and glistening.	Belladonna 200
• Bronchitis. Hacking, painful cough in the chest.	Bryonia 200
• With burning sensation while passing urine. Frequent urination.	Cantharis 200
• With body pain. Nose partially blocked. Steel band tightening on the skull.	Gelsemium 200
• On exposure to sun or heat.	Glonoine 200
• With pus, shooting and stabbing pain on empty swallowing in tonsils. Abscess with pain.	Hepar Sulph 200
• Abscess. Pus in tonsils.	Merc Sol 200
• Intermittent, unyielding fevers. Chronic malarial state.	Natrum Mur 200

Fissures anal

• Sensation of splinters piercing the anus. Constriction. Tenesmus. Burning. Foul oozing.	Nitric Acid 200
• Rectum feels as if full of broken glass. Burns for hours after stool.	Ratanhia 30. Mother tincture for local application.

Fits/Convulsions

• In children because of cerebral congestion.	Belladonna 200
• Convulsions. Limbs contorted.	Cicuta 200
• With cramps in epilepsy, cholera, whooping cough.	Cuprum Met 200
• During menstruation, or labour pains.	Hyoscymus 200

Flatulence
- In upper digestive tract with acidity.   Carbo Veg 200
- In central region. Abdomen bloated like   China 200
  a tent.
- With pressure downwards.   Lycopodium 200

Food poisoning.
- Unbearable pain. Burning, black, and   Arsenic Alb 200
  bloody diarrhoea.

Foreign bodies in the skin
- For expulsion of known or unknown   Hepar Sulph 200
  foreign body. Pus with stabbing pain.
- In chronic cases. Goes deep.   Silicea 200

Foreign body in the eye
- Injury caused by a foreign body.   Arnica 200
- Injury caused to nerves by a foreign object.   Hypericum 200

Do not rub the eye. Try to remove the foreign body with a soft wet tissue or by flushing the eyes with a lot of water.

Fracture
- Injury resulting in a fracture. Relieves pain   Arnica 200
  and swelling.
- Promotes repair and reunion of broken bones.   Calcarea Phos 30

Haemorrhoids/Piles
- Protruding like grapes with intense itching.   Aloe 200
- With continuous oozing of mucous.   Antim Crud 200
- Violently painful, red, swollen, inflamed.   Belladonna 200
- Profuse flow of dark blood.   Hamamelis 200.

Mother tincture for external application.

- Bleeding piles with anal fissures.   Nitric Acid 200
- Blind haemorrhoids. Intense itching.   Nux Vomica 200
- Fissures in anus. Burning and protruding   Ratanhia 200
  piles.

Hangover
- Head heavy in the morning. Tongue parched, Nux Vomica 200
  wooden. Results of excessive intake of alcohol.

Headache
- On exposure to dry cold air. Sudden. Burning. Aconite 30
- Caused by indigestion, overeating. Antim Crud 200
- Severe throbbing pain in carotids. Belladonna 200
  Face flushed.
- Frontal headache. Worse on motion. Bryonia 200
- In the base of the head with the sensation Gelsemium 200
  of a steel band tightening. Body pain.
  Tension headache.
- From exposure to sun or to light or to heat. Glonoine 200
  Because of sunstroke.
- With nausea. Ipecac 200
- In bones above eyebrows. In sinuses. Sinusitis. Kali Bi 200
- Chronic headache from sunrise to sunset. Natrum Mur 200
  Nausea. Face pale. Menstrual headache.
  Periodic headaches.
- Headache because of hangover or excessive Nux Vomica 200
  drinking.
- Caused by food heavy in fat. Pulsatilla 30
- Caused by eyestrain. Ruta 200

Heartburn
- Acidity with severe pain. Argentum Nit 200
- Acidity. Loss of appetite. Carbo Veg 200

Heart problems
- Angina pectoris attack. Arnica 200
- Angina pectoris with severe constriction, Cactus mother tincture, 10
  suffocation, cold sweat. drops in water, every 30
  minutes until condition
  stabilises.

- Collapse with coldness of external surfaces. Camphor mother tincture.
  10 drops on sugar every
  15 minutes. Drops on
  kerchief to smell.

• Arterial spasm with temporary loss of consciousness. Heart attack. **Get medical help at the earliest.**	Glonoine mother tincture 15 drops dose every few minutes.

Heat stroke
• With confusion, giddiness and fever.	Glonoine 200
• Cold sweat on forehead. Nausea. Throbbing arteries. Profuse, rice water, thin stool.	Veratrum Alb 200

Hiccup
• Violent. Spasmodic.	Cicuta 200 Cinnamon mother tincture, 5 drops on sugar every few minutes.

Hoarseness
• Loss of voice of professional singers.	Argentum Nitricum 200
• Because of overuse of voice.	Arnica 200
• Sudden, violent hoarseness. A raw, scraping feeling.	Belladonna 200
• On taking cold drinks or oily food followed by cold drinks.	Bryonia 200
• On taking cold drinks or oily food followed by cold drinks. Heaviness in the throat.	Ipecac 200
• Because of paralysis of vocal cords.	Lachesis 200

Indigestion
• Constriction in oesophagus. Nothing goes down. As if an egg is lodged.	Abies Nigra 200
• Because of overeating. Stinking belching. Foul flatus.	Antim Crud 200
• Cases of food poisoning.	Arsenic Alb 200
• Failure to digest even a small quantity of food. Acidity.	Carbo Veg 200
• With nausea being prominent.	Ipecac 200
• Pressure downwards. Wind passing with noise.	Lycopodium 200
• Because of irregular eating habits.	Nux Vomica 200
• Difficulty in digestion of milk, fruit, vegetables, heavy food.	Pulsatilla 30

Inflammation of gums
- Inflammation after tooth extraction.   Arnica 200
- Pus in gums with pulsation. Gums spongy,   Merc Sol 200
  swollen, bleeding. Breath stinks.

Influenza
- With profuse running nose.   Arsenic Alb 200
- With bronchitis. Severe hacking cough   Bryonia 200
  arising lower down in the centre of
  the ribs.
- With severe pain deep in bones.   Eupatorium Perf 200
- Body pain. Congestion in the forehead.   Gelsemium 200
  Skull feels tightened by a steel band.
  Sensation of cold going up the spine.
- Sluggishness
- With wheezing and nausea prominent.   Ipecac 200
- Uncontrollable flow from the nose.   Natrum Mur 200

**In addition, one dose of Influenzim 200
every day until a cure occurs.**

Injuries/Cuts/Wounds
- First medicine in any injury with or   Arnica 200
  without bleeding. Before and after surgery,   Calendula ointment for
  tooth extraction. In concussion of the brain.   external application on
                                                                          cuts and lacerations.

- Injury to part of the body rich in nerves like   Hypericum 200
  fingertips, spine.
- In punctured wounds. Avoids tetanus.   Ledum 200
- Wounds that do not heal.   Nitric Acid 200
- Injury to bones, cartilages. In sprains.   Ruta 200
  For eyestrain.

Insomnia
- Because of mental activity, flow of ideas.   Coffea 200
  Difficult to go to sleep in the early hours
  of the night.
- Inability to sleep after waking up around   Nux Vomica 200
  3.00 a.m.

Itching in the eye

• Intolerable itching. Burning tears.	Ambrosia 200
• Severe itching in the inner angles of the eyes.	Zincum Met 200

Menstrual problems

• Painful with labour like pains of short duration.	Belladonna 200
• Non-stop menstruation. Dark blood. Debility. One period runs into another.	Carbo Veg 200
• Profuse menstruation. Debilitating. Too early. Painful. Dark clots.	China 200
• Menstrual colic. Cramps. Pain ceases when flow starts.	Magnesia Phos 200
• Delayed otherwise than because of pregnancy. Scanty bleeding. Intermittent. Thick, dark, clotted blood.	Pulsatilla 30
• Scanty and irregular menstruation. Pain in the small of the back. Constant bearing down sensation as if the uterus would be pushed out.Sharp pain up the vagina.	Sepia 200

Milk diarrhoea

• Infant diarrhoea worse from milk.	Sepia 200

Motion sickness

• Nausea while travelling by any means of transport.	Cocculus 200

Muscular pain

• Worse on motion. With stiffness or without.	Bryonia 200
• Pain temporarily relieved on motion.	Rhus Tox 200

Nausea

• Vomit of bile, of blood, of brown black mucous. Result of food poisoning.	Arsenic Alb 200
• In morning. In pregnancy. Acidity. Weak digestion.	Carbo Veg 200
• Persistent nausea and vomiting. Vomit of bile, food, blood or mucous. Nausea in any sickness, for any reason.	Ipecac 200 **First medicine**

Numbness/Pins/Needles
- Numbness, tingling in face, in extremities. Aconite 30
  Caused by fear, anguish, sudden loss, or on
  exposure to dry cold air.
- With body ice-cold. Arsenic Alb 200
- In collapse, in cholera, with blue skin and Veratrum Alb 1000
  cold sweat. Unstoppable diarrhoea of rice
  water stools and retching.

Oesophagus-constriction of
- Difficulty in swallowing. Feels as if an egg Abies Nigra 200
  is lodged in the cardiac end of oesophagus.
  Nothing goes down.
- Because of acidity and poor digestion. Carbo Veg 200
- With persistent nausea and vomiting. Ipecac 200

Overeating
- Indigestion because of overeating. Foul Antim Crud 200
  eructation. Stinking flatus.
- Overeating of fatty food or too much fruit, Pulsatilla 30
  green vegetables or meat.

Pneumonia
- Acute, sudden inflammation with high Aconite Nap 30
  fever, dry, croupy cough. Mucous streaked Repeat at 30 minutes
  with blood. interval in acute stage.
  Later 4 doses a day.
- Rattling mucous difficult to take out. Antim Tart 200

Pyorrhoea
- Easily bleeding and retracted gums. Carbo Veg 200
- Ulcers in the mouth, on the gums. Merc Sol 200
  Foul smell. Pus pockets. Gums spongy.
  Severe itching.

Shock/Collapse
- Shock and collapse for any reason. Fainting. Camphor mother tincture,
  to smell.
- Surgical shock. Collapse in cholera. Veratrum Alb 200

Sinusitis-acute or chronic

- Chronic frontal sinusitis. Pain in the bones above the eyes also deep in the eyeballs. Thick, green mucous going down the throat, difficult to take out. Pain in ears. Early morning, persistent sneezing.   Kali Bi 200
- Old cold with smell lost. Bland, yellow, green mucous flowing outwards.   Pulsatilla 30

Sneezing

- Acute attack on exposure to dry, cold wind.   Aconite 30
- Without relief. Burning, excoriating discharge.   Arsenic Alb 200
- With body pain. Cold sensation up the spine. Steel band tightening around the skull.   Gelsemium 200
- With sinusitis. Pain in eyes, ears. Mucous difficult to take out.   Kali Bi 200
- When arsenic fails.   Merc Sol 200 or Natrum Mur 200

Sore throat

- Splinter like pain on swallowing.   Baryta Carb 200
- Angry looking congestion. Throat red, hot, burning, and swollen.   Belladonna 200
- Pus on the tonsils. Stabbing pain on empty swallowing. Fever.   Hepar Sulph 200
- Heaviness in the throat. Wheezing.   Ipecac 200
- Inflammation of the throat with purple colour.   Lachesis 200
- Pus formed without much pain.   Merc Sol 200
- Rough, scraping sensation in the throat.   Nux Vomica 200

Sprain

- Inflammation and swelling. Injury.   Arnica 200
  Alternate with Ruta 200

Stiffness of the back, of neck/Cervical spondylosis

- Stiffness with pain in the nape of the neck. Worse on movement. Stiffness and pain in cervical spondylosis.   Bryonia 200

- Stiffness of muscles with cervical spondylosis. Cicuta 200
- Stiffness and contraction in neck and back. Cimicifuga 200
  Cervical spondylosis. Severe pain. Giddiness. *A mixture of all these three*
  Numbness in fingers of the hand. Pain in *in equal measure does*
  shoulder blades. *wonders in cervical*
  spondylosis.

Strain

- Caused by injury. Arnica 200
- Caused by heavy lifting or severe muscular Rhus Tox 200
  exercise.

Stuffed nose

- On exposure to cold, wet weather. Dulcamara 200
- Body pain. Cold sensation up the spine. Gelsemium 200
  Onset of influenza. Steel band sensation
  around skull.
- With sinus pain, pain in the eyes. Tough Kali Bi 200
  mucous dripping inwards.
- Stuffed dry nose. Nux Vomica 200
- In old cold. Bland green mucous flows out Pulsatilla 30
  alternating with stuffed nose.

Sty

- Acute feeling of sand in the eyes. Lids Aconite 30
  swollen, dry, hot, and red.
- Swelling inside the eyelids which are red Apis 200
  and itching. Feeling of sand. Trachoma.
- Sty with piercing pain. Full of pus. Hepar Sulph 200
- Painful sty. Pulsatilla 30
- Recurring. Staphysagria 200

Surgery/Tooth extraction

- To prevent sepsis, to reduce pain, swelling, Arnica 200, before surgery
  for early healing of wounds. and after.

Swelling

- Because of insect bites, urticaria, or any Apis 200
  other cause. Red, puffed skin. Painful
  swelling.

- Because of injury.   Arnica 200

Urinary infection
- Scalding urine. Severe, cutting pain   Cantharis 200
  before, after, and during urination.
  Never-get-well feeling.
- Blood in urine with persistent tenesmus   Merc Cor 30
  of the bladder.

Wheezing
- In asthma, in bronchitis or for any other   Ipecac 200
  reason. Nausea present.
- Wheezing with rattling mucous difficult   Antim Tart 200, 1000
  to expectorate.

A TRAVELLER'S MEDICINE CHEST

In a small box, carry the following medicines wherever you go, with a copy of the chapter, '*A Short Circuit to Selection of Remedies/A Repertory for Instant Reference in Home, Office and for Travellers.*' [Page 555]. For most emergencies and common problems, these medicines will come handy. What is not included can be sourced at the local homoeopathic pharmacy.

Ask your chemist to pack your kit with one dram size bottles and prepare the medicines in pill size 20. Replenish from time to time.

1. Abies Nigra 200
2. Aconite 30
3. Aloe 200
4. Antim Tart 200
5. Apis 200
6. Arg Nit 200
7. Arnica 200
8. Arsenic Alb 200
9. Arundo 200
10. Belladonna 200
11. Bryonia 200
12. Calendula ointment
13. Cantharis 200. (For local application dissolve 20 pills in water and apply to affected surface.)
14. Carbo Veg 200
15. China 200

16.   Cimicifuga 200
17.   Cocculus 200
18.   Colocynthis 200
19.   Cuprum Met 200
20.   Dulcamara 200
21.   Euphrasia 200
22.   Gelsemium 200
23.   Glonoine 200
24.   Hamamelis 200
25.   Hepar Sulph 200
26.   Hypericum 200
27.   Ipecac 200
28.   Kali Bich 200
29.   Lachesis 200
30.   Ledum 200
31.   Lycopodium 200
32.   Merc Cor 30
33.   Merc Sol 200
34.   Nitric Acid 200
35.   Nux Vomica 200
36.   Podophyllum 200
37.   Pulsatilla 30
38.   Rhus Tox 200
39.   Ruta 200
40.   Silicea 200
41.   Sulphur 200
42.   Veratrum Alb 1000

Index